Lymphocyte Circulation

Lymphocyte Circulation

Experimental and Clinical Aspects

Maria de Sousa
Laboratory of Cell Ecology
Sloan-Kettering Institute for Cancer Research
New York, USA

with contributions by

A. S. G. Curtis
D. M. V. Parrott
Glasgow University
Scotland, UK

A Wiley–Interscience Publication

JOHN WILEY & SONS

Chichester · New York · Brisbane · Toronto

Copyright © 1981 by John Wiley & Sons Ltd.

All rights reserved.

No part of this book may be reproduced by any means, nor transmitted, nor translated into a machine language without the written permission of the publisher.

British Library Cataloguing in Publication Data:

De Sousa, Maria
   Lymphocyte circulation
   1. Lymphocytes
   2. Blood–Circulation
   I. Title
   II. Curtis, Adam Sebastian Geneviève
   III. Parrott, D. M. V.
   611'.0185   QP95.5   80-40848

ISBN 0 471 27854 8

Typeset in Great Britain by Pintail Studios Limited, Ringwood, Hants.
Printed by The Pitman Press, Bath, Avon.

Contents

Foreword ix

Preface xi

1. The Circuits 1

   1.1 Introduction 1
   1.2 Microvasculature of the spleen 3
   1.3 Microvasculature of the lymph node 4
   1.4 High endothelium venules (HEV) of the lymph node 6
      1.4.1 Ultrastructure 6
      1.4.2 Histochemistry and metabolic activity 7
      1.4.3 Permeability 8
      1.4.4 Morphology in T lymphocyte depleted animals 9
   1.5 Microcirculation and blood flow changes during the
       immune response 10
   1.6 Lymphatics 13

2. Methods and Their Sources 14

   2.1 Introduction 14
   2.2 The T6 chromosome marker 14
   2.3 Radioisotope markers 16
   2.4 Autoradiography 21
   2.5 The Ly system of isoantigens 24

**3. Areas of Lymphoid Cell Traffic within the Peripheral
Lymphoid Organs** 26

   3.1 Introduction 26
   3.2 Spleen 26
      3.2.1 Chicken 28
      3.2.2 Mouse, rat and human spleen 28
      3.2.3 White pulp 28
      3.2.4 Marginal zone 30
      3.2.5 Red pulp 31
   3.3 Lymph node 32

3.4	Peyer's patches and appendix	33
3.5	Application to the study of malignant lymphomas	35

4. Circulation of Lymphocytes within the Lymphoid System ... 37

4.1	Transit times in different species	37
4.2	Tempo of circulation of T and B lymphocytes	41
4.3	Migratory patterns of selected lymphoid cell populations: ecotaxis	45
	4.3.1 Bone marrow cells and bone marrow-derived cells	46
	4.3.2 Thymus cells and thymus-derived cells	49
	4.3.3 Bursa cells and bursa-derived cells	53
	4.3.4 Spleen cells and spleen-derived cells	53
	4.3.5 Lymph node cells	56
	4.3.6 Selected T and B lymphocytes	56
4.4	The effects of antigen	57
	4.4.1 Non-specific effects	57
	4.4.2 Specific recruitment of antigen-responsive cells	66
	4.4.3 Role in the initiation, propagation, and persistence (memory) of immunity	69
4.5	Factors other than antigen influencing lymphocyte circulation	75
	4.5.1 Phenotype	75
	4.5.2 Age	77
	4.5.3 Antibody	78
	4.5.4 Enzymes	79
	4.5.5 Non-specific mitogens	85
	4.5.6 Metal cations	90
	4.5.7 Agents that modify cell locomotion	91
	4.5.8 Irradiation	92
	4.5.9 ACTH	94
	4.5.10 *Bordetella Pertussis*	95
	4.5.11 Complement	96

5. Lymphocyte Circulation Outside the Lymphoid System ... 99
D. M. V. Parrott

5.1	Introduction	99
5.2	Migration of lymphocytes to non-mucosal sites	100
	5.2.1 Number and composition of cells in afferent lymph draining non-mucosal sites	100
	5.2.2 Alterations in afferent lymph following antigenic stimulation	102

	5.2.3	Vascular permeability and composition of lymphoid cells in non-lymphoid tissues	104
	5.2.4	Migration of inflammatory T blasts	104
	5.2.5	Lymphocyte traffic through the skin in CMI	106
	5.2.6	The role of blood flow in the delivery of lymphocytes	107
	5.2.7	Antigen-specific migration	107
	5.2.8	Role of chemoattractants and complement	108
5.3	Migration to mucosal sites		109
	5.3.1	Composition of lymphoid cells in the gut and other mucosal surfaces	109
	5.3.2	Identification of mucosal lymphocytes as effector cells	111

6. Lymphocyte Traffic in Disease ... 123

6.1	Lymphocyte traffic in experimental models of disease		123
	6.1.1	Thymic aplasia	123
	6.1.2	Autoimmunity	124
	6.1.3	NDV infection	126
	6.1.4	Murine leprosy	126
	6.1.5	Iron overload	129
6.2	Lymphocyte maldistribution syndromes in man		129
	6.2.1	Hodgkin's disease	130
	6.2.2	GI tract disease	134
	6.2.3	Chronic liver disease	136
	6.2.4	Skin diseases	139
	6.2.5	Connective tissue diseases	143
	6.2.6	CNS diseases	149
	6.2.7	Pulmonary diseases with pleurisy	152
	6.2.8	Solid tumours	152
	6.2.9	Leukaemia	155
	6.2.10	Thoracic duct drainage as a therapeutic tool	161
	6.2.11	Glomerulonephritis (GLN)	161
	6.2.12	Rheumatoid arthritis	162
	6.2.13	SLE	162

7. Clues, Concepts, and Possible Answers from other Systems ... 163
A. S. G. Curtis

7.1	Introduction	163
7.2	Cell–cell recognition systems	163
7.3	Patterning systems – is there specific control of the movement of cells?	166

7.4	Effector systems for cell positioning and cell behaviour	170
7.5	Experimental demonstration of selectivity in cell adhesions	174
7.6	Patterning possibilities in recognition systems	177
7.7	Interaction modulation and the control of cell positioning	182
	7.7.1 Evidence for the interaction modulation theory	182
	7.7.2 Examples of positioning systems	184
	7.7.3 Initial evidence for the existence of lymphocyte IMFs	186
	7.7.4 *In vivo* effects of IMFs	190
	7.7.5 Effects of IMFs on T:B interactions *in vivo*	193
	7.7.6 Allogeneic effects of IMF's histocompatibility restriction and cell interactions	193
7.8	Reinterpretation of findings on suppression	195
7.9	Envoi	195

8. A Circulation of Lymphocytes: Reflections on the Questions of How and Why ... 197

8.1	A circulation of lymphocytes: how?	198
8.2	A circulation of lymphocytes: why?	201
	8.2.1 Detectable Fe, other cations, and iron-binding proteins in sites of physiological and pathological lymphocyte migration	202
	8.2.2 Aspects and implications of the association of iron-binding proteins with cells of the immune system	212
8.3	Concluding remarks	216

References ... 218

Index ... 253

Foreword

EDWARD A. BOYSE MD FRS

Memorial Sloan-Kettering Cancer Center, 1275 York Avenue,
New York, N.Y. 10021

'If you understand *E. coli* you can explain an elephant'. Monod's words belong among those heady slogans of victory over which critics brood when the mood of intoxication has passed. But doubtless he was not advocating the exclusive study of *E. coli* as the best approach to all biological questions.

No one has explicitly said: 'If you understand lymphocytes you can explain a human being', but the thought is implicit in contemporary writings: and not all such authors would count themselves immunologists.

Prospectors of the terrain that divides bacteria from mammals have staked claims in the vicinity of *E. coli* or near the elephant – very near in fact, because mouse, man, and elephant were bedfellows in very recent evolutionary times – and have registered their claims by the models they chose to study.

The former parties can show notable successes with the slime mould Dictyostelium and other 'simple' organisms that are flirting with the metazoan mode. Indeed one need go no further than pack-hunting Myxobacteria to find examples of refined societal interplay coordinated by a veritable Signals Corps of genes.

From such vantage points, the tasks of other investigators, among them displaced medical persons, tackling allied questions with animals of such seemingly inextricable complexity as mouse or man, may have seemed insuperable. But look at the matter this way:

No one to my knowledge subscribes to any theory of Special Creation of lymphocytes, even of the human variety (though there may be a sect devoted to such a cause in California). *Omnis cellula a cellula*; and likewise surely for the exquisite genetic programs that dictate the identity of each cell set. Thus, the argument runs, 'If you understand lymphocytes you may explain a great deal about all cell sets that compose a mammal'. For '*E. coli*', in the context above, read 'lymphocytes', not 'mouse'.

Why lymphocytes? Rather than any other cell set? That can be regarded as a matter of convenience. Lymphocytes, comprising subpopulations that represent sequential and divergent steps in ontogeny, are obligingly accessible, either in transit or at the several sites on their itinerary.

Phylogenetic implications aside, lymphocytes are still a seemingly inexhaustible source of inspiration. The more spectacular aspects of lymphocyte research are sufficiently familiar, but others undoubtedly are neglected. This volume has a special place in that regard, because its theme – where lymphocytes go, and how, and why – entails the bringing to light of many facets of lymphocyte physiology and pathology that easily escape notice or have yet to see their day. Thus it has much to offer its readers, from beginners to the more experienced. Immunological novices, especially those without medical training, will profit from the broad perspective it affords, and many a seasoned physician may be surprised to find how many diseases may be interpretable in terms of the rules of lymphocyte traffic and penalties for their violation.

Preface

Work in immunology during the past 20 years has transformed our understanding of the lymphocyte from a cell whose function was manifestly unclear in 1958 (Florey and Gowans, 1958) to two major lymphocyte populations consisting of different sets of morphologically similar cells, whose functional variety and importance to the development and regulation of the immune response constitute the central subject of attention in current immunological research.

The work that led to the characterization of the two major T and B lymphocyte populations was done largely in experimental models *in vivo*; much of the later work dissecting further functional and differentiation cell sets within each of the two major lymphocyte classes has been done *in vitro*. For a cell to carry its functional commitment to help, suppress or kill other cells *in vivo*, it is a pre-requisite that such a cell should migrate to the site where its function is needed. Persistence, or sequestration, in the wrong site of a cell required to act at a tumour or infection site will influence considerably the way in which the host will allow progression or regression of such a tumour or infection. Persistence, or sequestration, of circulating cell sets at any point of the recirculating pathway will also create an apparent state of immunodeficiency in other compartments, similar to the anaemia created by sequestration of sensitized circulating red blood cells in the spleen or liver. Lymphoid cells, however, differ from red blood cells, in that they have a much more complex functional machinery; whereas the fate of a sequestered red cell in the spleen or liver is to be engulfed and broken down by splenic or hepatic macrophages, the fate of a sequestered T cell is to determine the function, or threaten the life, of its surrounding neighbour cells.

Thus, lymphocyte maldistribution may be seriously implicated in the pathogenesis of numerous diseases whose basic aetiology still escapes us, such as rheumatoid arthritis, scleroderma, mycosis fungoides, etc. Lymphocyte maldistribution may also be implicated in clinical instances of immunodeficiency diagnosed on the basis of peripheral blood tests, when the functionally effective cells are probably to be found misplaced elsewhere in the recirculatory pathway.

This book is an attempt to bring together experimental work on factors influencing and controlling normal lymphocyte circulation (Chapters 1, 3, and 4) and distribution to non-lymphoid sites (Chapter 5) and clinical work illustrating the existence, and some of the consequences, of lymphocyte maldistribution in disease (Chapter 6). In Chapter 2, the original work in manipulating the tools that have come to be universally used in studies of lymphocyte circulation is reviewed.

The basic questions of specific cell migration and positioning are not exclusive of lymphocyte circulation; in Chapter 7, A. S. G. Curtis reviews those questions in light of knowledge derived from other biological systems. In spite of all that is already known, there is much we do not know; in Chapter 8 I speculate on how and why lymphocytes circulate.

I am indebted to my colleagues D. M. V. Parrott (Departments of Bacteriology and Immunology) and A. S. G. Curtis (Department of Cell Biology), both of the University of Glasgow, for the writing of Chapters 5 and 7, respectively, and for their helpful suggestions and comments made during the preparation of the manuscript.

I am most grateful to my friends I. Canto and M. R. Pires Marques for the use of their summer house as my writing quarters in three successive summers (and to the children for keeping quiet). The completion of this book was made possible, however, by the understanding of my colleagues K. Nishiya and C. G. Munn, who kept the day-to-day affairs of the laboratory going and accepted kindly my irregular appearances in the last three months. Finally, I wish to acknowledge my assistant T. Holden, for her invaluable help in the last revisions of the text and preparation of the bibliography. The illustrations are the work of Ms. K. Ferris and were photographed by Ms. J. Kempa. I warmly acknowledge the help of Ms. H. Doumas and Ms. M. Doumas in preparing the typescript.

New York *Maria de Sousa*
1980

Chapter 1

The Circuits

1.1 INTRODUCTION

The gross anatomy of the three major circuits utilized by cells in traffic – the systemic, the pulmonary, and the lymphatic circuits – is represented diagrammatically in Fig. 1.1. In mammals, where the majority of the experiments on lymphoid cell traffic *in vivo* have been done, the blood leaves the left ventricle of the heart oxygenated, goes into the systemic circuit, and returns to the right atrium and right ventricle to enter the pulmonary circuit deoxygenated. After oxygenation in this circuit, the blood reenters the left atrium, the left ventricle, and the systemic circuit. A cell injected intravenously joins the blood in the systemic circuit on its way to the pulmonary circuit; progress of circulating cells in the

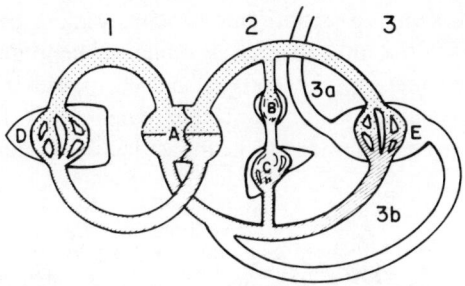

Figure 1.1 Diagram illustrating the pulmonary (1) and systemic (2) blood circuits and the peripheral (3a) and central (3b) lymph circuits utilized by red and white cells in the mammal. Oxygenated blood (▨) leaves the heart (A) into the systemic circuit, which includes the spleen (B), the liver (C), and the total mass of the peripheral lymphoid tissue (E). From the periphery the deoxygenated blood (▨) returns to the heart *via* the lungs (D). The peripheral lymphoid tissues, in addition to receiving lymphocytes from the blood (see Plate 3), also act as lymph filters *via* the afferent lymphatics (3a); the efferent lymphatics eventually drain into major lymphatic ducts (3b). From de Sousa (1976)

1

blood circuit is likely to be influenced by velocity of flow and structure of the capillary wall in addition to the gross anatomical and geometrical arrangement of the blood vessels.

Velocity of flow varies in an inverse relationship to the cross-sectional area of the vessels; for example, in man, the velocity of flow is slowest in the capillary vessel region (0.07 cm/sec), which has a cross-sectional area of approximately 5,000 cm^2 in contrast with the much smaller cross-sectional area of the largest arteries and veins (20–30 cm^2) where the velocity of blood flow is as high as 50 cm/sec in the arteries and 40 cm/sec in the veins (Fig. 1.2). Accordingly, in autoradiographs of lungs removed from mice killed shortly (within the first hour) after injection of radioisotopically labelled lymphocytes, the labelled cells are found in the alveolar capillary bed. Later, the numbers of normal lymphocytes found in the lungs start to decrease and slowly all injected cells accumulate in the spleen, lymph nodes, and Peyer's patches. As we will see later, however, this is not a general rule, and different kinds of lymphocytes spend different lengths of time in the pulmonary circuit (Chapter 4.2) depending presumably on the nature of their surface characteristics and resulting interaction with the capillary endothelium.

Studies of the ultrastructure of the microvascular bed (Rhodin, 1973) have shown some morphological differences between the endothelial walls of capillaries in different organs; these differences are not so marked that they alone can account for the differences observed in cell distribution.

Basically, four types of endothelium have been described: (1) continuous thick, found in cardiac, skeletal and smooth muscle, consisting of endothelial cells with an average thickness of 0.2 μm and a basal lamina; (2) continuous thin, consisting of endothelial cells with an average thickness of 0.1 μm, with a basal lamina in the lung and without a basal lamina in the spleen, lymph nodes, thymus, and lymph capillaries; (3) fenestrated thin, found in the endocrine organs, urinary system,

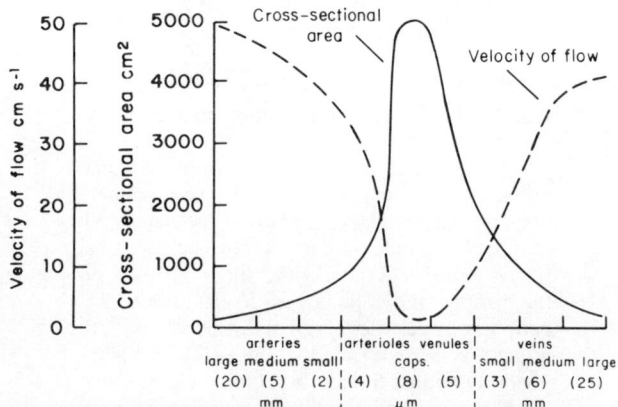

Figure 1.2 Diagrammatic representation of the relationship between cross-sectional area and blood flow at different levels of the systemic blood circuit. Modified from Berne and Levey (1972) and Navaratnam (1975).

choroid plexus of the brain, ciliary body of the eye, venous capillaries of the dermis, and lamina propria of the intestinal mucosa, characterized by endothelial cells 800 Å thick on average, with round fenestrations having a diameter of about 600 Å closed by a single layer of membrane derived from the fusion of the basal and laminal plasma membranes; (4) discontinuous, found in the sinusoids of the liver parenchyma, containing cytoplasmic holes with a diameter ranging between 0.5 and 2 μm. The holes are rarely closed and there no basal lamina is present.

Therefore, if morphology of the capillary wall alone was to guide cell 'diffusion' from the blood circuit into an organ, circulating cells should be expected to penetrate the liver parenchyma, in large numbers. Although lymphocytes are present in the liver (see Chapter 5, Table 5.1), the largest number of normal lymphocytes pass the pulmonary, portal and hepatic circuits on their way to the spleen, lymph nodes, and Peyer's patches. Within the spleen they are first found in the red pulp and marginal zone sinus, and in the lymph nodes and Peyer's patches in and around postcapillary venules; eventually they leave the blood circuit in these organs to occupy clearcut sites within the white pulp of the spleen, the outer and mid-cortex of the lymph nodes, and the interfollicular and nodular areas of the Peyer's patches (see Chapter 3). Does the actual microvasculature of the peripheral lymphoid organs take them there?

1.2 MICROVASCULATURE OF THE SPLEEN

The splenic microcirculation has been studied extensively using reconstruction models from serial histological sections (Burke and Simon, 1970; MacNeal, 1929; Snook, 1946; Weiss, 1965), *in vivo* transillumination (Knisley, 1936; McKenzie *et al.*, 1951; Peck and Hoerr, 1951), and microangiography based on injection of coloured or radiopaque substances followed by histologic or microradiographic analysis (van Rooisen, 1972; Dubreuil *et al.*, 1975). A diagrammatic representation of the modes of microcirculation of the white pulp, based on the microcirculation study of the rat spleen by Dubreuil *et al.* (1975), is presented in Fig. 1.3.

The loosely arranged capillaries leave the central arteries supplying the continuous white pulp lymphoid masses aggregated round the arteries. On the periphery of the white pulp masses, these capillaries are connected to a dense, thick vascular network whose venous drainage is not clear. This vascular network occupies the zone corresponding histologically to the marginal zone (Fig. 1.3, see Plate 5). The morphology of the microcirculation in this zone with such a large sectional area indicates a slow blood flow. Lymphocytes, however, do not stay in it for long and generally between 3 and 6 hr after injection migrate into the substance of the white pulp. As mentioned earlier, the venous drainage of this area is not clear, and from the study of Dubreuil *et al.* (1975) the only other way out for a cell which migrated from the marginal zone across the white pulp substance is the lymphatic drainage originating in large lymphatic channels surrounding the central artery (Plate 1). The exit route from the marginal sinus thus remains

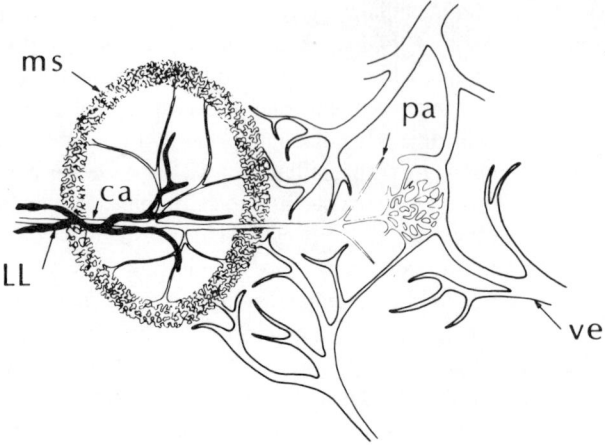

Fig. 1.3 Diagrammatic representation of the white pulp microcirculation. ca, central artery; ms, marginal sinus, close anastomosing irregular channels filling from capillaries branching off the ca; ve, veins of the red pulp: note few direct connections between the marginal sinus and the red pulp veins; LL, lymphatic channels around the central artery; pa, penicillae arteries originating at the central artery. Data from Dubreuil et al. (1975), courtesy P. G. Herman

unknown, since large numbers of perfused cells were recovered in the splenic vein in a separate study of the fate of labelled lymphocytes in the perfused rat spleen (Ford, 1969). Although it seems conceivable that the lymphatic channels observed by Dubreuil et al. (1975) in the substance of the white pulp drain into the splenic vein at a point undetectable by their technique and located in the venous circuit at a point earlier than the point used for cannulation by Ford (1969), there is at present no evidence to confirm it.

1.3 MICROVASCULATURE OF THE LYMPH NODE

The microvasculature of the lymph node (Fig. 1.4) consists of a system of arteries with average diameters varying from 20–40 μm in the rabbit popliteal node (Herman et al., 1972) to 50–70 μm in the axillary nodes of the rat (Anderson and Anderson, 1975), branching into a capillary network most prominent under the subcapsular sinus and in the medullary cords. Some of these branches terminate in small clusters of arterioles and capillaries which form basket-like plexuses around germinal centres. Few capillaries are seen without the outer B cell nodules (see Chapter 3, Plate 9 for details of lymph node ecology) and germinal centres appear relatively avascular. Arteriovenous communications were described beneath the subcapsular sinus in the rat axillary nodes (Anderson and Anderson, 1975) forming loops which joined directly with postcapillary (high endothelial) venules (Plate 2). The existence of arteriovenous anastomoses has also been

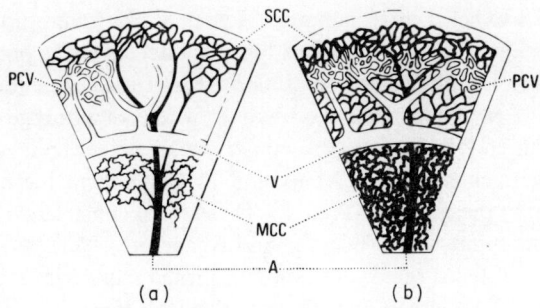

Figure 1.4 (a) Diagram of normal microvasculature. SCC, subcapsular capillaries; PCV, postcapillary venule; MCC, medullary cord capillaries; A, artery; V, vein. (b) Diagram at height of microvasculature changes following antigen stimulation (4–5 days). Courtesy P. G. Herman, from Herman et al. (1972)

demonstrated in a study of the regional blood flow of the lymph node measured with microspheres of different diameters (Table 1.1, Herman et al., 1979). Because the diameters of the capillaries and the arteriovenous anastomoses are different within the same organ, by injecting microspheres of different sizes the blood flow through capillaries and arteriovenous anastomoses can be separated and measured (Herman et al., 1979).

In this study (Herman et al., 1979) the regional blood flow of the lymph node measured with the 15 μm spheres was almost twice as high as that measured with 9 μm spheres (Table 1.1). This indicates that a significant number of the smaller microspheres were not trapped in the capillary bed but were shunted through arteriovenous anastomoses.

Capillaries with an average diameter of 11 μm get together in groups of two to five capillaries to form the postcapillary venules with an average diameter of 15–30 μm. Postcapillary venules are most numerous in those areas of the cortex with a rich capillary supply, namely the subcapsular region, although they are found uniformly disseminated throughout the cortex, forming intricate venous plexuses in the deep cortex. The majority of the postcapillary venules do not have

Table 1.1 Blood flow to kidneys, the unchallenged lymph node, and the cardiac output as measured with 9 μm and 15 μm microspheres. Data from Herman et al. (1979)

Organ	ml/g/min		Difference (%)
	15 μm	9 μm	15 μm − 9 μm
Right kidney	4.36 ± 0.26*	4.26 ± 0.26	2
Left kidney	4.32 ± 0.26	4.22 ± 0.26	2
Right lymph node	0.46 ± 0.07	0.26 ± 0.03	43
Cardiac output (ml)	373 ± 10	361 ± 0.19	3

*Data expressed as mean ± standard error of the mean.

unusually high endothelia. High endothelial venules are found mostly in the mid-cortex at the section of the node utilized by lymphocytes in the process of circulation from blood to lymph. The luminal diameters of the high endothelial venules increase as the vessels approach the medulla where they merge into segmental veins lined by flat endothelium. Focal constrictions were seen in venular walls at the junctions between segmental veins and at sites where these vessels joined larger veins deep in the medulla (Plate 2). These focal constrictions are caused by contracted venous sphincters (Anderson and Anderson, 1975).

Rich networks of fenestrated and non-fenestrated capillaries are present in the cortex and medulla (Anderson and Anderson, 1975). Fenestrae are present along segments of alternated endothelial cell cytoplasm where they are covered only by basement membrane. Postcapillary venules are lined with two to four low endothelial cells and are surrounded by a delicate basement membrane. In the mid-cortex postcapillary venules connect with high endothelium venules, and mitotic figures are seen occasionally at the junctions where there is an abrupt transition from flat to cuboidal endothelium. High endothelium venules are surrounded by a complex reticular sheath which appears to spiral about these vessels as they traverse the lymph node cortex. This sheath consists of two to three layers of overlapping cytoplasmic plates derived from reticular cells. In addition, collagen bundles and amorphous ground substance are seen separating layers of the perivenular sheath.

1.4 HIGH ENDOTHELIUM VENULES (HEV) OF THE LYMPH NODE

Since the observation that small lymphocytes leave the bloodstream and enter the lymph circuit through a section of the postcapillary venules localized in the mid-cortex of the lymph node and characterized in normal rats and mice (Plate 3a) by the presence of high endothelial cuboidal cells (Gowans and Knight, 1964; Marchesi and Gowans, 1964), interest has developed in the interaction of lymphocytes with endothelial cells at this point, and on the histology, histochemistry, and ultrastructure of HEV (Smith and Henon, 1959; Sugimura, 1964; Soderstrom, 1967; Schoefl and Miles 1972; Van Deurs and Ropke, 1975; Anderson *et al.*, 1976; Mikata and Niki, 1971; Sordat *et al.*, 1971; Ford *et al.*, 1978; Andrews *et al.*, 1980; and Stamper Woodruff, 1978).

1.4.1 Ultrastructure

In animals with the normal quota of circulating lymphocytes, the endothelial cells are tall, cuboidal and contain well-developed organelles. The Golgi area contains prominent vesicles. Electron-dense mitochondria are present, often clustering together in one section of the cytoplasm. They contain many free ribosomes occasionally forming polysomes. The nucleus is round or slightly elongated containing light chromatin, the nucleolus is small.

Lymphocytes were at first thought to cross HEV by passing through channels inside the endothelial cells (Marchesi and Gowans, 1964). Later studies, however, have indicated that lymphocytes cross HEV utilizing intercellular spaces (Schoefl and Miles 1972; van Ewijk et al., 1975; Anderson et al., 1976).

1.4.2 Histochemistry and metabolic activity

A summary of enzyme and other metabolic activities of high endothelial cells of lymph nodes is presented in Table 1.2. Like other types of endothelium, HEV show moderate to intense staining for lactic dehydrogenase, isocitric dehydrogenase, and ATPase activity. In addition, they have enzyme and metabolic activities which are not seen in other endothelia, namely acetyl esterase activity, light to intense staining for acid phosphatase, and β-glucuronidase activity (Smith and Henon, 1959; Mikata et al., 1968; Anderson et al., 1976). They also have the singular ability to incorporate ^{35}S-sulphate, which shows maximum autoradiographic labelling at 15–30 min after footpad injection of the labelled sulphate and is almost exclusively confined to the Golgi apparatus (Andrews et al., 1980). Experiments on the incorporation of labelled sugars *in vitro* using lymph node slices have demonstrated that HEV selectively incorporate glucosamine, glucuronic acid, and mannose, but not galactose, fructose, and glucose (Andrews et al., 1980).

The exact significance of the sulphate uptake by HEV is not fully understood at present. Experiments injecting partially purified sulphated material from lymph nodes into the skin of rats indicated that this material induced an increased localization of recirculating lymphocytes to the site of injection. It is possible that this sulphated molecule which is secreted by the endothelial cells (Ford, personal communication) acts as a signal of lymphocyte migration to HEV; this possibility will be discussed in more detail later (Chapter 8.1).

Table 1.2 Comparative enzymatic activities of the endothelium in lymph node blood vessels. Data from Anderson et al. (1976)

Enzymes	Intensity of reaction*			
	High endothelial venule	Medullary veins	Capillaries	Arterioles
Lactic dehydrogenase	++	++	++	++
Isocitric dehydrogenase	++	++	++	++
Adenosine triphosphatase	+	++	++	++
Alkaline phosphatase	0	0	++	+++
Acetyl esterase	+++	0	0	0
Acid phosphatase	+	0	0	0
β-glucuronidase	+	0	0	0
Cytoplasmic RNA	++	0	0	0

*Recorded as ++++ intense activity, +++ strong activity, ++ moderate activity, + weak activity, and 0 no activity.

1.4.3 Permeability

Thorotrast particles of about 70 Å in diameter and carbon particles of much larger sizes (350–450 Å) have been used to investigate the permeability of lymph node HEV in the mouse (Mikata and Niki, 1971). Shortly (5 min) after an intravenous injection of thorotrast solution, particles were seen in the lumen of HEV and in narrow intercellular spaces between endothelial cells. Later, at 10–30 min after injection, thorotrast particles were seen between endothelial cells, between endothelial cells and neighbouring lymphocytes, and between the endothelial cells and the basement membrane near sites of lymphocyte emigration from the venules.

The larger carbon particles were also seen in the lumen of HEV at 5–10 min after intravenous injection, and between endothelial cells and crossing lymphocytes. At the early times after injection, occasional small phagocytic

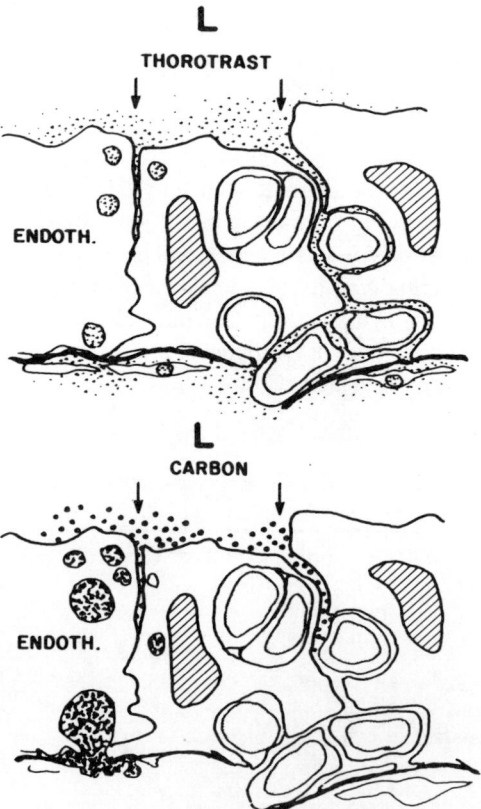

Figure 1.5 Schematic drawing showing pathways of thorotrast and carbon particles through high endothelium venule, after injection into vein. L, lumen. Modified from Mikata and Niki (1971)

vacuoles containing carbon particles were seen in the luminal portion of the endothelial cytoplasm. Later, by 30 min, these phagocytic vacuoles coalesced, forming large intracytoplasmic vesicles containing clusters of carbon particles. This was more evident in samples taken at 2–24 hr after carbon injection.

The pathways utilized by thorotrast and carbon particles within HEV are represented schematically in Fig. 1.5. According to Mikata and Niki, their observations indicate that 'lymphocyte emigration across HEV provides a suitable pathway for exudation of noncellular elements of the blood'. It is clear also from their study that if such exudation takes place, it is not random, since many more thorotrast than carbon particles were found to cross the HEV.

1.4.4 Morphology in T lymphocyte depleted animals

The question whether the sections of the postcapillary venules at which lympocytes enter the nodes are specialized or appear to become specialized as lymphocytes penetrate them has been the subject of some controversy. The reason for this question stems from two main observations: (a) microangiographic studies of lymph nodes, showing that in normal animals the section of the postcapillary venule with high endothelium is confined to the mid- and deep-cortex of the lymph nodes (Herman et al., 1972); (b) studies of the morphology of the postcapillary venule in animals depleted of circulating T cells have given conflicting results. In some instances no changes were observed (Anderson et al., 1976), but others have shown that in the absence of the major part of the recirculating pool of lymphocytes, the endothelium of the postcapillary venule is low and ill-defined (Parrott et al., 1966; de Sousa, 1969; de Sousa et al., 1969; Goldschneider and McGregor, 1968a; Fossum et al., 1980).

The usual morphology of the postcapillary venule in the lymph nodes of T cell depleted mice and rats is illustrated in Plate 3b. The venules are barely detectable with the ordinary stains and are more readily detected by the use of a reticulin stain. The lumen is well delineated, venules are therefore not collapsed, and it is the endothelium that under these circumstances is very low and ill-defined, in contrast with the usual high endothelium of the venules in normal lymph nodes (Plate 3a). The low endothelium, however, can change to the high endothelium form in response to the injection of recirculating lymphocytes (Goldschneider and McGregor, 1968a), antigens, and thymus grafts (de Sousa and Pritchard, 1974; Parrott and de Sousa, 1967). It is not clear whether the response to the administration of an antigen is due directly to the unusual capacity of this endothelium to phagocytoze certain particles (Mikata and Niki, 1971) or indirectly as a result of increased lymphocyte mobilization into the circulation.

The point that must be borne in mind is that most likely the high endothelial cells of those sections of the lymph node postcapillary venules through which lymphocytes cross into the lymph node substance are a 'special' reflection rather than the 'specialized' cause of selective lymphocyte entry. Additional support for this view derives from the finding of similar changes from low to high endothelium in venules present in non-lymphoid sites in conditions of increased lymphocyte migration (Smith et al., 1970; Graham and Shannon, 1972).

1.5 MICROCIRCULATION AND BLOOD FLOW CHANGES DURING THE IMMUNE RESPONSE

It is clear from the studies of the microvascular beds of the spleen and lymph node that the reasons why white cells leave a circuit are not determined exclusively by the anatomy or structure of the circuit. Anatomical and structural factors seem to operate and influence cell traffic mainly as regulators of flow volume and flow velocity, reflecting the extreme flexibility of the geometry of the blood microcirculation. This flexibility is best illustrated by the blood flow changes that occur in lymph nodes during an immune response.

Determination of blood flow to various organs has been achieved by examining the distribution of radioactive microspheres. When the number or total radioactivity of the microspheres introduced in the arterial circulation *via* catheters positioned in the ascending aorta injected is known, the distribution to the different organs can be considered to reflect the cardiac output of the animal to that organ. In Table 1.3 a summary of data for blood flow to organs of sheep, rabbit, and mouse is presented (Hay and Hobbs, 1977; Herman et al., 1979; Ottaway and Parrott, 1979). On a weight basis, the blood flow to a lymph node was found to be equivalent to the blood flow to an equal weight of spleen. The lowest flow per gramme of tissue in sheep was to the thymus. The mean blood flow to the lymph nodes (per gramme) was 0.012% of the cardiac output. The average weight of the popliteal and prefemoral nodes was 1.2 g in sheep.

Based on the estimation of Hales (1973) of an average cardiac output of sheep, 4–8 month old, of 3.3 l/min, Hay and Hobbs estimated that the blood flow to a lymph node weighing 1 g was 3.3 l/min x 0.012%, thus equalling 0.396 ml/min, or 24.06 ml/hr (Hay and Hobbs, 1977). The estimated numbers of lymphocytes entering a node from the blood per hour equalled 1.12×10^8; the efferent lymph output of cells derived from the blood is 2.85×10^7/hr. Therefore, such a lymph node removes the equivalent of one in four lymphocytes that enter the blood. The remaining three of the four lymphocytes presumably leave the lymph node in the venous blood.

Following the administration of antigens, marked changes take place both in blood flow (Hay and Hobbs, 1977) and in microvasculature of lymph nodes (Herman et al., 1972).

Herman et al. (1972), in a study of the blood microcirculation in the rabbit popliteal lymph node during a primary immune response, compared microangiograms prepared at different times following injection of an antigen in the footpad with control microangiograms of the contralateral node draining the uninjected footpad.

The first changes after antigen administration in the footpad were observed at 6 hr and characterized by slight increases in the diameter of the capillaries in the

Table 1.3 Blood flow to lymphoid organs based on percentage of microspheres administered (% of cardiac output)*

Reference	Method	Experimental animal	Spleen	Thymus	Lymph nodes
Hay & Hobbs (1977)	Microspheres (15 μm)	Sheep	1.8 ± 0.3	0.051 ± 0.015	0.012 ± 0.001
		Rabbit	0.32 ± 0.11	—	0.011 ± 0.004
		Mouse	1 ± 0.13	—	—
Herman et al. (1979)*	Microspheres (15 μm)	Rabbit	—	—	*
	Microspheres (9 μm)	Rabbit	—	—	*
Ottaway & Parrott (1979)	86RbCl	Mouse	0.36 ± 0.08	—	0.10 ± 0.02

*See data in Table 1.1.

submarginal sinus region. At 24 hr both the capillary diameter and the density of distribution of the capillaries had increased; by 48 hr an increasingly dense capillary network was observed virtually without avascular areas in the draining node (Fig. 1.4). The medullary cord capillaries had at this time an average diameter of 15–20 μm. By the fifth day many capillaries in the medullary cords had a diameter of 25 μm, an increase of over 100% compared with the average diameter of 11 μm in the resting state. A diagram summarizing these findings is represented in Fig. 1.4.

In separate studies of the blood flow to the popliteal lymph node in the rabbit during a primary immune response to keyhole limpet haemocyanin (KLH), Hay and Hobbs (1977) found that the blood flow was significantly increased ($p < 0.05$) within 1.5 hr after injection. The flow continued to increase until 14 hr and then decreased until near 24 hr. During the subsequent 3 days of the immune response it increased again, averaging three times the normal flow.

Similar results were observed in sheep following challenges with PPD or allogeneic lymphocytes (Table 1.4). The stimulated lymph nodes all had a larger number of trapped microspheres even when compared to the contralateral nodes on an equal weight basis. Stimulated nodes weigh on average 1.42 times the control, and the microsphere localization per gramme was 4.18 times the control.

By comparing the changes in blood flow measured with 15 μm and 9 μm microspheres following antigenic stimulation, Herman et al. concluded that the marked increase in blood flow was largely due to increased shunt flow (Herman et al., 1979). Thus, following antigenic stimulation, the differential flow measured with 15 μm spheres at 16 hr increased significantly compared with the resting node, while the flow measured by the smaller 9 μm microspheres increased only slightly.

In an additional experiment comparing microsphere localization and lymphocyte output from a sheep popliteal lymph node responding to the subcutaneous injection of allogeneic lymphocytes, Hay and Hobbs demonstrated that the increased blood flow coincided with increased lymphocyte traffic through the regional lymph node and suggested that the increase in lymphocyte traffic is a direct consequence of the increase in blood flow. In a simultaneous study of blood

Table 1.4 Blood flow: comparison of stimulated nodes and contralateral unstimulated nodes. Data from Hay and Hobbs (1977)

Antigen	Ratio of stimulated nodes to contralateral controlled nodes	
	Weight	Microsphere count
Tuberculin, day 3	1.65	3.99
Allogeneic lymphocytes, day 5	1.44	6.48
Allogeneic lymphocytes, day 4	1.70	4.66
Allogeneic lymphocytes, day 5	0.87	4.26
Allogeneic lymphocytes, day 6	1.43	1.59
Mean	1.42	4.18

flow and lymph node cell migration, Ottaway and Parrott demonstrated the existence of a significant correlation between the two (Ottaway and Parrott, 1979). This correlation is sometimes disrupted. In *T. spiralis* infected mice, increased blast cell migration to the small intestine occurred in the absence of detectable changes in blood flow (Ottaway and Parrott, personal communication).

1.6 LYMPHATICS

Finally, lymphocytes after entering the lymph nodes from the blood join the lymph circuit. Unlike the mystery that surrounds the lymphatic drainage of cells from the spleen, the entry of lymphocytes into the lymphatic circuit from a lymph node is well documented (Hall and Morris, 1963, 1964, 1965). But the existence of lymph nodes is not an indispensable prerequisite for blood to lymph circulation of cells to occur since it takes place in birds and fish, species in which lymph nodes are not present (Bell and Lafferty, 1972; Ellis and de Sousa, 1974).

According to the studies of Casley Smith (1970, 1971, 1973), the development of a true lymphatic system in phylogeny, i.e. of a separate system of vessels not containing blood, occurred in the torpedoes and teleosts coinciding with a marked increase in venous blood pressure. Such an event in the evolution of the blood circulation required the junctions in the venous vessels to be permanently closed, thus preventing material from reentering the blood vessels by body movements and creating the conditions for a separate system to develop.

The lymphatic system has been divided, on the basis of functional reasoning (Casley Smith, 1970), into initial lymphatics and collecting lymphatics. The initial lymphatics have the function of removing material from the tissues. They are usually flattened in normal tissues, 100–500 µm long. In areas of inflammation they are greatly dilated and after mild injuries, i.e. heat, light, touch, etc., have characteristically many open junctions (Casley Smith, 1973). The collecting lymphatics perform the function of transporting the material removed by the initial lymphatics, have fewer open junctions and an overall structure resembling that of the great veins.

In mammals, in which most experiments on the circulation of lymphocytes have been done, the major collecting lymphatics, after draining into and from lymph nodes, coalesce to form four major lymph trunks: the jugular, the subclavian, the mediastinal and the lumbar lymphatic trunks. All the collecting lymphatics of the lower part of the body and left upper half drain into the thoracic duct, and the lymphatics from the right upper half regions drain into the right lymph duct. Both major lymph ducts drain in turn into the large thoracic veins.

Chapter 2

Methods and Their Sources

2.1 INTRODUCTION

The reasons why some methods become the methods of choice in a particular field cannot be discerned from their technical detail; such reasons lie in the conceptual rather than the pragmatic history of the subject. The purpose of this chapter is twofold: (a) to review the original papers in which chromosome markers, radioisotope labelling, autoradiography and detection of surface isoantigens were first applied to the study of lymphocytes; (b) to illustrate how the development and timely application of a new technique contributed to end decisively an ongoing controversy (Ford et al., 1956; Gowans, 1959) or to provide substantial evidence in favour of a new fact (Parrott et al., 1966; Boyse et al., 1968). In both cases a considerable body of work followed, adopting the same methods, confirming the original observations, and expanding the number of questions first posed by the availability of the new tool.

2.2 THE T6 CHROMOSOME MARKER AND THE CONTROVERSY SURROUNDING THE THERAPEUTIC EFFECT OF HAEMOPOIETIC CELLS GIVEN TO LETHALLY X-IRRADIATED RECIPIENTS
(C. E. Ford *et al.*, 1956)

In those papers in which the use of a new method contributed decisively to end a major controversy of the time, a description of the controversy is usually found in the introduction. Ford *et al.*'s paper on the 'Cytological identification of radiation chimaeras' published in *Nature* in March 1956 is no exception:

> 'it has been shown by Jacobsen *et al.* (1951) and soon after by Lorenz *et al.* (1951), that adult mice irradiated with an expectedly lethal dose of X-rays could recover if grafted or injected with haemopoietic tissue from a normal mouse. Consequently, it was not surprising that they postulated recovery to be due to a "humoral" or chemical factor in the material given, rather than to replacement of the damaged tissues of the host by the foreign cells.'

The controversy thus revolved round two alternatives: (a) of donor factors acting on host cells; (b) of donor cells themselves repopulating the host tissues. At the time indirect evidence could be produced in favour of both (Cole *et al.*, 1953;

Lindsley et al., 1955; Main and Prehn, 1955). The irony is that, 20 years later, we know that success of bone marrow transplantation still depends on the complex interplay of unclear humoral factors and clearly defined cell populations. To decide definitively between the two alternatives at the time, a tool had to be available that would enable the unquestionable identification of *dividing* donor cells in host tissues.

Such a tool became available in the Harwell Laboratories in 1955; its discovery is also described in the *Nature* paper:

> . . . 'in the course of a survey of the cytological properties of a series of semisterile stocks raised by Carter, Lyon, and Phillips (1955), the stock (T6) was found to be heterozygous for a very unequal reciprocal translocation between two of the smallest members of the normal chromosome set. One of the two rearranged chromosomes was thus much smaller than any of the normal complement and showed up prominently in spermatological metaphases. A potential marker having been obtained the next step was to develop a really satisfactory technique for making preparations of bone marrow. This proved more successful than had been anticipated and will be described elsewhere. It is sufficient to say here that it is an adaptation of the Feulgen squash method, in which colchicine pretreatment is used and the tissue is handled as a cell suspension. The small marker chromosome was found to be even more distinctive in bone marrow cells than in spermatogonia (Plate 4). It usually appears as three dots arranged in a triangle, suggesting the presence of an under-stained ('heterochromatic') region close to the centromes.'

Transfer of bone marrow cells containing the T6 chromosome marker would make it possible to demonstrate decisively their presence in irradiated hosts. And in all animals killed in the original experiments at 5, 14, 19, 28, and 49 days after injection, the characteristic T6 marker chromosome was indeed found in spleen, lymph node, and thymus, suggesting 'that the situation in these organs is essentially the same, that is, virtually complete replacement of the host's tissue by donor cells.

> 'The possible applications of the chromosome marker technique are worth noting. In principle, it provides a biological "tracer" method which should be applicable to all questions where the origin in development or regeneration of a particular group of cells is at issue, provided the cells concerned undergo mitosis naturally, or can be persuaded to do so.'

Application of the method in the ways then predicted led first the Harwell group and later others to define the major pathways of cell traffic within the lymphomyeloid system. These were represented diagrammatically 10 years later by the same group (Micklem et al., 1966) as an inspired summary of 'present knowledge and ignorance, and as a basis for future experiment' (Fig. 2.1).

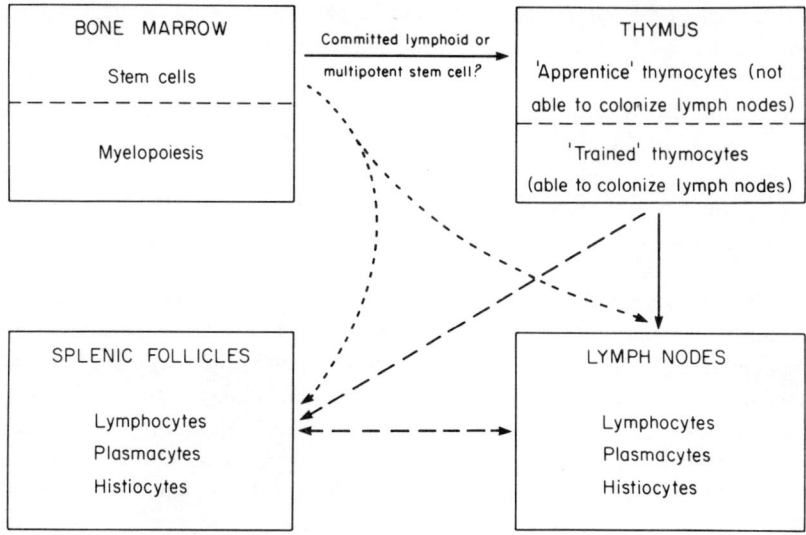

Figure 2.1 Diagram of cell migration pathways in the lymphomyeloid complex as envisaged by Micklem *et al.*, in 1966

Later experiments fully confirmed that summary of knowledge and ignorance.

Multipotent stem cells from the bone marrow colonize the thymus and other lymphoid tissues (this second alternative not excluded in the original diagram); those which enter the thymus acquire therein surface characteristics specific to themselves (see Section 2.4) and a considerable proportion (the 'trained' thymocytes in the diagram, Fig. 2.1) leave the thymus, enter the blood circulation, and dwell in the peripheral lymphoid organs.

Parallel experiments making use of radioisotope markers tell us that from specific sites within the peripheral lymphoid organs, lymphocytes find their way to the lymph. The role played by the availability of radioisotopes to end another major controversy of the fifties is illustrated in the following section.

2.3 RADIOISOTOPE MARKERS AND THE CONTROVERSY SURROUNDING THE RAPID TURNOVER OF LYMPHOCYTES IN THE BLOOD (Gowans, 1959)

Any physiologist educated in the first half of this century would have accepted Virchow's views on the origin of the large numbers of lymphocytes flowing from a thoracic duct fistula (Virchow, 1858). Virchow had suggested that the peripheral lymphoid organs, in addition to their patent filtering function, were major sites of lymphocytopoiesis. Accordingly lymphocytes made in these organs would enter the lymph in numbers that sufficed to replace several times per day the lymphocytes in the blood. How could this rapid turnover of lymphocytes be explained? Did lymphocytes in the blood die and were constantly replaced by newly formed cells derived from the lymph? Did they 'hide'? Where? (Fichtelius, 1953; Trowell, 1958; Florey and Gowans, 1958).

It was known that drainage from a lymph duct without simultaneous reinfusion of lymphocytes from the blood resulted in a progressive depletion of the lymphocytes recovered in the lymph (Mann and Higgins, 1950). Moreover, this depletion could not be obviated by the simultaneous infusion of cell-free lymph (Gowans, 1959). To integrate these two separate lines of evidence by suggesting that lymphocytes continuously circulated between the blood and lymph compartments seemed inconceivable. Such a suggestion was resisted for some time, in spite of precise experimental evidence (Yoffey, 1960; Jansen et al., 1962).

Such experimental support had to derive from the use of a technique enabling the tracing of cells from point of entry to point of exit; if it was suspected that these were not newly formed rapidly dividing cells, the use of chromosome markers was ruled out.

'The possibility that the intravenous transfusion of lymphocytes had initiated the production of new lymphocytes in the recipient animal was tested by infusing tritium-labelled thymidine into one femoral vein of a rat while lymphocytes were transfused simultaneously into the other. Autoradiographs were prepared from successive 4-hour samples of lymphocytes collected from the thoracic duct of the recipient. If the extra lymphocytes collected from the thoracic duct had been formed after the start of the transfusion, their DNA would have become labelled. The results of the experiment are shown in Fig. 2.2 and Table 2.1. During the rising

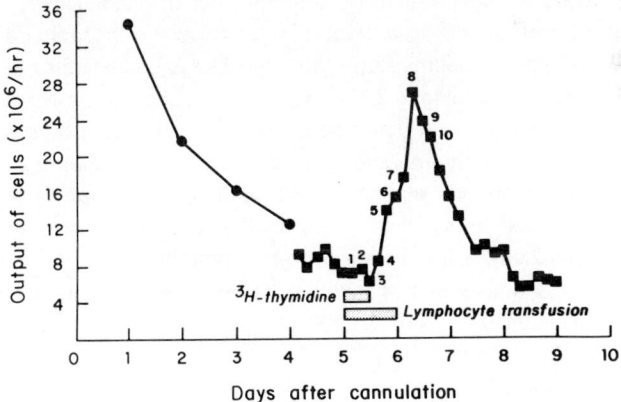

Figure 2.2 Output of lymphocytes from the thoracic duct of a rat which received an intravenous transfusion of lymphocytes during the sixth day after cannulation. Tritium-labelled thymidine was infused intravenously at 20 µc/hr during the first 12 hr of the transfusion. Mean output of cells per hour for successive 24 hr (●──●) and 4 hr (■──■) collections of lymph. 1–10, successive 4 hr collections of lymphocytes from which autoradiographs were prepared. See Table 2.1. Data from Gowans (1959)

Table 2.1 Proportion of small lymphocytes and of tritium-labelled lymphocytes in autoradiographs prepared from collections of lymphocytes. Data from Gowans (1959)

Collection no.	Small lymphocytes (%)	Labelled lymphocytes*	
		Small (%)	Medium and large (%)
1	88.8	0	40
2	88.8	0.1	66
3	92.4	0.4	88
4	93.0	2.0	93
5	94.3	0.9	97
6	96.7	1.2	97
7	94.9	1.6	93
8	97.0	0.4	91
9	95.6	1.1	91
10	94.3	1.0	77

*Percentage derived from counts on 1,000 small lymphocytes and 100 large and medium lymphocytes in each collection.

phase of the output (collections 4–8) more than 90% of the cells in the lymph were small lymphocytes; 2% or less of these contained labelled DNA. This very low proportion of labelled small lymphocytes was not due to an inadequate level of tritium-labelled thymidine in the animal, since, during the same period, more than 90% of the larger lymphocytes which are known to divide in the thoracic duct lymph, became labelled. It was concluded that almost all the small lymphocytes from the thoracic duct of the recipient were 'old' cells in the sense that their DNA had been formed before the start of the transfusion. This experiment rules out mechanisms 1) chemical substances derived from the transfused cells might be essential for the formation of new lymphocytes in the lymph nodes of the recipient animal. 2) The transfused cells might repopulate the lymph nodes of the recipient animal and by successive cell divisions, give rise to a progeny of new lymphocytes unless it is held that "new" lymphocytes can be produced by some process that does not involve the synthesis of new DNA at any stage' (Gowans, 1959).

No such process is known to exist.

Having discarded mechanisms 1 and 2, Gowans proceeded to demonstrate the existence of a *re*circulation of lymphocytes, by following the fate of ^{32}P-labelled lymphocytes into a cannulated rat and measuring the radioactivity in the lymph cells emerging from the thoracic duct (Fig. 2.3). Table 2.2 (Gowans, 1959) shows the relation between the radioactivity in the lymphocyte fractions entering the blood and that recovered in the cell fraction from the thoracic duct. About 20% of the total radioactivity and about 40% of the radioactivity-labelled lipid in the transfused cells were recovered in the lymphocyte fraction from the thoracic duct.

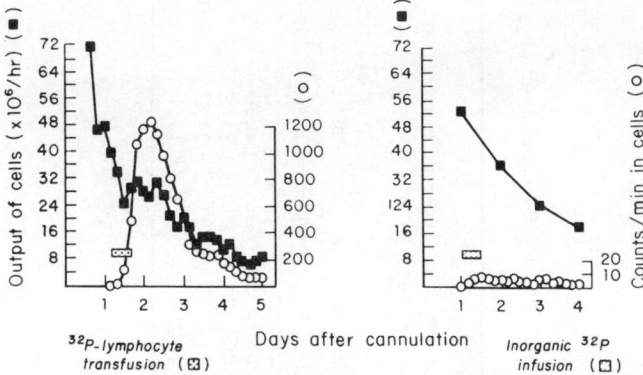

Figure 2.3 Comparison between the amount of radioactivity recovered in the thoracic duct lymph following a transfusion of ^{32}P-labelled lymphocytes (left: total counts/min in transfused cells = 47,500) and the amount of radioactivity recovered following an infusion of a comparable amount of inorganic ^{32}P (right: total counts/min in infused phosphate = 48,800). Data from Gowans (1959)

It could be argued that the radioactivity in the thoracic duct lymphocytes was due to leakage of ^{32}P from the transfused cells and its uptake by the recipient rat's own lymphocytes. The measure of radioactivity in the lipid provides some control against this (Table 2.2). In addition, when the amount of radioactivity which had been transfused into a rat as ^{32}P-labelled lymphocytes was infused into another rat as inorganic phosphate (Fig. 2.3), the cells from the thoracic duct contained a negligible amount of radioactivity (Gowans, 1959).

With these experiments the foundations of a new era in lymphocyte physiology were laid and, I believe, the invaluable contribution of radioisotope labelling well illustrated.

^{32}P is no longer used as a tracer in lymphocyte traffic experiments. DNA or RNA (or both) precursors are the tracers used most frequently nowadays, particularly in experiments involving the use of autoradiography and transfer of non-dividing cells. IudR (Iododeoxiuridine ^{125}IudR) is also being frequently used as a label of dividing cells, enabling the simultaneous quantitative analysis of distribution of the cells by scintillation counting and precise analysis of the distribution of the labelled cells in tissues by autoradiography. ^{51}Cr and more recently ^{111}In are also being used in quantitative studies of lymphocyte distribution (Rannie, Thakur and Ford, 1977).

One must not forget that all the expansion in the use of radioisotopes as markers and cell tracers has its roots in Gowans' first use of ^{32}P and ^{3}H-thymidine. One must also remember that in those days, lymphocytes were believed to come from the site Virchow had indicated, i.e. the lymph nodes, and that in the Harwell group's summary of cell traffic within the lymphomyeloid system (Fig. 2.1) cells originating in the bone marrow, passing or not through the thymus, did not go beyond the lymph nodes.

Table 2.2 Recovery of radioactivity in lymphocytes from thoracic duct after the intravenous transfusion of ^{32}P-labelled lymphocytes. Data from Gowans (1959)

Rat no.	Period of lymph drainage before start of transfusion (days)	No. of cells transfused (×10^6)	Duration of transfusion (hr)	Duration of expt from start of transfusion (hr)	Counts/min in transfused cells		Radioactivity recovered in cells from thoracic duct		As % of counts/min transfused	
							Counts/min			
					Total	Lipid	Total	Lipid	Total	Lipid
149	1	708	14	108	82,800	—	16,680	—	20.1	—*
153	1	444	12	92	47,400	—	10,000	—	21.0	—*
157	5	496	15	120	14,700	1,730	3,310	656	22.5	38.0†
167	5	604	16	84	18,800	1,210	3,270	456	17.4	37.7†

*Radioactive assays, on planchets.
†In liquid counter.

In the next section we shall analyse how the use of autoradiography to trace the fate of radioisotopically labelled lymphocytes in tissues contributed to integrate in the sixties what were separate pieces of the puzzle of lymphocyte circulation in the late fifties.

2.4 AUTORADIOGRAPHY AND THE SPECIFIC POSITIONING OF LYMPHOID CELL POPULATIONS
(Parrott *et al.*, 1966)

Gowans' conclusions in 1959 still met with some criticism, in spite of being supported by the most thorough and impeccable experimental work. Genuine reservations were expressed by the group who discovered that heparin causes a marked lymphocytosis in the blood and an increase in the numbers of lymphocytes in the lymph of the rat (Jansen *et al.*, 1962), suggesting the heparin administered to Gowans' cannulated rats might have caused the appearance of large numbers of lymphocytes in the lymph. 'Historical' criticism was expressed by others.

I call 'historical' criticism the kind of criticism that is expressed by those highly committed to long-lasting controversies suddenly ended by the presentation of new self-evident experimental data. An example that comes to mind is the sudden reduction in the numbers of members of the Flat Earth Society reported by the London *Times* at the time the first American spacecraft reached the moon and produced striking pictures of an unmistakably round earth.

Unlike the American astronauts, who perhaps never heard of the existence of such a peculiar twentieth century society, Gowans acknowledged those who said that so far the evidence for a recirculation of lymphocytes was indirect and that individual small lymphocytes had never been seen in detail along their supposed route from blood to lymph, and produced coloured pictures of autoradiographs of labelled lymphocytes in the lymph nodes, pictures as definitive in the field of lymphocyte physiology as the pictures of a round earth taken from the moon (Gowans and Knight, 1964).

Small lymphocytes not only recirculated from blood to lymph but did so mostly through well-defined areas of the spleen and lymph nodes. Autoradiographs of the spleen and lymph nodes of rats that received intravenous infusions of thoracic duct lymphocytes labelled *in vitro* with ^{3}H-adenosine showed that at 24 hr 'the labelled cells occupied the mid and deep zones of the cortex; they did not penetrate into the germinal centres nor into the cuff of small lymphocytes which sometimes surrounds them'. In the spleen, more labelled small lymphocytes were found in the red pulp of the spleen than in the white pulp. 'However, by 24 they had left the red pulp and appeared in large numbers into the lymphoid follicles, where they localised very precisely around the central arteriole. At no time did labelled cells penetrate into the germinal centres' (Gowans and Knight, 1964).

No reference is made in this paper to the length of exposure time of the autoradiographs; in a more recent paper from Gowans' laboratory (Howard *et al.*, 1972) it has been shown that there are cells in a thoracic duct lymphocyte inoculum which do penetrate the zones round the germinal centres both in lymph nodes and spleen. Their metabolic rate is, however, different from that of the cells found in the original autoradiographs and therefore they were not detected then.

The presence of an additional lymphoid cell population, morphologically indistinguishable from that occupying the periarteriolar sheath in the splenic white pulp and the mid and deep cortical zones in the lymph nodes, was detected for the first time in the peripheral layer of the white pulp follicles in the spleen and in the primary nodules of the lymph nodes, in a study of the migratory patterns of ^{3}H-adenosine-labelled thymus and spleen cells in the mouse (Parrott et al., 1966).

Technically, the tracing methods used in these experiments were identical to those pioneered by Gowans, i.e. *in vitro* labelling with ^{3}H-adenosine and the 'dipping' autoradiography technique modified by Kopriwa and Leblond (1962). Their design, however, was very different. They were not designed to end, or start, a major controversy; equipped with the acute awareness that two independent lines of lymphoid cell differentiation existed (Good and Gabrielsen, 1964), they were designed to demonstrate that the positioning of different classes of lymphoid cells in the peripheral lymphoid organs was a morphological and dynamic reflection of that dichotomy, whose functional implications were expressed in the different abilities of thymus and spleen cells to correct the impaired immunological responses of neonatally thymectomized mice (Parrott and East, 1964).

The tedious counting of the numbers of labelled cells in different areas of spleen and lymph nodes led to the discovery that labelled thymus cells migrated predominantly to the areas where Gowans and Knight (1964) had found labelled thoracic duct lymphocytes to be located. Spleen cells were found in addition in the periphery of the white pulp follicles and in the lymph node primary nodules (Table 2.3).

From these observations it was concluded:

'that the normal thymus produces throughout life, but particularly in the neonatal period, large numbers of cells which contribute directly to the "mobilisable pool" of lymphocytes. The results suggest that there also exists another system primarily responsible for production of the plasma cell series, comparable to the Bursa of Fabricius in chickens, but as yet unidentified in mammals (Peterson *et al.* 1965). Nevertheless, these two systems function synergistically so that diminution or absence of the thymus-dependent population of lymphocytes will cause aberrant activity of the plasma cell series. The thymus may thus, directly or indirectly, control the balance of cell populations within the body, a conclusion which receives additional support from recent studies using the "autoimmune" strain of New Zealand Black mice (East *et al.*, 1965) (Parrott *et al.*, 1966).'

Relatively simple morphological methods had led to the discovery of cell migration differences between otherwise identical cells, a phenomenon later called

Table 2.3 Destination of ³H-adenosine-labelled thymus and spleen cells in the spleen of thymectomized and intact mice. Data from Parrott et al. (1966)

Time after injection hr	min	Inoculum	No. of mice	No. of sections counted*	No. of labelled cells/area RP	MZ	B	T
0	15	Thymus cells	1 Tx	2	87, 133	21, 30	0, 0	0, 0
0	15	Thymus cells	1 Intact	3	96, 91, 90	38, 68, 72	0, 0	0, 0, 0
1	15	Thymus cells	2 Tx	4	3, 0, 2, 1	61, 10, 12, 2	5, 0, 0, 0	0, 0, 0, 0
5–6		Thymus cells	3 Tx	12	1 (0–3)	0	1 (0–3)	2 (0–10)
		Thymus cells	1 Intact	1	0	1	2	9
24		Thymus cells	3 Tx	8	1 (0–4)	0	8 (0–16)	51 (18–90)
		Thymus cells	2 Intact	3	0, 0, 0	0, 0, 0	2, 8, 38	20, 42, 120
62		Thymus cells	1 Tx	1	0	2	9	145
0	15	Spleen cells	1 Tx	4	1, 0, 0, 0	0, 1, 2, 0	0, 0, 0, 0	0, 0, 0, 0
0	15	Spleen cells	1 Intact	4	1, 5, 1, 1	7, 6, 0, 1	0, 3, 0, 0	0, 0, 0, 0
1	15	Spleen cells	2 Tx	5	8 (1–24)	1 (0–1)	1 (0–2)	1 (0–1)
5–6		Spleen cells	2 Tx	3	4, 5, 4	0, 2, 0	99, 67, 38	47, 49, 22
		Spleen cells	3 Intact	3	7, 13, 22	0, 2, 4	56, 188, 113	22, 140, 113
24		Spleen cells	3 Tx	3	1, 16, 2	1, 1, 0	176, 349, 54	63, 90, 24
		Spleen cells	2 Intact	2	0, 9	0, 5	224, 425	38, 97
62		Spleen cells	2 Tx	2	6, 14	6, 11	258, 239	90, 116

*The mean number and range of labelled cells counted is indicated when more than four sections were scanned.
RP = red pulp; MZ = marginal zone; B = cell area; T = T cell area (see plate 5); Tx = thymectomized.

ecotaxis (de Sousa, 1971). There were no clues at the time that more subtle differences existed within each of the two major lymphoid cell populations. Detection of these differences depended on the availability of yet another set of discriminating tools. The discovery of these is described in the following section.

2.5 THE Ly SYSTEM OF LYMPHOCYTE ISOANTIGENS IN THE MOUSE
(Boyse et al., 1968)

The description of the discovery of cytotoxic antibodies specific to lymphocytes (thymic and peripheral) shares many features with the description of the discovery of the T6 chromosome. Both discoveries seem to have occurred 'in the course' of another study, their use permits the following of the distribution of donor cells in the lymphoid tissues of X-irradiated recipients, and their application has turned out to be crucial to the understanding of lymphoid cell participation in the development and control of the immune response (Cantor and Boyse, 1975).

The existence of isoantigens specific to lymphocytes was discovered in the course of studies of the G (Gross) and the ML (mammary leukaemia) mouse leukaemia antigens (Old et al., 1963; Stück et al., 1964):

'the cytotoxic typing sera used in analyzing these systems were found to contain additional unidentified cytotoxic antibodies, distinct from the leukaemia antibodies anti-G and anti-ML. Further investigation of these additional antibodies has revealed the existence of two hitherto unrecognized systems of isoantigens which appear to be confined to lymphocytes

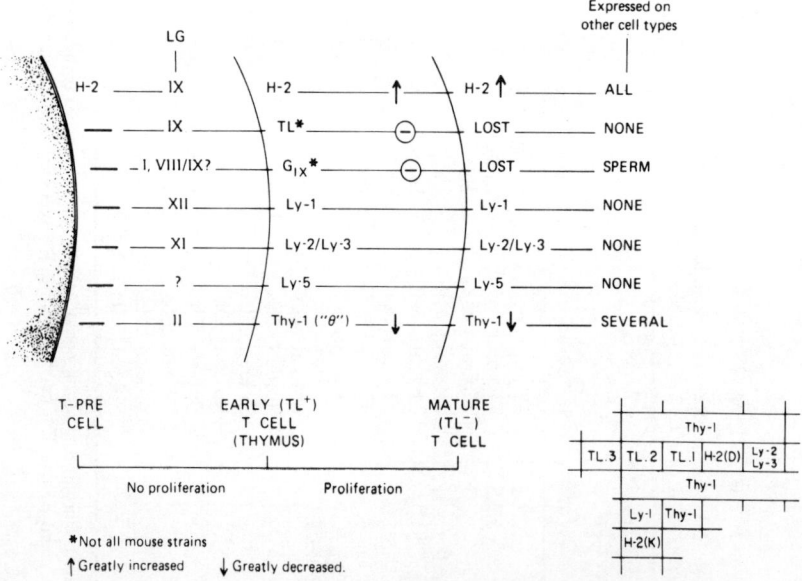

Figure 2.4 Differentiation of T cells (courtesy E. A. Boyse)

including thymic lymphocytes. The designations Ly-A and Ly-B (Ly = lymphocyte) seem appropriate for isoantigens of these two systems, in view of the finding that the antigens are not demonstrable on cells other than lymphocytes. Both systems appear to be simple, each mouse strain possessing one of two alternative alleles for each system. The genetic loci will be designated Ly-A and Ly-B' (Boyse et al., 1968).

This new development in the methodology of lymphocyte identification is most important; it shares with the chromosome marker technique the attraction of making possible the finding of a cell at any time following cell transfer, and with the radioisotope labelling technique the attraction of detecting non-dividing cells. A summary of the updated termination describing the presently known T lymphoid cell differentiation antigens is presented in Fig. 2.4.

From the absorption capacity of various tissues for Ly antibodies and from assays of the cytotoxic activity of the antibodies (Boyse et al., 1968; Cantor and Boyse, 1975), it is now known that the Ly antigens are expressed only in thymus-derived lymphocytes and that their relative proportions in the spleen and lymph nodes differ (Table 2.4).

Table 2.4 Distribution of Ly-bearing T cells. Data from Beverley (1977)

Ly phenotype†	Percentage of T cells in*				
	Thymus	CRT	Spleen	Lymph node	TDL
1^+‡	>10	35–45	30–40	35–45	40–60
$2^+ 3^+$	>10	10–20	10–20	5–15	2–10
$1^+ 2^+ 3^+$	>90	40–55	45–55	40–50	35–55

*Based on numbers of cells killed by anti-Ly sera expressed as a percentage of cells killed by anti-Thy 1.
†Data for C57B1/6 except for TDL in CBA/CA (Sprent and Beverley, unpublished).
‡Number of Ly 1^+ cells obtained by subtracting number killed by anti 2.3 antiserum from 100%.
CRT, cortisone-resistant thymocytes; TDL, thoracic duct lymphocytes.

Chapter 3

Areas of Lymphoid Cell Traffic within the Peripheral Lymphoid Organs

3.1 INTRODUCTION

Detailed descriptions of the morphology of the peripheral lymphoid organs, of the arrangement of lymphoid cell populations in major T and B cells areas, and of morphological changes taking place in those areas during the development of cell mediated or humoral immunity responses have been the subject of numerous reviews and chapters published elsewhere (Parrott, 1967; Parrott and de Sousa, 1971; de Sousa and Anderson, 1970; Weiss, 1972; de Sousa, 1973; Turk, 1973; Weissman *et al.*, 1974; Weissman, 1975, 1976; de Sousa, 1978a; de Sousa and Good, 1978; Weissman *et al.*, 1978). In addition, updated illustrations of lymph node and spleen morphology have become part of standard histology and immunology textbooks (Ham, 1979; Roitt, 1977). The purpose of this chapter is to remind the reader briefly of the distribution in the peripheral lymphoid organs of the major areas of lymphoid cell traffic and to bring to his attention some ultrastructural and cytochemical aspects of these areas that may contribute to the control of the different patterns of migration exhibited by distinct lymphomyeloid cell populations.

3.2 SPLEEN

The main microenvironments found in the chicken and mammalian spleen are represented diagramatically in Fig. 3.1 and Plate 5. In fish, lymphoid tissue is present in the spleen and in the kidney pronephros and mesonephros. Both in the pronephros and mesonephros and in the spleen, the organization of lymphoid cells in fish is much less complex than that seen in the chicken and in mammalian spleens. In all cases, macroscopically the spleen can be divided into two major components, the red and the white pulps. The white pulp consists of firm, whitish nodules dispersed among the spongy mass of the red pulp. Malpighi (1686), in a series of experiments aimed at separating and characterizing the two pulps, demonstrated that the white pulp nodules were connected like bunches of grapes,

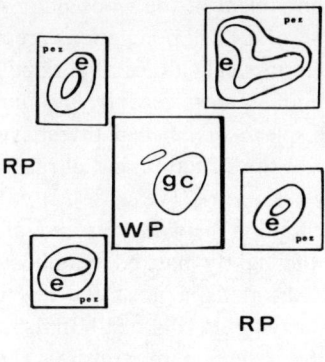

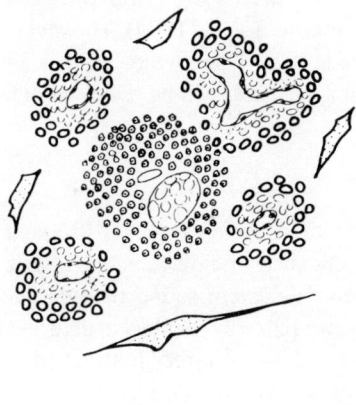

Figure 3.1 Diagrammatic representation (a) of the main areas of the chicken spleen drawn from a tissue section (b). The white pulp (WP) consists of thymus-derived lymphocytes occupying the periarteriolar sheath, and of well-delineated germinal centres (gc) containing lymphoblasts of bursa origin. At the interface between white and red pulp (RP) ellipsoids (e) can be found. The lymphoid cells surrounding the ellipsoids constitute the periellipsoidal zone (pez) and contain mostly bursa-derived cells

and since then the term 'Malpighian follicle' or 'Malpighian body' has been used widely to define the main component of the white pulp. A technique to separate white and red pulp for analysis of the cell populations present in the two pulps was developed by Fagraeus in her classical studies of antibody production by plasma cells (Fagraeus, 1948) and applied more recently by Durkin *et al.* (1978) to the study of distribution in the spleen of labelled thymocytes and thymus-derived cells. For an extensive study of the structure and ultrastructure of the spleen, the reader is invited to consult Weiss's work (Weiss, 1972).

Histologically, the differentiation between the red and white pulps is comparatively easy insofar as the tightly packed lymphocytes that constitute the Malpighian body stand out distinctly against the less well-organized sheet of haemopoietic cells found in the red pulp (Plate 5b). In fish, the ratio of red to white pulp is greater than 1; the white pulp consists simply of aggregates of melanomacrophages (rich in iron and melanin) and lymphocytes. Plaice labelled neural duct lymphocytes were found to migrate selectively to the lymphoid macrophage aggregates of the splenic white pulp, indicating that the phenomenon of non-random migration of circulating lymphoid cells is apparent at an early stage in evolution (Ellis and de Sousa, 1974). However, the specific migration of lymphoid cells to selected sites of the white pulp is much more striking in the chicken and in the rodent spleen and will be reviewed in detail later (Chapter 4).

3.2.1. Chicken (Fig. 3.1)

The white pulp in the chicken spleen consists of three major components: the lymphoid area immediately surrounding the central arterioles, containing mostly thymus-derived cells; well delineated, round or oval germinal centres containing bursa-derived cells; and specialized vascular structures, the ellipsoids, positioned at the interface between white and red pulps and surrounded by a cuff of lymphoid cells derived mostly from the bursa of Fabricus.

3.2.2 Mouse, rat and human spleen (Plate 5)

Most detailed experimental studies of the structure and ultrastructure of the lymphoid microenvironments of the spleen have been done in the mouse and the rat. With the exception of the fact that haemopoiesis takes place in the mouse spleen red pulp (which does not occur in other rodents or in the human spleen), most of the observations made in the mouse are applicable to the analysis and understanding of spleen structure in other mammalian species including man.

3.2.3 White pulp

The white pulp consists of lymphoid nodules aggregated around branches of the splenic artery (for details of microvasculature, see Fig. 1.3) distributed along the major axis of the spleen. Each nodule can be further subdivided into two lymphoid areas: a thymus-dependent area located in the periarteriolar sheath, normally occupied by lymphocytes derived from the thymus, and a thymus-independent area located in the outer zone of the Malpighian nodule, normally occupied by lymphocytes of thymus-independent derivation (Plate 6). With the generalization of the use of the terms T and B cells to designate lymphocyte populations of thymus-dependent or thymus-independent derivation, the use of the terms T and B cell areas or domains has also become generalized. The presence of cells other than lymphocytes, namely plasma cells and polymorphs in splenic T cell areas, has been reported in pathological situations of transient or permanent T cell depletion, such as in old neonatally thymectomized mice (Parrott et al., 1966) following whole body X-irradiation (van Ewijk et al., 1974), during certain types of systemic infections (Turk, 1973), and in splenic B cell lymphomas (de Sousa, unpublished observations). But normally T and B cell areas contain separate circulating lymphoid cell populations. Furthermore, studies of the origin of lymphoid cells reconstituting the depleted lymphoid organs of animals that received whole body irradiation have confirmed the selective reconstitution of B cell regions with B cells or cells of bone marrow derivation (Gutman and Weissman, 1973; van Ewijk et al., 1974) and of thymus-dependent areas with T cells or cells of thymus derivation (van Ewijk et al., 1974).

Other studies attempting to define further differences between the two areas that could constitute the basis for the selective migration of distinct lymphoid cell populations have shown that the reticulum cells occupying these two areas have distinct ultrastructural and histochemical properties (Veerman, 1974; van Ewijk et al., 1974; Müller-Hermelink, 1974; Müller-Hermelink et al., 1976; Lennert et al., 1978). A summary of these findings is presented in Tables 3.1 and 3.2.

The ultrastructure of the reticulum cell found in T cell areas was first described in detail by Veldman in a study of the rabbit lymph node (Veldman, 1970) and was designated by this author as interdigitating reticulum cell (IDC). IDCs are present in splenic and lymph node T cell areas in close contact with small lymphocytes. They have a very low electron density of the cytoplasm, containing only a few mitochondria, poorly developed granular endoplasmic reticulum, and

Table 3.1 Enzyme histochemical patterns of different reticulum cells in human lymphatic tissue. Data from Müller-Hermelink et al. (1976)

Reticulum cells	Localization	Non-spec. esterase	Acid phosphat.	Alkaline phosphat.	5'-n'ase	ATPase
Dendritic	B cell region	+	–	–	+	–
Interdigitating	T cell region	((+))	(+)	–	–	+
Fibroblastic	Esp. border of T cell region	(+)	(+)	+	–	–/+
Histiocytic	Uncharacteristic	+++	+++	–	–	–/+

Table 3.2 Ontogenetic appearance of different reticulum cells in human lymphatic tissue. Data from Müller-Hermelink et al. (1976)

Gestational age	Thymus	Lymph node	Spleen
8–9 weeks	First appearance of IDC in perivascular spaces		
12–14 weeks	Demarcation of medulla. IDC ++	Haemopoiesis, esp. myelopoiesis, first lymphatic cells	
16 weeks	'Normal'	IDC ++, typical T cell region	
20 weeks	'Normal'	IDC ++, typical T cell region	First lymphocytes in periarteriolar region. IDC +/−
26–30 weeks	'Normal'	In some: B cell region with DRC	B cell and T cell regions with IDC and DRC

numerous large empty vacuoles about 1 μ in diameter. They also contain small tubular vesicles about 800 Å in diameter and microtubules, 330 Å in diameter, mostly close to the nucleus. They contain few phagosomes, and therefore are thought not to be actively phagocytizing. The nucleus is generally very irregular with deep indentations (van Ewijk et al., 1974). An illustration of the ultrastructure of an IDC is shown in Plate 7.

Histochemically, IDCs are ATPase positive, alkaline phosphatase negative and 5'-n'ase negative. They appear first in the human spleen at 20 weeks of gestation (Müller-Hermelink et al., 1976).

The ultrastructure of the reticulum cell present in B cell areas was also first described by Veldman (1970) and designated dendritic reticulum cell (DRC). The dendritic reticulum cell (Plate 8) has long, fine cytoplasmic projections which are often connected by desmosomes. It has very few lysosomes and no evidence of phagocytosis is seen in association with this cell.

3.2.4 Marginal zone

The marginal zone surrounds the white pulp nodules at the interface between white and red pulps (Plate 5c). As shown earlier (see Fig. 1.3), the microvasculature in this region has a large sectional area and thus blood flow is correspondingly slow therein. Intravenously injected cells, antigenic or nonantigenic materials, are found predominantly in this area within seconds of injection (Plate 5c). Labelled cells stay in the marginal zone up to 5 hr following injection, before migrating to selected areas within the white pulp. This is, therefore, a route of entry into spleen, an area of 'non-specific' cell, antigen or particle traffic, probably the most important area within the spleen, in which interactions between different macrophage, lymphocyte and granulocyte populations take place.

Table 3.3 Some distinguishing features between marginal zone and red pulp macrophages. Data from Humphrey (1980)

Fluorescent polysaccharide	Spleen zone	Uptake	Lymphocyte adhesion
S3	Red pulp	High	+
	Marginal zone	Low	+++
Ficoll and hydroxyethyl starch	Red pulp	Very low	+
	Marginal zone	High	+++

Morphological and autoradiographic studies indicate that following the administration of antigens or adjuvants, cell traffic through this area is delayed (de Sousa, unpublished observations; Freitas and de Sousa, 1977). This is also the area to which significant numbers of cells derived from the thymus cortex migrate, following antigen stimulation (Durkin et al., 1978).

Thus, many of the important processes of regulation of the immune response, involving antigen presentation to lymphocytes by antigen-bearing macrophages, interaction between suppressor lymphocytes and macrophages, etc., could take place in this region. It is, therefore, of considerable importance to find means of characterizing the macrophage populations in it. This has been done, in part, recently in a study of the distribution of fluorescent polysaccharides within the spleen. Humphrey (1980) was able to establish distinguishing features between marginal zone macrophages and macrophages found in other splenic sites. A summary of these features is presented in Table 3.3.

Pneumococcal polysaccharide type 3 (S3) was present in all red pulp macrophages and in some but not all marginal zone macrophages. Ficoll and hydroxyethyl starch, on the other hand, were highly concentrated in and confined to large cells in the marginal zone. In this study, marginal zone macrophages (detected by Ficoll or hydroxyethyl starch phagocytosis) were isolated from spleen cell suspension and examined in cytocentrifuge preparations. They were generally larger than red pulp macrophages and had as the most characteristic feature several lymphocytes adhering to them. They stain strongly for cytoplasmic acid phosphatase and non-specific esterase and have both Fc and C3 receptors.

Finally, this is also the zone through which granulocytes appear to circulate in large numbers, both shortly after the administration of antigens and in some forms of disease, i.e. Hodgkin's disease (de Sousa, Smithyman, and Tan, 1978) and chronic myeloid leukaemia.

3.2.5 Red pulp (Plate 5a and b)

The red pulp is largely occupied by circulating erythrocytes and most light microscopy and ultrastructural studies of this spleen zone have been concerned with its microcirculation and with the interactions occurring therein between erythrocytes and macrophages. Lymphoid cell aggregates, however, are also found in the red pulp as cuffs round the trabeculae and as scattered aggregates, not as well defined as those constituting the white pulp. In addition, during the development of an immune response these are the sites of maturation of antibody-producing cells. Plasma cells are found in the peritrabecular cuffs and frequently in small groups close to the marginal zone.

In addition, in the mouse, the red pulp is also an active haemopoietic environment. Curry and Trentin (1967) delineated the specific microscopic localization of erythroid, granulocytic and megakaryocytic colonies in X-irradiated mice 8–9 days following reconstitution with small numbers of bone marrow cells. Erythroid colonies appear anywhere within the red pulp, avoiding the atrophic white pulp follicles. Granulocytic colonies are usually found growing along the trabeculae or in subcapsular sheets. Megakaryocytes occur in aggregates by themselves or mixed within colonies of other cell types. They are usually found under the splenic capsule (Curry and Tentin, 1967).

3.3 LYMPH NODE

Histologically, the lymph node is divided into two major compartments: the cortex and the medulla, which, in most lymph nodes, can be easily differentiated as a result of the arrangement of the medulla in cords and sinuses in contrast with the more uniform appearance of the cortex (Plate 9). Moreover, the medulla contains a much wider variety of cells (including lymphocytes, plasma cells, macrophages, and mast cells) than the cortex, where the predominating cell, in an unstimulated node, is the small lymphocyte. In the periphery of the cortex, immediately under the marginal sinus, lymphocytes of bone marrow or foetal liver origin are aggregated in well-defined nodules (primary nodules) constituting the B cell area (Plate 9); the rest of the cortex consists of a diffuse sheet of small lymphocytes (Plate 9) amongst which prominent, high endothelium venules are present. In the lymph nodes of thymus-deprived animals, a selective depletion of lymphocytes occurs in the mid-cortex, also designated paracortex; lymphocytes remain in the primary nodules and in the border between cortex and medulla (cortico-medullary junction) and in the medulla. As illustrated earlier (Plate 3), postcapillary venules in T cell depleted nodes are ill-defined and often difficult to locate. In normal sheep lymph nodes, venules with high endothelium are infrequent (Fahy et al., 1980). In the pig, the relative arrangement of the two lymph node areas is inverted, with a central cortical region and peripheral medulla which lacks typical sinuses and cords (reviewed by Binns, 1980).

In most other species, the medulla consists of cords and sinuses (Plate 10). In an unstimulated lymph node the cords are occupied mostly by B lymphoid cells; after antigen stimulation, at the time of antibody production, plasma cells occupy the medullary cords. Normally, there are very few cells present in the lymph node medullary sinuses. There are, however, situations both in mice and in man in which the sinuses appear choked by large numbers of macrophages and histiocytes. In experimental animals, sinus histiocytosis is frequently associated with continuous high antigen stimulation, such as that necessary for the development of high zone tolerance (de Sousa et al., 1971). In terms of cell traffic, the cortex is the zone preferentially utilized by cells leaving the bloodstream and entering the lymph circuit. Both T and B lymphocytes enter the lymph nodes through postcapillary venules located in the mid-cortex. Once in the substance of the node, T cells circulate through the T cell area and B cells, somehow, find their way to the outer cortical region (Plates 9 and 12).

Analyses of the ultrastructural and cytochemical features of reticulum cells in the two major lymph node areas have yielded results identical to those described earlier for splenic regions (Table 3.1).

Recent studies of the cellular composition of afferent lymph have given some clues to the possible origin of the interdigitating reticulum cell (IDC) characteristically found in lymph node thymus-dependent areas (Plate 7). Evidence from the recent work of Hendriks (1978) and Kelly and co-workers (Kelly et al., 1978) indicates that the T cell region IDC derives from the so-called 'veiled' cell in afferent lymph. Veiled cells constitute 8–30% of the total cell population of afferent lymph draining the skin. They are present in all species examined thus far (man, rabbit, pig, sheep). They are not found in the blood or efferent lymph.

Kelly et al. (1978) followed the fate of ^{3}H-adenosine-labelled veiled cells reinfused in afferent lymph and found that they distribute in the mid-cortical T cell region. Hendriks, in the reverse type of experiment, observed the disappearance of lymph node interdigitating cells at 6 weeks of ligation of the afferent lymphatics (Hendriks, 1978). Further similarities between the two cell types include the recent demonstration that veiled cells in lymph and IDC in lymph node and spleen T cell areas are strongly Ia positive (Lampert et al., 1979).

The interaction of circulating T and B lymphocytes with IDC and DRC distributed in separate lymph node regions may constitute part of the basis for the selective distribution of the two major lymphoid cell populations within lymph nodes and spleen. In addition to having distinct destinations within the tissues, T and B lymphocytes have also different tempos of circulation from blood to lymph (see Chapter 4.2) and T lymphocytes are more easily mobilizable from lymphoid tissues into lymph than B lymphocytes (Cottier et al., 1980). It has been speculated that the open arrangement of the reticular framework in the thymus-dependent area (de Sousa, 1969) allows the easier mobilization of cells in this area, whereas the closer reticular patterns of the medullary cords (Plate 10a) might lead to a greater degree of cell sequestration.

It seems unlikely, however, that reticular arrangement alone should participate in the control of lymphoid cell mobilization, since the primary nodules, consisting predominantly of B lymphocytes, are virtually devoid of reticular fibres. Cell adhesion and other physical and immunological properties of the circulating cells must also contribute to their different mobilization properties.

3.4 PEYER'S PATCHES AND APPENDIX

It has been stated by Reynolds that 'it is important to emphasize that Peyer's patches are not mere goose pimples in the wall of the intestine' (Reynolds, 1980).

In small rodents, Peyer's patches appear as isolated round whitish patches along the intestine wall, predominantly along the small intestine. But, for example, in the three month lamb, one Peyer's patch alone extends for about 1.5 m along the distal end of the small intestine (Reynolds, 1980). In sheep, Peyer's patches reach their maximum size in two month-old lambs, then they get smaller, and by 15 months are macroscopically involuted.

Detailed descriptions of the structure and function of Peyer's patches in the development of IgA-producing cells will be given in Chapter 5 (p. 112).

Briefly, Peyer's patches can be be divided into three major microenvironments represented schematically in Plate 11. They are a nodular or follicular area occupied largely by B cells, the interfollicular area normally containing thymus-derived lymphocytes, and the dome area facing the intestinal luminal side in a region of non-villous intestinal epithelium. In animals that have been neonatally thymectomized or born without a thymus, a clear depletion of lymphocytes can be seen selectively along the interfollicular, thymus-dependent area (Plate 11c).

In mice, Peyer's patches at birth have the histological appearance of primitive lymphoid organs consisting largely of reticular, endothelial and histiocytic cells. Within 1–3 days after birth, however, the number of lymphocytes increases markedly, and by day 4, lymphocytes constitute 90–95% of the cells present in Peyer's patches (Joel *et al.*, 1972). The majority of these lymphocytes have been

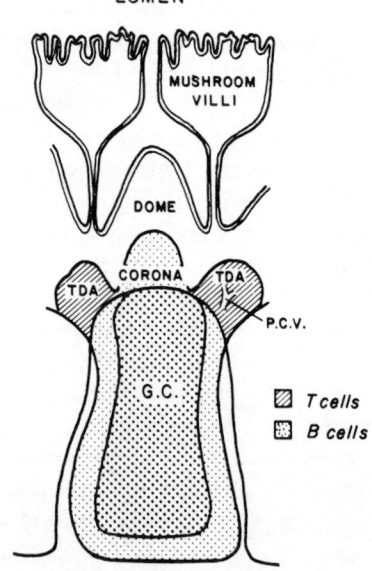

Figure 3.2 Diagrammatic representation of the distribution of T and B cells in the appendix. G.C., germinal centre; TDA, thymus-dependent area. From Parrott (1976a,b)

shown to derive from the thymus (Joel et al., 1972). The greater expansion observed in the growth patterns and lymphoid cell population of Peyer's patches (and the mesenteric node) than in peripheral lymph nodes in the neonatal period has been attributed to antigenic stimulation from the intestinal flora which develops during this period (Joel et al., 1972). It has been pointed out that Peyer's patches are located at a strategic site which becomes highly exposed to antigens after birth. This is also the section of the intestine where iron absorption takes place. The possibility that the extensive migration of T cells to the small intestine shortly after birth is also related to the absorption of Fe is raised and discussed later (Chapter 8.2).

T and B cell regions have also been delineated in the appendix (Waksman et al., 1973; Parrott, 1976a,b) and are represented diagrammatically in Fig. 3.2. Briefly, the T cell region is diamond-shaped and localized between the upper ends of adjacent B cell nodules consisting of germinal centres surrounded by small B lymphocytes.

3.5 APPLICATION TO THE STUDY OF MALIGNANT LYMPHOMAS

The histochemical and ultrastructural characterization of the reticulum cells of T and B cell areas has been of value in the study of some lymph node diseases (Goos and Kaiserling, 1975; Rausch et al., 1977) and malignant lymphomas (Lennert et al., 1978).

In low-grade malignant lymphomas of germinal centre origin (follicular lymphoma) non-specific esterase positive cells, with the ultrastructural features of DRC, have been found associated with the follicular areas of the lymphoma (Lennert et al., 1978). Interdigitating reticulum cells, on the other hand, have been

Table 3.4 Occurrence of specific reticulum cells in low-grade non-Hodgkin's lymphomas. Data from Lennert et al. (1978)

Low-grade malignant lymphoma	Dendritic reticulum cells	Interdigitating reticulum cells	No characteristic pattern
Lymphocytic			
B-CLL			+
T-CLL		+	
Hairy-cell leukaemia			+
Mycosis fungoides and Sézary syndrome		+	
T-zone lymphoma		+	
Lymphoplasmacytic/lymphoplasmacytoid (LP immunocytoma)			+
Plasmacytic			+
Centrocytic	+		
Centroblastic/centrocytic	+		

There is no characteristic reticulum-cell pattern in high-grade non-Hodgkin's lymphomas.

identified in association with low-grade malignancy T cell lymphomas in thymus-dependent areas of lymph nodes (Rausch *et al.*, 1977; Lennert *et al.*, 1978) and in skin of patients with mycosis fungoides (Goos *et al.*, 1976). A summary of the findings of Lennert and his co-workers on the distribution of dendritic and interdigitating reticulum cells in non-Hodgkin's lymphomas is presented in Table 3.4. It is intriguing that both in T and B cell lymphomas of high-grade malignancy, only occasional reticulum cells were detected (Lennert *et al.*, 1978).

Chapter 4

Circulation of Lymphocytes within the Lymphoid System

4.1 TRANSIT TIMES IN DIFFERENT SPECIES

The first demonstration of a continuous circulation of lymphocytes between blood and lymph (Gowans, 1959) was described earlier (Chapter 2.2). The existence of a blood to lymph circulation of small lymphocytes has since been widely confirmed in the rat (reviewed by Ford and Gowans, 1969; Ford, 1975) and other experimental animals investigated, namely plaice (Ellis and de Sousa, 1974), duck (Bell and Lafferty, 1972), sheep (Frost *et al.*, 1975; Hall and Morris, 1965; Pearson *et al.*, 1976), mouse (Sprent, 1973), and in man (Tilney and Murray, 1968). In experiments of design essentially similar to that of Gowans' (1959) and Gowans and Knight's (1964), we have enlarged considerably the detail of our knowledge about the route, time, ontogeny, and phylogeny of lymphocyte recirculation and, but for one lonely voice (Sainte-Marie, 1975), the original conclusions of Gowans have remained undisputed.

In the original study, little significance was attributed to the finding of large numbers of labelled small lymphocytes in the lungs at the early times after intravenous injection, and it was almost inferred that the finding of small lymphocytes at this time in the lungs was unphysiological (Gowans and Knight, 1964). Subsequent quantitative studies of the distribution of intravenously infused [^{3}H]-uridine- or [^{3}H]-adenosine-labelled lymphocytes have confirmed, however, that the physiological route of migration for labelled cells injected intravenously is indeed through the pulmonary capillary network in the mammals and through the gills in fish.

In Figs. 4.1a and b, graphs of the distribution of labelled rat thoracic duct and plaice neural duct lymphocytes at different times after injection are presented. At the early times after injection (10 min and $\frac{1}{2}$ hr) a considerable proportion of recovered TCA-insoluble radioactivity is present in the lungs and gill. By 24 hr, the majority of recovered radioactivity is present in the peripheral lymphoid organs, i.e. spleen and lymph nodes in the rat and spleen and kidney lymphoid tissue in plaice (Fig. 4.1).

The transit time of lymphocyte circulation clearly differs from species to species, and, within the same species, with age. The first estimations of transit

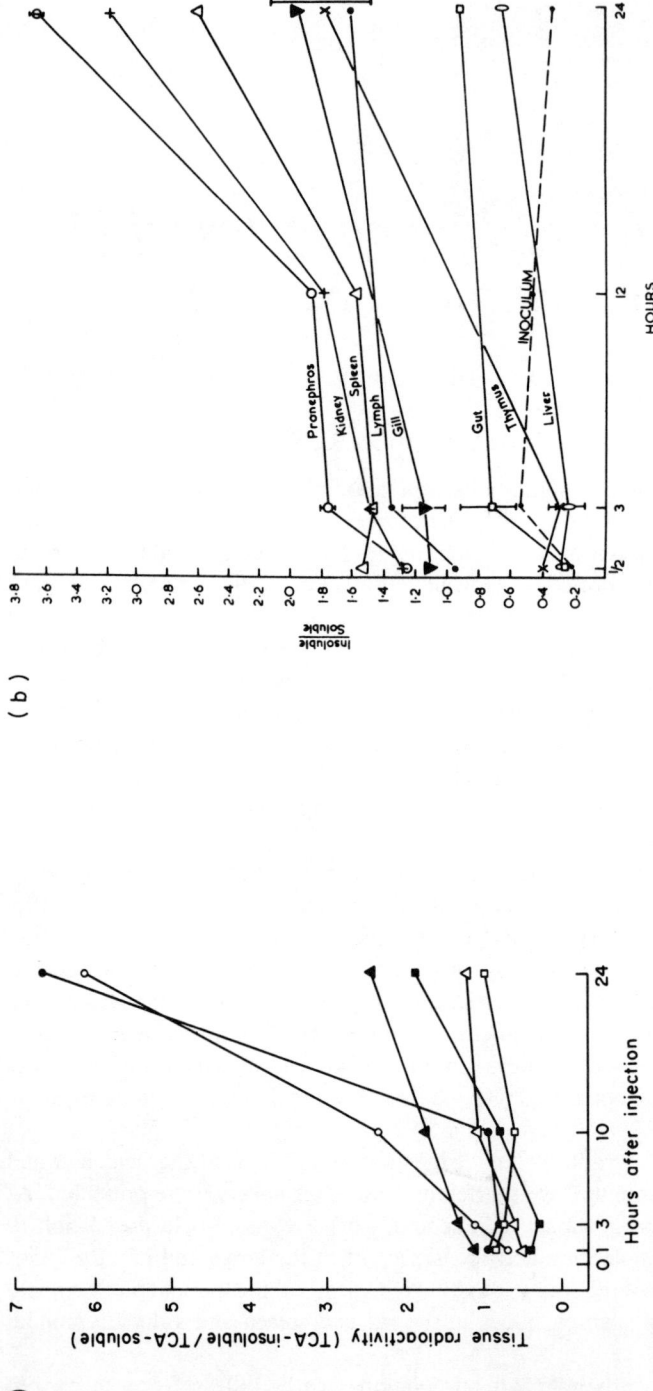

Figure 4.1 (a) Radioactivity in samples of lungs (▲——▲), spleen (○——○), mesenteric lymph node (●——●), thymus (△——△), liver (□——□), and intestine (■——■) from rats injected intravenously with 10^6 [H^3]-5-uridine-labelled thoracic duct lymphocytes per gramme of body weight. Between 1 and 21 hr, there was a relative increase in radioactivity in the trichloroacetic acid (TCA)-insoluble fraction of spleen and mesenteric lymph node. Little or no increase occurred in other tissues. Data from Goldschneider and McGregor (1968a). (b) Pattern of the change in TCA-soluble: TCA-insoluble ratio over a 24 hr period after injection of 10^5 neural duct lymphocytes per gramme of body weight labelled in vitro with [^{3}H]-uridine reinjected intravenously into the renal portal vein (plaice). In this period of time there was a relative increase in radioactivity in the TCA-insoluble fraction of pronephoros, kidney, and spleen. Little or no increase occurred in other tissues. Data from Ellis and de Sousa (1974)

Table 4.1 Estimated transit times through the main compartments of the blood to lymph circuit in the rat. Data from Ford and Gowans (1969)

Compartment	Total no. of small lymphocytes		Average transit time (hr)
	Recirculating ($\times 10^6$)	Other ($\times 10^6$)	
Blood	100	15	0.6
Spleen	450	300–600	5–6
Lymph nodes			
Above diaphragm	600	Negligible	15–20
Below diaphragm	600	Negligible	15–20

times of the circulation of lymphocytes through the different compartments of the blood to lymph circuit were published by Ford and Gowans (1969) for the male rat (Table 4.1). Small lymphocytes spend less than one hour (0.6 hr) in the blood and take 5–6 hr to migrate through the spleen and 15–20 hr through the lymph nodes. The time small lymphocytes infused intravenously take to reach the lymph (Table 4.2) is much shorter in plaice (0.5 hr) and duck (0.5–11 hr), approximately the same in the adult mouse (18–24 hr), and longer in the adult sheep (27–36 hr) but shorter in young sheep. Pearson *et al.* (1976), in perhaps technically the most remarkable study of lymphocyte recirculation, cannulated the thoracic duct in lambs *in utero* and determined the time labelled foetal lamb thoracic duct lymphocytes infused intravenously take to reach the thoracic duct lymph. In the foetal lamb, the time is shorter (12–18 hr) than in the young or the adult sheep.

One important aspect of this work, besides its obvious technical achievement, is the demonstration that the recirculation of lymphocytes between blood and lymph is an inherent component of the physiology of the lymphoid system, which clearly antecedes any interaction of the circulating cells with antigen. A detailed summary of the changes observed in lymph flow and in numbers of small lymphocytes reaching the lymph during foetal life is included in Table 4.3.

Table 4.2 Comparison between the times of arrival of labelled cells to lymph following intravenous injection

Author	Animal	Peak arrival time to lymph (hr)
Ellis and de Sousa (1974)	Plaice	0.5
Bell and Lafferty (1972)	Duck	9.5–11
Pearson *et al.* (1976)	Foetal lamb	12–18
Ford *et al.* (1976)	Young lamb	18–24
Ford and Gowans (1969)	Adult rat	15–20
Sprent (1973)	Adult mouse	18–24
Frost *et al.* (1975)	Adult sheep	27–36

Table 4.3 The concentration of cells, the rate of flow, and the output of cells in the thoracic duct lymph of normal sheep foetuses 70–150 days of gestational age as predicted by regression equations relating ln cell concentration and $\log_e$ lymph flow to the foetal age.* Data from Pearson et al. (1976)

Days	Cells/ml × 10^{-6}†	ml/hr†	Cells/hr × 10^{-6}†
70	2.0 (1.7–2.4)	0.7 (0.2–2.5)	1.5 (0.4–6.0)
80	2.4 (2.0–2.9)	1.1 (0.3–3.7)	2.7 (0.7–10.6)
90	2.9 (2.5–3.4)	1.7 (0.5–5.4)	5.1 (1.4–18.7)
100	3.5 (3.0–4.1)	2.6 (0.9–8.1)	9.3 (2.6–33.7)
110	4.3 (3.6–5.0)	4.1 (1.3–12.3)	17.3 (4.9–61.5)
120	5.1 (4.4–6.0)	6.2 (2.0–18.9)	32.0 (9.0–113.9)
130	6.2 (5.3–7.3)	9.5 (3.1–29.5)	59.3 (16.4–214.4)
140	7.5 (6.4–8.8)	14.6 (4.6–46.4)	109.7 (29.4–409.4)
150	9.0 (7.6–10.7)	22.4 (6.8–74.1)	203.0 (52.0–792.9)

*The calculated regression equations were ln cells/hr = $0.062X - 3.920$ and $\log_e$ ml/hr = $0.043X - 3.302$, where X = days of gestation (standard errors for B were 0.006 and 0.006, respectively).
†95% confidence interval, in parentheses.

The design of all the experiments mentioned thus far has been similar to the one first used by Gowans, i.e. collection of cells from a major lymph duct, labelling *in vitro* with a radioisotope, intravenous infusion, and collection of the labelled cells from a major lymph duct.

One other set of experiments that gave substantial support to the idea that the

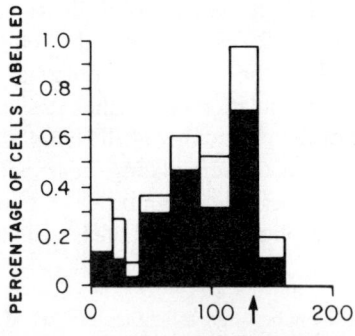

Figure 4.2 The appearance of labelled lymphocytes in the efferent lymph from an unstimulated popliteal node during its continuous perfusion *via* an afferent lymphatic with a solution containing [³H]-thymidine. The proportion of the labelled cells which was made up of large, immature lymphocytes is shown by the blocked area. ↑ = perfusion stopped. Modified from Hall and Morris (1965)

majority of lymphocytes in the lymph had circulated from the blood and were not being constantly made in the lymph nodes were those of Hall and Morris, on the origin of the cells in the efferent lymph from a single lymph node (Hall and Morris, 1965). If the large numbers of lymphocytes found in the lymph were the progeny of cells made in the lymph nodes, infusion of [^{3}H]-thymidine in the afferent lymphatic would result in the labelling of the majority of cells made within the node and detection of the newly formed cells in the efferent lymph. From the analysis of the proportion of labelled lymphocytes present in the efferent lymphatic of a lymph node, which had been perfused with [^{3}H]-thymidine *via* the afferent lymphatic, it was concluded that at the most a lymph node contributed 2–4% of newly formed lymphocytes, generally large lymphocytes, that entered the efferent lymph (Fig. 4.2). In lymph nodes where accidental antigen stimulation occurred, large numbers of cells of the plasma cell series appeared labelled.

4.2 TEMPO OF CIRCULATION OF T AND B LYMPHOCYTES

As mentioned earlier (Chapter 2, p. 17), the controversy over the finding of large numbers of lymphocytes in the lymph centred around the question of lifespan rather than that of origin. There were no clues in the late fifties about the dual origin of the two major classes of lymphocytes (Greaves *et al.*, 1974) and the criteria used by those concerned with the study of lymphocyte recirculation were strictly morphological. There were small (<8 µm in diameter) lymphocytes (Gowans, 1959; Gowans and Knight, 1964), of which some, after thoracic duct drainage, could be easily mobilized and collected in the lymph, 'the mobilisable lymphocyte pool', and others not, the 'non-mobilisable or sessile' lymphocytes (Caffrey *et al.*, 1962). After the elegant work of Hall and Morris (1965), it was clear that the majority of small lymphocytes found in lymph were not made in the lymph nodes (Fig. 4.2).

The first indication that the majority of small lymphocytes in the lymph had their origin in the thymus derived from the observations of Scholley and Kelly (1964) in thymectomized rats. The output of thoracic duct lymphocytes in rats thymectomized at birth was reduced by a factor of 3.8 (Table 4.4). Moreover, following prolonged thoracic duct drainage, the sequence of morphological changes in the spleen and lymph nodes pointed to the thymus-dependency of the easily mobilizable pool and to the thymus-independent nature of the sessile pool of lymphocytes, i.e. lymphocyte depletion was first observed in those areas of the spleen and lymph nodes (McGregor and Gowans, 1962) later defined as thymus-dependent (Parrott *et al.*, 1966).

All this, however, was circumstantial evidence for the existence of a recirculation of T and B lymphocytes, and the use of the general term 'small lymphocyte' persisted in the lymphocyte circulation literature until the early seventies. In two separate studies of the recirculation of pure B lymphocyte populations in the rat and the mouse, Howard (1972) and Sprent (1973) demonstrated that the recirculatory pool of lymphocytes contains both major classes of cells.

T cell depleted or B animals were prepared by adult thymectomy, irradiation,

Table 4.4 Output of thoracic duct lymphocytes (TDL) in normal and thymectomized animals

Author	Species	T cell depletion	No. of animals	Lymphocyte output x 10^6/hr
Scholley & Kelly (1964)	Rat	Neonatal thymectomy	11	3.10 ± 1.0*
		Sham thymectomy	12	11.7 ± 1.4*
Howard (1972)	Rat	Tx, irradiation, BM reconstitution	17	5.05 (1.98–9.27)†
			10	6.53 (4.01–10)
			6	8.49 (5.27–11)
		Normal	23	26.6 (16–40.5)
				No. collected over 24 hr ($\times 10^{-6}$)
Sprent (1973)	Mouse	Neonatal thymectomy	15	3.9 (0.9–6.8)‡
		Tx, irradiation, BM reconstitution	8	15 (8–25)
		Athymic *nu nu*	13	23 (12–45)
		Control CBA	17	131 (111–165)
		nu nu littermates	6	140 (105–170)

*Standard error of the mean.
†Mean and range from first 12 hr collection after thoracic duct cannulation.
‡TDL collected over first 24 hr of drainage, mean and range.

Tx, thymectomy; BM, bone marrow.

Table 4.5 Percentages of T and B lymphocytes in thoracic duct lymph of normal or T cell depleted animals

Author	Species	Source of TDL		Detection of TDL origin Alloantisera			
				HO anti-AO	AO anti-HO	HO anti-DA	DA anti-HO
Howard (1972)	Rat	Normal rats	HO	1	99	2	100
			(HO × AO)F$_1$	92	97	–	–
			(HO × DA)F$_1$	–	–	100	100
		B rats*	(HO × AO)F$_1$ → HO	91	96	–	–
			(HO × DA)F$_1$ → HO	–	–	100	100
				anti-Thy-1 antiserum		Binding complexes	
Sprent (1973)	Mouse	Normal CBA		82 (75–89)		16 (13–18)	
		N Tx CBA		16 (15–19)		70 (67–72)	
		Tx BM CBA		14 (8–17)		73 (66–83)	
		nu nu		0		97 (95–98)	
		nu nu littermates		78 (75–81)		20 (16–24)	

*Thymectomized, irradiated HO rats received 2 × 10^8 marrow cells from (HO × AO)F$_1$ or (HO × DA)F$_1$ donors, before thoracic duct cannulation.
N Tx, neonatally thymectomized; Tx BM, thymectomized, reconstituted with bone marrow (BM).

and reconstitution with syngeneic bone marrow cells in the case of the mice and F_1 hybrid marrow cells in the case of the rat; nude, congenitally athymic mice were also used in Sprent's experiments (Sprent, 1973).

A summary of the effect of T cell depletion on the output of T and B lymphocytes from the thoracic duct in mice and rats is presented in Table 4.5. The bone marrow origin of the circulating cells in Howard's experiments was established by the use of alloantisera against specific histocompatibility antigens of the donor inoculum. B lymphocytes in Sprent's experiments were identified by their capacity to bind radiolabelled immune complexes (Basten *et al.*, 1972).

In addition, in the mouse experiments, the number of T cells in the thoracic duct lymph was positively identified by the use of an anti-Thy-1 antiserum. This enabled the follow-up, not only of the small changes in cell output, but of the precise participation of the T cell and the B cell pools in those overall changes (Fig. 4.3). Whereas the numbers of T cells decreased sharply during the first few days of thoracic duct drainage, the decline in B cells over the same time was negligible. Over longer periods of thoracic duct drainage in nude mice, the decline in cell output was also slight, i.e. from $14 \times 10^6/12$ hr at 2 days to $5 \times 10^6/12$ hr at 10 days, thus providing direct evidence for the T cell population being easily 'mobilizable' and the B cell population being less easily mobilizable, or sessile. In both studies (Howard, 1972; Sprent, 1973), the lifespan of the cells emerging in the thoracic duct lymph of B lymphocytes recovered in the thoracic duct lymph of

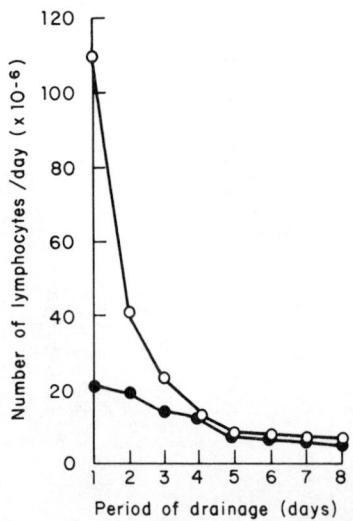

Figure 4.3 Numbers of T lymphocytes (O———O) and B lymphocytes (●———●) collected over intervals of 24 hr from normal CBA mice. Each point represents the arithmetic mean of data pooled from one to seven mice. Data from Sprent (1973)

B animals was estimated and it was concluded that the lifespan of B lymphocytes recovered in the thoracic duct lymph is not essentially different from that of its total normal population of small lymphocytes, i.e. longer than 10 days. In the mouse, B cells in the thoracic duct lymph consist of a single population with an average lifespan of 5–7 weeks; the estimated average lifespan of mouse thoracic duct T lymphocytes is longer, 4–6 months (Sprent and Basten, 1973).

One major difference between the recirculation of T and B lymphocytes is their tempo of circulation. The first appearance of labelled B lymphocytes in the thoracic duct lymph following an intravenous infusion is delayed relative to lymphocytes from normal donors both in the rat (Howard, 1972) and the mouse (Sprent, 1973) and in the foetal lamb (Pearson et al., 1976).

A summary of the values of recoveries of B and normal lymphocytes in rats and mice is included in Table 4.5. Over a 48 hr period, in the rat, the values for the total recovery of B and normal labelled lymphocytes were 19.5% and 33.0%, respectively. In mice, these differences were even more striking. The percentage of labelled cells in recipients of normal thoracic duct lymphocytes rose rapidly within the first 24 hr. In contrast, only 0.3% of labelled B cells were present at the same time after injection.

Over a period of 48 hr, 39–65% of normal lymphocytes were recovered, in contrast with the much lower values of 1–3% recovered in the recipients of thoracic duct lymphocytes of thymectomized, irradiated and bone marrow reconstituted donors and 2–4% in the recipients of injected labelled nude mouse thoracic duct cells.

The failure of large numbers of injected B cells to reach the lymph rapidly is reflected by their slower migration through the lungs (Freitas and de Sousa, 1975) and spleen (Sprent, 1973). Removal of the spleen, therefore, should increase the numbers of B lymphocytes that reach the lymph nodes and thus the lymph. Sprent, investigating the recovery in the thoracic duct lymph of labelled B lymphocytes, obtained from splenectomized or non-splenectomized donors, increased recovery from 4–6% (in the recipients of cells from non-splenectomized donors) to 7–11% (in the recipients of cells from splenectomized donors). The finding of this minimal change led Sprent to suggest that B cells lack some cell membrane constituent or 'receptor' which would be specific for a cell's recognition of the lymph node postcapillary venule endothelium, and thus regulate admittance or non-admittance into the lymph circuit. This interpretation has not been substantiated by more recent studies of the adhesion of rat T and B lymphocytes to high endothelial venules in vitro, in which the two cell types were found to adhere equally well to the venules (Kuttner and Woodruff, 1979).

4.3 MIGRATORY PATTERNS OF SELECTED LYMPHOID CELL POPULATIONS: ECOTAXIS

Many experiments on the tissue distribution of labelled lymphoid cells other than thoracic duct lymphocytes followed experimental designs essentially similar to the one first adopted by Gowans and Knight (1964). In addition, the fate of cells derived from one organ labelled *in situ* with [³H]-thymidine to other organs has also been traced by means of autoradiography.

From the results of early studies comparing the distribution of [³H]-adenosine-labelled mouse thymus, spleen and bone marrow cells, it became apparent that there is a considerable heterogeneity of lymphoid cell distribution and that distinct cell populations migrate to distinct regions of the peripheral lymphoid organs (Parrott *et al.*, 1966; Parrott and de Sousa, 1971; de Sousa, 1971). The ability of separate cell populations to migrate and arrange themselves within separate microenvironments of the peripheral lymphoid organs was designated ecotaxis (de Sousa, 1971). A detailed account of the numerous instances of ecotaxis within the lymphoid system in the mouse and other experimental animals is presented below; a distinction is made between experiments using radioactively labelled cell suspensions prepared from one organ, i.e. bone marrow cells or thymus cells, and experiments tracing the fate of cells leaving an organ which was previously labelled with [³H]-thymidine, i.e. bone marrow *derived* on thymus-*derived* cells.

4.3.1 Bone marrow cells and bone marrow-derived cells

The fate of radioisotopically labelled bone marrow cells has been traced in the mouse, guinea pig, and the rabbit. In the mouse and the rabbit, the distribution of

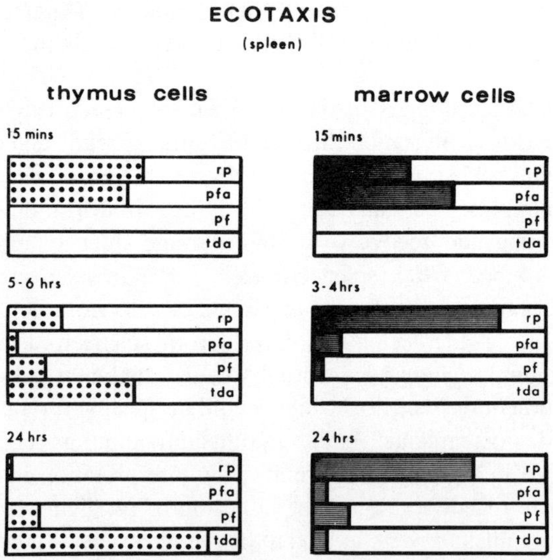

Figure 4.4 Percentage distribution of thymus and marrow cells found in the various spleen compartments at several times following intravenous injection of [³H]-adenosine-labelled cells. Whole spleen section counts done under a × 1,000 magnification; cells with 10 or more silver grains were counted and their position in the various spleen compartments recorded: rp, red pulp; pfa, perifollicular or marginal zone; pf, periphery of Malpighian follicle (B cell area); tda, thymus-dependent area (T cell area). From de Sousa (1971)

unselected bone marrow cells labelled *in vitro* with [³H]-adenosine was studied (de Sousa, 1971; Parrott and de Sousa, 1971). In the guinea pig, two types of studies have been carried out: those tracing the fate of labelled cells leaving the bone marrow labelled *in situ* with [³H]-thymidine (Brahim and Osmond, 1970, 1973, 1976) and those tracing suspensions of lymphoid cell enriched fractions from [³H]-thymidine-labelled bone marrow separated in linear sucrose gradients (Yoshida and Osmond, 1978).

In the experiments tracing the suspensions of [³H]-adenosine-labelled unfractionated mouse bone marrow cells (de Sousa, 1971), most cells, at the early times (15 min) after intravenous injection, were found in the lungs and in the spleen, in the marginal zone and red pulp (Fig. 4.4). Later (at 3–4 hr and at 24 hr), the majority of labelled bone marrow cells were present in the spleen, in the red pulp and outer regions of the Malpighian body (Fig. 4.4). Cells were also seen in the lymph node at 24 hr, predominantly in the medullary cords and primary nodules (Fig. 4.5). Small proportions of the labelled cells were always found in the thymus-dependent area and cortico-medullary junction.

In the guinea pig experiments using [³H]-thymidine-labelled fractionated bone marrow cells (Yoshida and Osmond, 1978), a comparison was drawn between the

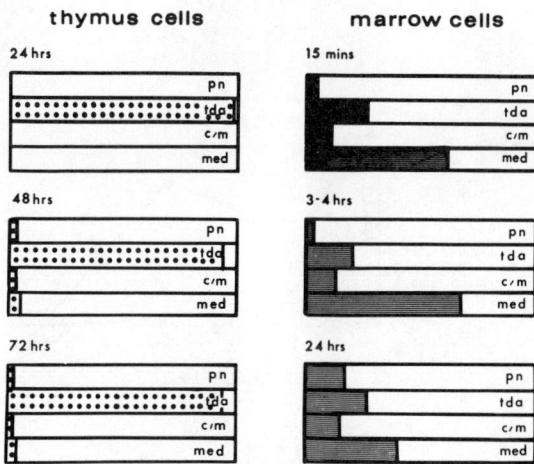

Figure 4.5 Percentage distribution of thymus and marrow cells in the various lymph node compartments at several times following intravenous injection of [³H]-adenosine-labelled cells. Whole lymph node section counts done under a x 1,000 magnification; cells with 10 or more silver grains were counted and their position in the various lymph node compartments recorded: pn, primary nodule (B cell area); tda, thymus-dependent area (T cell area); cm, cortico-medullary junction; med, medulla. From de Sousa (1971)

fates of granulocytes, small lymphocytes, and large lymphoid cells in lethally x-irradiated recipients. From 1 to 6 hr after transfusion, radiolabelled granulocytes and small lymphocytes disappeared from the blood and appeared in the recipient's bone marrow and spleen (Fig. 4.6). For the first 24 hr after injection, labelled granulocytes were the predominant labelled cells found in the bone marrow; much smaller numbers of granulocytes were found in the spleen. After the first day, the number of labelled granulocytes fell progressively. In contrast, the proportions of

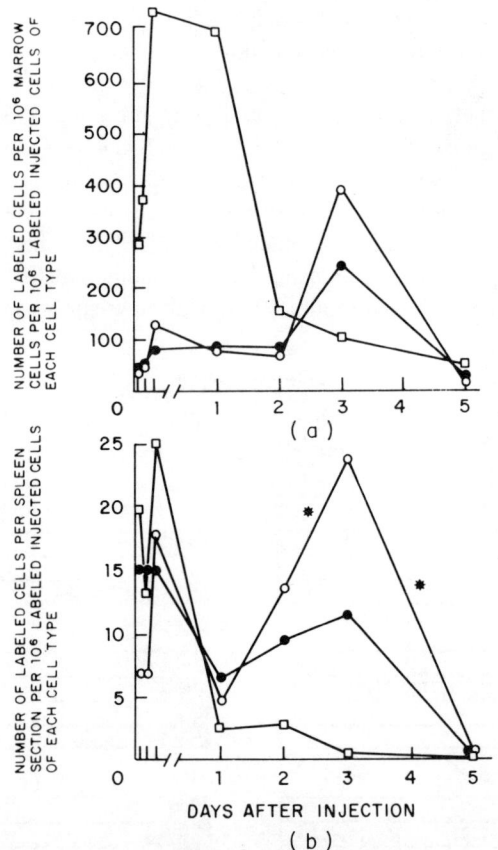

Figure 4.6 Numbers of labelled small lymphocytes (●———●), large lymphoid (O———O) or large mononuclear (O—*—O) and mature granulocytes (□———□) in the bone marrow (a) and spleen (b) of irradiated recipients after transfusion of labelled lymphocyte-rich bone marrow fractions. Numbers of labelled cells in bone marrow (a) expressed per 10^6 cells. Numbers in spleen expressed per transverse section (b). Data from Yoshida and Osmond (1978)

Table 4.6 Numbers of fractionated labelled bone marrow lymphoid cells in spleen, mesenteric lymph node, Peyer's patches, and thymus.* Data from Yoshida and Osmond (1978)

		Time after injection					
		Hours			Days		
Cell fraction	Organ	1	2.5	6	1	2	3
Small lymphocytes	Spleen	268	290	232	142	97	192
	MLN	14	4	11	5	11	120
	PP	4	5	3	6	9	10
	Thymus	1	0	1	1	0	4
Large mononuclear†	Spleen	28	40	70	50	38	60
	MLN	0	0	0	1	3	10
	PP	0	0	0	1	1	1
	Thymus	0	0	0	1	0	0

*Number of labelled cells per whole transverse section.
†The majority of mononuclear cells had lymphoid morphology in sections.

labelled small lymphocytes and large lymphoid cells found in the marrow and spleen increased from 2–3 days. Very few labelled cells were present in the bone marrow by 5 days after injection (Fig. 4.6). Both in marrow and spleen, labelled large mononuclear cells were present in the highest relative frequency. Bone marrow cells, in addition to showing preference for organ destination, i.e. many more labelled cells were found in bone marrow and spleen than in lymph nodes, thymus or Peyer's patches (Table 4.6), also showed some preferential migration to specific regions within the spleen. Thus, within the first 6 hr after infusion, labelled cells were located mainly in the red pulp. At 1–3 days, the numbers of large lymphoid cells and small lymphocytes decreased in the red pulp and increased in the white pulp. Within the white pulp, large mononuclear cells were always found to predominate in areas outside germinal centres and the T cell area; small proportions of small lymphocytes were always found in the T cell area, although the majority at 4 and at 3 days after injection were present outside the T cell area, within germinal centres and in the remainder of the white pulp.

Following intramyeloid labelling with [^{3}H]-thymidine (Brahim and Osmond, 1973), bone marrow-derived labelled small lymphocytes were found in popliteal lymph nodes at 3–4 days following [^{3}H]-thymidine administration, in the subcapsular sinus, in the B cell areas, within the wall or lumen of postcapillary venules in the deep cortex, and in the medullary cords. Well-labelled small lymphocytes were also seen in the white pulp of the spleen. After 5–6 days, the overall number of labelled cells declined, indicating that the majority of the labelled bone marrow-derived cells found in the tissues were short-lived.

4.3.2 Thymus cells and thymus-derived cells

Unfractionated thymocytes recirculate poorly in comparison with peripheral T lymphocytes (Fig. 4.7). They filter through the lung capillaries more slowly than

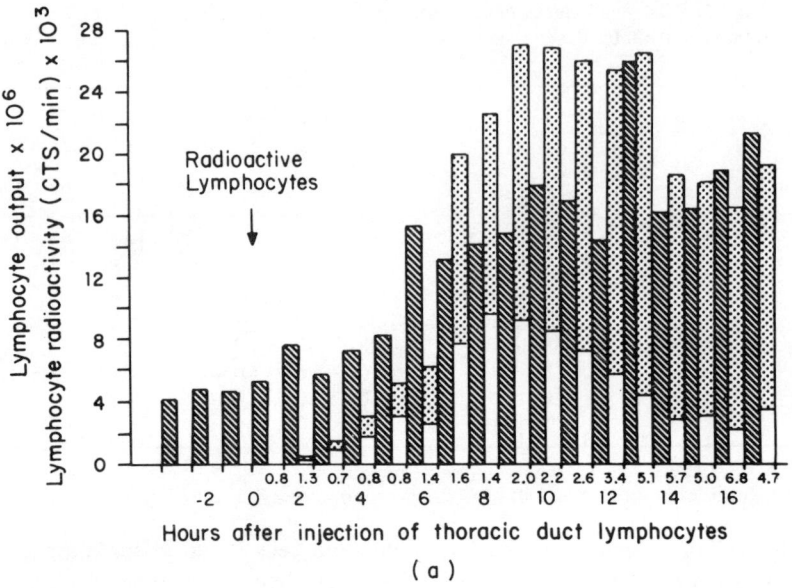

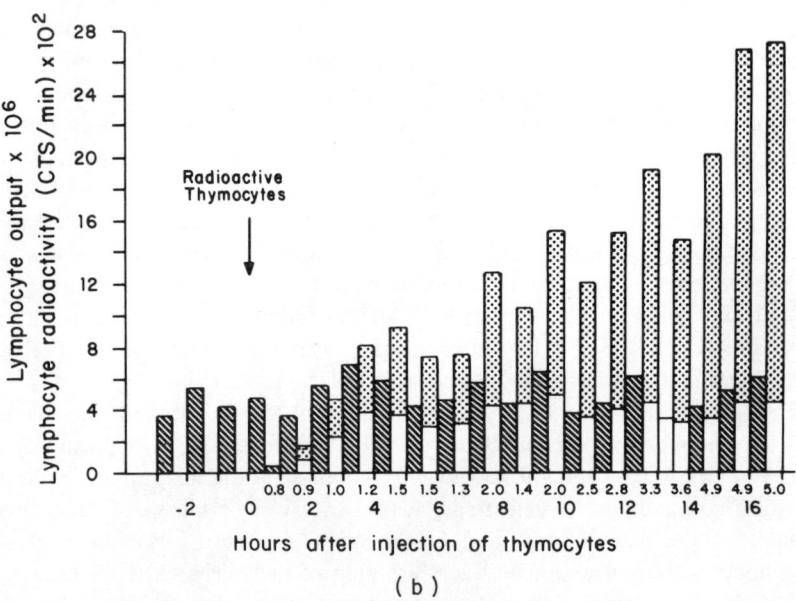

Figure 4.7 Lymphocyte output (▨) and radioactivity in cells from the thoracic duct of two lymphocyte-depleted rats injected intravenously with $1,031 \times 10^6$ ^{3}[H]-uridine-labelled thoracic duct lymphocytes (result shown in a) or $1,053 \times 10^6$ ^{3}[H]-uridine-labelled thymocytes (result shown in b). The number below each composite bar is the ratio of radioactivity in the trichloroacetic acid (TCA)-insoluble cell fraction (▨) to that in the TCA-soluble fraction (☐). Data from Goldschneider and McGregor (1968b)

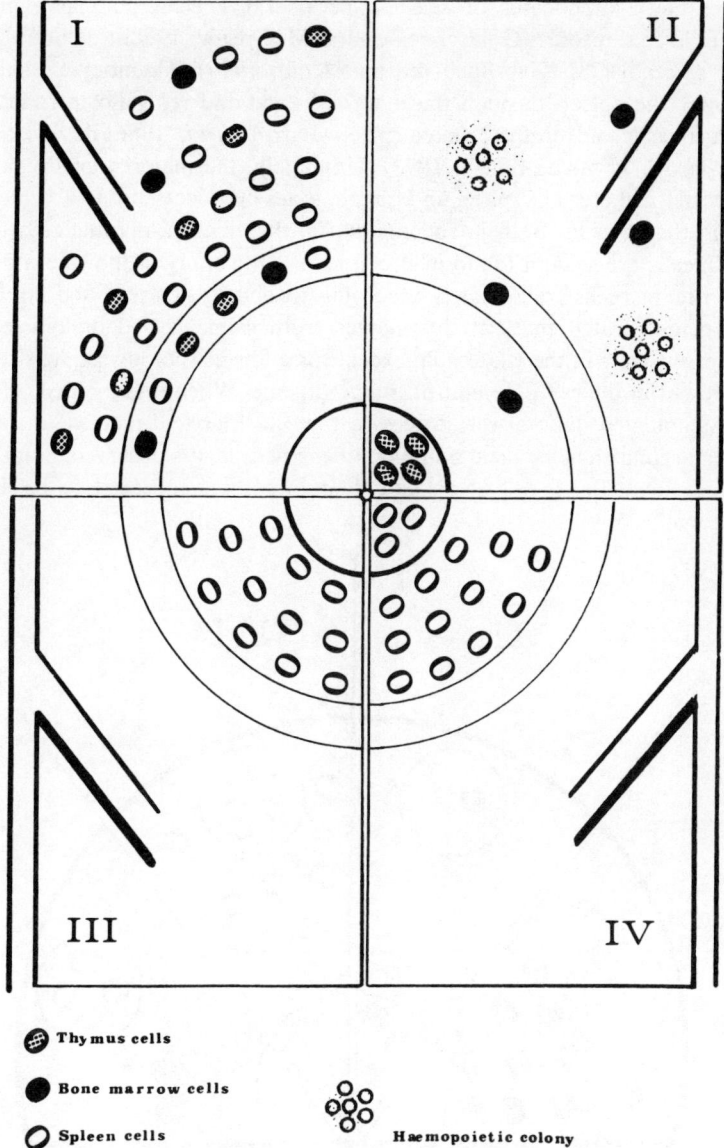

Figure 4.8 Diagrammatic representation of lymphoid cell ecotaxis in the spleen. After using similar routes of entry, namely the red pulp and marginal zone, at the early times after injection (I), thymus and thymus-derived cells and bone marrow or bone marrow-derived cells (II) ultimately migrate to clearly distinct sites of the red and white pulps. Selected B lymphocytes migrate to the outer layer of the Malpighian body (III); suspensions of mixed T and B lymphocytes, such as a spleen cell suspension (IV), are found both in T and B cell areas. For details of spleen microenvironments see Chapter 3, Plate 5

thoracic duct lymphocytes or selected peripheral T cells, and large numbers persist in liver sinusoids (Goldschneider and McGregor, 1968b; de Sousa, 1971; Durkin *et al.*, 1978; Kolb-Bachofen and Kolb, 1979). Thymocytes, like other cells, enter the spleen through the marginal zone and red pulp in rodents and through the ellipsoids in the chicken spleen (Parrott *et al.*, 1966; de Sousa, 1971; Durkin *et al.*, 1978; de Sousa, 1973). Ultimately, the majority of thymus cells migrate to T cell areas of spleen and lymph nodes in rodents and to T cell areas of spleen in the chicken. Both in rodents and in the chicken, thymus cells or peripheral T cells are seldom found in B cell areas. In a study of the spleen distribution of thymus cells fractionated according to density, Durkin and co-workers (1978) demonstrated that rat thymocytes from saline-treated donors localized almost exclusively in the white pulp except for a few cells of lowest density which were present in the red pulp and/or marginal zone. When fractionated cells from antigen-stimulated donors were traced, a three to four fold increase in red pulp and/or marginal zone localization of light density cells was observed. Small, dense cells were found in T cell areas and their migration appeared to be antigen-independent.

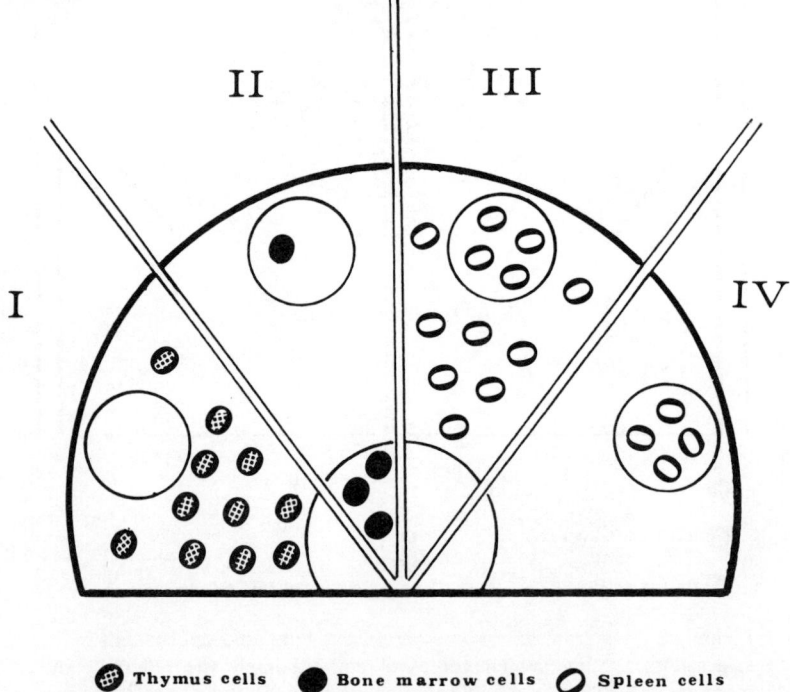

Figure 4.9 Diagrammatic representation of lymphoid cell ecotaxis in the lymph node. After entering the lymph nodes through sections of the postcapillary venules located in the mid-cortex, thymus or thymus-derived cells (I), bone marrow or bone marrow-derived cells (II), selected B lymphocytes (IV) or mixtures of T and B lymphocytes (III) migrate to distinct lymph node regions. For details of lymph node microenvironments see Chapter 3, Plate 9

Experiments tracing cells derived from the thymus labelled *in vivo* with [^{3}H]-thymidine have demonstrated a substantial emigration of newly formed cells from the thymus in the neonatal period (Weissman, 1967; Joel *et al.*, 1972) destined predominantly to Peyer's patches and the mesenteric lymph node (Joel *et al.*, 1972; Waksman, 1973). In the adult, [^{3}H]-thymidine or ^{125}IuDR thymus-derived cells continue to be detected in peripheral lymphoid organs (Chanana *et al.*, 1973; Laissue *et al.*, 1976); previous administration of antigen appears to double the number of cells reaching the spleen (Durkin *et al.*, 1978).

Recently, Scollay *et al.* (1979) have determined the proportion of Lyt cell migrants found in the peripheral lymphoid organs shortly (at 3 hr) after *in situ* labelling of the thymus with an intrathymic injection of a solution of fluorescein isothiocyanate (FITC). Although the number of fluorescein-positive cells counted in the periphery is small, the results are clearcut. About 75% of peripheral FITC-labelled cells are Lyt-1 and 25% are Lyt 1, 2; Lyt-2 cells are extremely rare. No obvious difference was found in these experiments between the relative proportions of Lyt cell sets in spleen and lymph nodes (see for comparison Table 2.4).

The ultimate destination of thymocytes and thymus-derived cells in the spleen (Fig. 4.8), lymph nodes (Fig. 4.9), and Peyer's patches is essentially similar: the majority of the injected cells are found in the thymus-dependent areas, i.e. round the central arteriole in the spleen, in the mid-cortex of the lymph node, and in the interfollicular zone and dome area of the Peyer's patches. Numerically, however, more peripheral T cells than thymocytes reach the peripheral lymphoid organs (Goldschneider and McGregor, 1968a; Mitchell, 1972) and lymph (Goldschneider and McGregor, 1968b; Fig. 4.7).

4.3.3 Bursa cells and bursa-derived cells

Bursa cells migrate preferentially to the spleen, both as labelled cell suspensions (de Kruyff *et al.*, 1975) and following *in situ* labelling of the bursa of Fabricius with [^{3}H]-thymidine (Fig. 4.10); negligible proportions of bursa cells (less than 5% of injected cells) are also found in the thymus, bursa, liver, and lung. At early times after intravenous injection, labelled bursa cells are seen in the lumen and around the splenic ellipsoids; later (at 24 hr after injection), the cells localize as aggregates within well-defined germinal centres and are also found scattered within the cuff of lymphoid cells surrounding the ellipsoids. Following *in situ* labelling with [^{3}H]-thymidine a similar distribution pattern has been observed (Fig. 4.10).

4.3.4 Spleen cells and spleen-derived cells

Experiments tracing the fate of spleen cells include unseparated spleen cells and spleen cell suspensions labelled *in vitro*, selected according to origin, antigen binding (Mitchell, 1972; Parrott and de Sousa, 1971; de Sousa *et al.*, 1973), and lifespan (Parrott and de Sousa, 1971). The fate of spleen cells released from [^{3}H]-

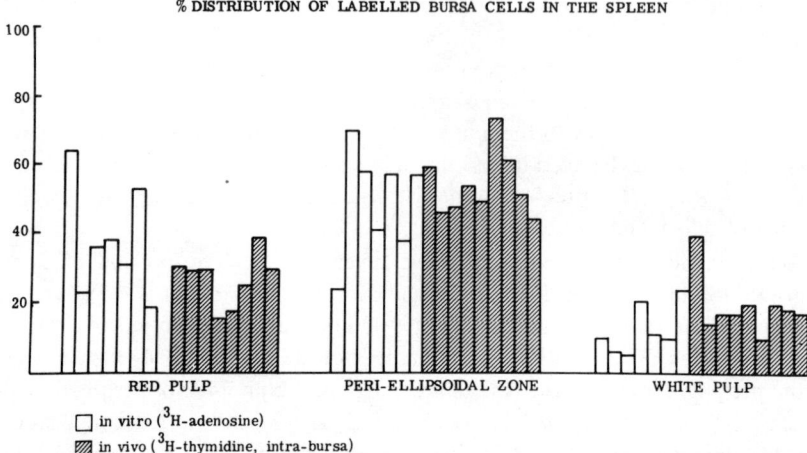

Figure 4.10 Distribution profiles of labelled bursa (☐) or bursa-derived (▨) cells in the chicken spleen following intravenous injection of cells labelled *in vitro* with [^{3}H]-adenosine or following *in vivo* labelling of the bursa with [^{3}H]-thymidine. Autologous cells were used after surgical bursectomy and labelled *in vitro* at a concentration of 10µCi/ml. For the *in vivo* labelling, the bursa was exposed, and a volume of 0.1–0.2 ml PBS containing 40 µCi of [^{3}H]-thymidine was injected into its substance. Immediately after intrabursal injection, 0.5 ml of a cold thymidine solution containing 0.5 mg [^{1}H] was flushed over the exposed surface of the bursa and 2.5 mg of the cold thymidine injected intraperitoneally (de Sousa, Eslami and White, unpublished data). For chicken spleen areas see Fig. 3.1

thymidine-labelled spleen grafts has also been studied in the rat (Parrott *et al.*, 1975) and in the pig (Pabst *et al.*, 1977).

In vitro labelled spleen cells utilize routes of entry into the spleen and lymph nodes similar to those used by other cells, i.e. the marginal zone and red pulp in the spleen (Fig. 4.8), the postcapillary venules in the lymph nodes, and Peyer's patches. After using common routes of entry, T spleen cells are found predominantly in T areas, B spleen cells in B areas, namely the periphery of the Malpighian bodies in the spleen (Fig. 4.8), the primary nodules in the lymph nodes (Fig. 4.9), and Peyer's patches. B spleen cells rarely penetrate germinal centres; antigen-binding cells, however, are found frequently within germinal centres (Mitchell, 1972).

Spleen cells selected according to lifespan differ in their final pattern of distribution in the spleen (Table 4.7a): long-lived cells have a distribution pattern similar to that of *in vitro* labelled cells, i.e. the majority of the labelled cells are present in the T and B areas of the Malpighian bodies, whereas a lot more short-lived cells (near 50%) are found in the red pulp and marginal zone at 24 hr after injection.

Similarly, when labelled cells were allowed to leave a grafted [^{3}H]-thymidine-labelled spleen (Parrott *et al.*, 1975), there was not a clearcut exclusive migration to the white pulp of the recipient spleen; in addition, large dividing ([^{3}H]-thymidine-labelled) cells were found in the recipients' intestine wall. From the

Table 4.7a Distribution of [³H]-thymidine-labelled spleen cells from adult donors in the spleen. Data from Parrott and de Sousa (1971)

Labelling regime	Time (days)	Dose	No. of recipients	Total‡	RP	PFA	PF	TDA
Short-term*	1	5 × 10⁷	1	873	46.8	10	27	16
	4	5 × 10⁷	4	101	15.8	19.9	42.4	19.7
	6	5 × 10⁷	2	110	14.9	14.5	58.6	11.8
	8	5 × 10⁷	2	31	17.7	16.1	51.6	14.5
Long-term†	1	5 × 10⁷	2	1,309	19.8	7.8	53.9	19.1
	3	5 × 10⁷	1	231	5.6	3	61	30.3
	6–7	5 × 10⁷	3	250	1.6	3.0	54.5	40.8

Table 4.7b Distribution patterns of short-lived and long-lived lymph node cells in the spleen. Data from Parrott and de Sousa (1971)

Labelling regime	Time (days)	Dose	No. of recipients	Total‡	RP	PFA	PF	TDA
Short-term*	1	1.5–1.8 × 10⁷	2	39.3	12.1	18.4	30.5	38.8
	2	1.5–1.8 × 10⁷	2	73	18.8	16.4	36.9	27.7
	3	1.5–1.8 × 10⁷	1	18	22.2	22.2	27.7	27.7
	4	1.5–1.8 × 10⁷	2	29.7	22.6	17.6	33.3	26.0
	8	1.5–1.8 × 10⁷	2	4.8	20.8	3.3	33.3	37.4
	14	1.5–1.8 × 10⁷	1	7.5	6.6	19.9	33.3	39.9
Long-term†	2	1.5–1.8 × 10⁷	2	129	19.5	6.9	17.7	55.8
	3	1.5–1.8 × 10⁷	1	60	6.0	3.1	5.9	84.9
	4–5	1.5–1.8 × 10⁷	3	83.3	5.6	2	18.0	74.4
	8	1.5–1.8 × 10⁷	1	99	12.6	5.3	6.1	75.7
	14	1.5–1.8 × 10⁷	1	44.5	12.3	5.6	6.7	75.2

*Intraperitoneal [³H] thymidine injections (0.5 μCi/gbw) twice daily for 3 days.
†Intraperitoneal [³H] thymidine injections (0.5 μCi/gbw) twice daily for 28 days, stopped for 3 days before transfer.
‡Mean total number of cells/section. Autoradiographs exposed for 9–11 weeks.

study of the destination of labelled cells derived from the spleen of young pigs selectively labelled with [³H]-thymidine (Pabst et al., 1977), it was deduced that about 15% of all splenic lymphocytes are newly produced per day, and that about 17% of these leave the spleen within the first day of labelling. In this study too a considerable proportion of spleen-borne lymphocytes was found in the gut-associated lymphoid tissue. Newly formed spleen-derived labelled lymphocytes were seen at 24 hr in mesenteric, cervical and inguinal lymph nodes, in the bone marrow and in the blood (Pabst et al., 1977).

4.3.5 Lymph node cells

Populations of unseparated lymph node cells labelled *in vitro* with radioisotopes have migration patterns which are very similar to those of thoracic duct lymphocytes (Austin, 1968). After using similar routes of entry in the spleen and lymph nodes, the labelled cells are found predominantly in the T areas of the spleen and lymph nodes, but also in the B areas (Table 4.7b). Lymph node cells selected for short lifespan by short-term labelling with [³H]-thymidine, however, do not show such a clearcut form of migration; short-lived lymph node cells are found virtually equally distributed over the four main splenic areas, i.e. red pulp, marginal zone, B and T areas. Long-lived cells, on the other hand, have a distribution pattern which is identical to that of *in vitro* labelled lymph node cells, i.e. most cells at 24 and 48 hr after injection are confined to the T and B areas of the white pulp.

4.3.6 Selected T and B lymphocytes

Suspensions of selected populations of peripheral T or B lymphocytes in cell traffic experiments have been obtained from numerous sources, namely the spleen, lymph nodes, and the thoracic duct lymph in mice and rats (de Sousa *et al.*, 1973; Gutman and Weissman, 1973; Nieuwenhuis and Ford, 1976; Freitas and de Sousa, 1975; Howard, 1972; Sprent, 1973). T and B lymphocytes, regardless of source or species studied, have clearly distinct migratory patterns in spleen, lymph nodes, Peyer's patches, and appendix. After using common routes of entry into the peripheral lymphoid organs, i.e. the marginal zone and red pulp in the spleen and the mid-cortical or interfollicular postcapillary venules in the lymph node and Peyer's patches, T cells migrate predominantly to T cell areas whereas B cells are found mostly in B cell areas (Figs. 4.8, 4.9, Plates 12–14).

Suspensions of unselected lymph node or thoracic duct lymphocytes contain both T and B lymphocytes and this is reflected in the migration of labelled cells to both T and B cell areas after transfer.

In the mouse, *in vitro* labelling with [³H]-adenosine or [³H]-uridine of thoracic duct lymphocytes results in the equal labelling of the two major lymphocyte classes; in the rat, however, B cells seemingly incorporate much less uridine than T cells (Howard *et al.*, 1972). This is reflected in the distribution of lightly labelled lymphocytes in the B areas of the spleen and lymph nodes and the finding of heavily labelled lymphocytes in the T areas.

This finding of Howard *et al.* (1972) and a similar earlier finding of Austin (1968), who observed that lightly labelled lymph node cells (labelled *in vitro* with [^{3}H]-uridine) localized preferentially in lymph node B areas, constitute the explanation for the earlier description of the route recirculation of lymphocytes in the rat being confined to the T areas. Indeed, a careful reexamination of the original autoradiographs of lymphoid tissue after transfusion of [^{3}H]-adenosine-labelled lymphocytes prepared in the experiments of Gowans and Knight (1964) has revealed that there are indeed lighly labelled cells in areas corresponding to those illustrated in Plates 13 and 14 (Howard *et al.*, 1972).

4.4 THE EFFECTS OF ANTIGEN

4.4.1 Non-specific effects

The idea of specificity in immunology is strongly related to antigen specificity; by 'non-specific' effects of antigen are meant those changes influencing the whole of the recirculating pool and not just the cells specifically committed in the response to the antigen administered. Effects which are 'non-specific' in a more general sense than just the immunological one include the induction of increased blood flow to the draining lymph node (mentioned in detail earlier, Chapter 1, p. 10) and the concomitant delay observed in the lymphocyte circulation through the draining organ.

The observation that administration of some antigens causes a transient delay in lymphocyte traffic through the organ draining the site of antigen injection was first reported by Hall and Morris (1962, 1963, 1965) in a study of lymph flow and cell output from the efferent lymphatic of the popliteal lymph node in sheep.

Following the subcutaneous injection of a number of antigens, namely human serum globulins, bovine serum albumin, human serum albumin, ovalbumin, killed *Salmonella typhi* 'O' organisms, chicken red cells, *Listeria monocytogenes*, and an extract of *Ascaris lumbricoides*, the cell output from the efferent duct of the draining popliteal node fell by 50% within 30 min of injecting the antigen (Fig. 4.11). This fall continued so that the cell output had reached a minimum value of less than 20% of the original output 2 hr after the injection of the antigen. The cell output then fell more gradually and within 5 hr of the injection returned to its original levels. The injection of non-antigenic material had no effect on the cell output from the popliteal node.

Experiments in which one single lymph node is analysed give no information about the overall changes occurring concomitantly in other compartments of the circulating system. Moreover, the cause or causes of the observed decrease in cell output from the draining lymph node remain unclear. Such fall in cell output could be due (a) to accumulation of incoming lymphocytes in the substance of the draining lymph node, (b) to the failure of lymphocytes already in the lymph node to leave it, or (c) to the fall of lymphocyte input into the node.

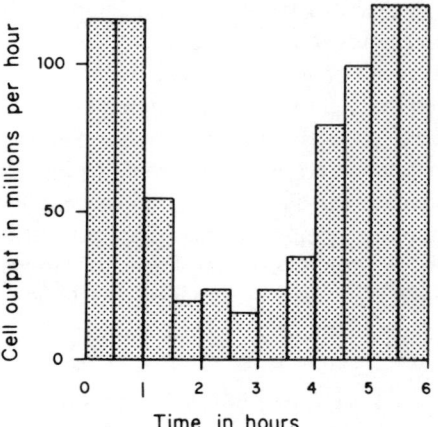

Figure 4.11 The fall in the output of lymphocytes in the efferent lymph from a popliteal node following the injection of an antigen (human serum globulin) into the lower part of the leg of a sheep. Slightly modified from Hall and Morris (1965)

Clarification of these various alternatives has developed through the years from the early work of Ford (1968) on the kinetics of lymphocyte circulation through the spleen and of Dresser *et al.* (1970) on the effect of localized injection of adjuvant materials and sheep red blood cells on lymphocyte circulation in the mouse to the recent work of Cahill *et al.* (1976) on the effect of antigen on migration of recirculating lymphocytes through single lymph nodes in sheep.

Ford (1969), studying the migration of thoracic duct lymphocytes through the perfused rat spleen, verified that addition of a high dose of sheep red blood cells to the perfusate (0.2 ml of a 50% suspension), but not of swine influenza virus, $1\frac{1}{2}$ hr after the addition of labelled lymphocytes failed to reduce the lymphocyte input into the spleen, but inhibited the release of lymphocytes (Fig. 4.12). This was interpreted as the result of delayed transit of the lymphocytes recently migrated into the spleen through the splenic structure.

The possible relevance of such a mechanism of slowing down lymphocyte circulation through an organ draining the site of antigen injection to the initiation of the immune response was first discussed in detail by Dresser *et al.* (1970) in a study of the effect of administration of adjuvant materials and sheep red blood cells on the migration of ^{51}Cr-labelled lymph node cells to the lymph nodes draining the site of injection of the adjuvant or antigen. Mice injected subcutaneously in the footpad with *Bordetella pertussis*, sheep red blood cells, syngeneic red blood cells, alum or vitamin A received 3 or 6 days later an intravenous injection of ^{51}Cr-labelled syngeneic lymph node cells and were killed 24 hr after the cell injection; the radioactivity recovered in the peripheral nodes, mesenteric nodes, and

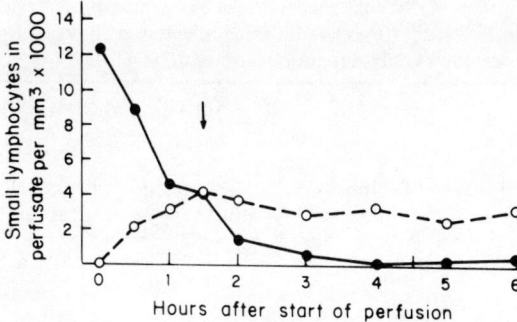

Figure 4.12 Effect of antigen on circulation of lymphocytes through the perfused spleen in the rat. Sheep erythrocytes were added after $1\frac{1}{2}$ hr of perfusion (indicated by arrow). ●──● concentration of original small lymphocytes; OO concentration of splenic small lymphocytes. Compared to perfusions in which no antigen was added, the concentration of original small lymphocytes fell at the same rate to a lower nadir and after 6 hr showed less recovery. This indicates that the antigen did not inhibit the migration of labelled lymphocytes into the spleen but delayed their transit through the splenic tissue. Slightly modified from W. L. Ford (1969)

draining and non-draining nodes was estimated and expressed as percentage of the injected radioactivity. From the results summarized in Table 4.8, it is clear that much higher amounts of radioactivity were recovered from the draining lymph nodes than from the control nodes, and that the increases observed in the popliteal lymph nodes occurred concomitantly with decreases in the mesenteric and other peripheral lymph nodes. A significant increase in draining lymph node weight was also observed and interpreted as the result of increased cell influx. Dresser et al. (1970) proposed that 'the observed enlargement can be due to one of two possible mechanisms: (1) a change in the physical structure of the node which results in an increase in the efficiency of the mechanical trapping of circulating lymphocytes and also perhaps changes that make space available for circulating cells to settle down; and (2) the secretion of a chemotactic agent which actively stimulates the cells to migrate to and settle down in a draining node'.

In this study, an analysis of the fate of intravenously injected ^{51}Cr-labelled syngeneic red blood cells failed to demonstrate any change in vascularity or increase in blood volume of the draining node, a result slightly different from more precise studies of the blood flow during the immune response (Hay and Hobbs, 1977; Herman et al., 1979). Dresser et al. (1970) concluded that 'stimulation of the migration of a population of cells likely to be rich in antigen-sensitive cells to a site in close proximity to an antigen trapping mechanism (Balfour and Humphrey,

Table 4.8 Distribution of ^{51}Cr-labelled normal syngeneic mesenteric lymph node cells after intravenous injection of 10^7 cells into mice injected in the right footpad with various substances 6 days previously. Data from Dresser et al. (1970)

Substance injected into right footpad (day − 6)	Activity (%) (day + 1)			
			Popliteal lymph nodes	
	Peripheral nodes	Mesenteric nodes	Right (draining)	Left (control)
Nil (control)	5.2 (7.9−3.5)	8.7 (15.1−5.0)	0.23 (1.7−0.03)	0.34 (1.1−0.11)
2.5 x 10^8 pertussis	3.7 (5.4−2.6)	7.0 (10.7−4.7)	1.66 (2.8−1.0)	0.22 (2.2−0.02)
5 x 10^6 sheep RBC	4.9 (7.4−3.2)	7.6 (10.7−5.5)	1.21 (2.3−0.63)	0.38 (1.05−0.14)
5 x 10^6 CBA mouse RBC	5.0 (6.9−3.6)	7.7 (10.2−5.9)	0.56 (0.62−0.51)	0.39 (0.58−0.28)
Alum particles without antigen	4.5 (6.2−3.2)	7.4 (10.2−5.4)	1.05 (1.2−0.91)	0.39 (0.78−0.20)

Numbers in parentheses are 95% confidence limits.

1966; Humphrey, 1969) immediately prior to the initiation of division of antigen-sensitive cells, would teleologically speaking be an optimal situation for the stimulation of an immune response'.

The possible value of the existence of a 'non-specific' so-called 'lymphocyte trapping' mechanism in antigen-draining lymphoid organs was more extensively investigated by Zatz and Lance (1971), who coined the expression 'lymphocyte trapping'.

In a thorough study of the distribution of ^{51}Cr-labelled lymph node lymphocytes in mice immunized at different times before cell injection, utilizing different routes of immunization, i.e. intravenous, intraperitoneal and subcutaneous, with various antigens, namely sheep red blood cells, S. typhi H, Keyhole limpet haemocyanin (KLH), and allogeneic and xenogeneic skin grafts, during the primary and secondary immune responses, Zatz and Lance (1971) observed that at 20–24 hr after lymphocyte injection there is an increased localization of the labelled cells in the spleen after intravenous or intraperitoneal immunization, in draining lymph nodes after subcutaneous injection or skin grafting. Moreover, the increased localization of the labelled lymphocytes, which the authors designated 'lymphocyte trapping', is dependent on the dose of antigen administered (Fig. 4.13) and occurs at 1–6 hr after the intravenous injection of antigen and at 24 hr after subcutaneous injection. It is a transient phenomenon, and more readily induced with lower concentrations of antigen in primed animals.

In these experiments too, increased recovery of radioactivity from one organ

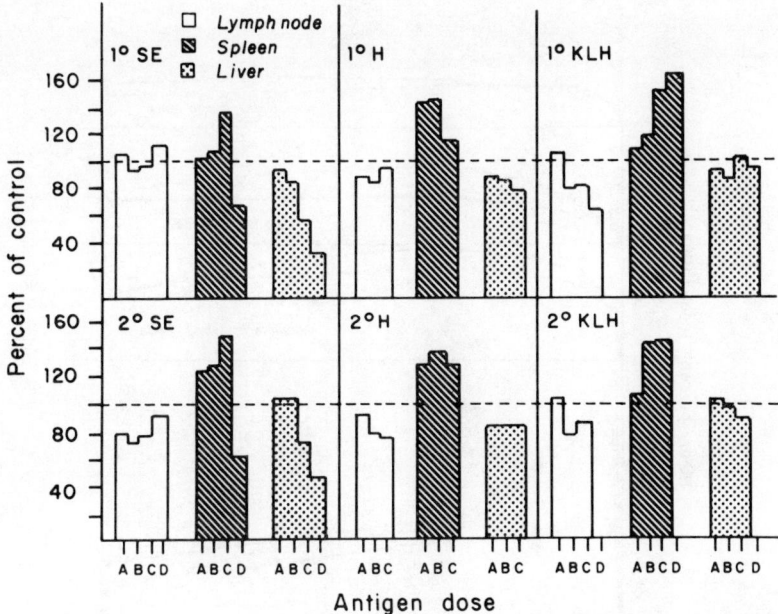

Figure 4.13 Effect of antigen dose on lymphocyte distribution in normal and presensitized recipients 1 hr after intravenous injection of various doses of SE, H, or KLH. After 24 hr the mean per cent of organ localization was determined in experimental and control (no antigen) groups. The results were expressed as per cent of control organ localization. Dose A = 5×10^6 SE, 0.1 x H, or 1 μg KLH; B = 5×10^7 SE, 1.0 x H, or 10 μg KLH; C = 5×10^8 SE, 10.0 x H, or 100 μg KLH; D = 5×10^9 SE, or 1,000 μg KLH. Slightly modified from Zatz and Lance (1971)

occurred 'at the cost' of lower recoveries from other organs, i.e. after subcutaneous injection of antigen, 'lymphocyte trapping' in the draining node occurred concomitantly with decreased lymphocyte migration to the contralateral non-injected lymph node and the mesenteric lymph node (Fig. 4.14).

Recoveries of high amounts of radioactivity from lymphoid organs draining the site of administration of antigens and adjuvants indicate that there is no inhibition of cell influx into the organ. They give, however, no indication about the degree of quantitative change in cell influx and they do not tell whether the lymphocytes are truly 'trapped', as the term 'lymphocyte trapping' implies, or simply transiting through the organ in much higher numbers than through control, unstimulated organs. Such questions can only be answered by studies of lymphocyte circulation through single organs.

In a recent study of the action of antigens on cell input and output from the popliteal and prefemoral lymph nodes in sheep, Cahill et al. (1976) defined the precise quantitative changes occurring in cell influx as well as cell output following antigen stimulation with six different antigens, namely human influenza virus, pokeweed mitogen (PWM), bacteriophage φX174, purified protein derivative

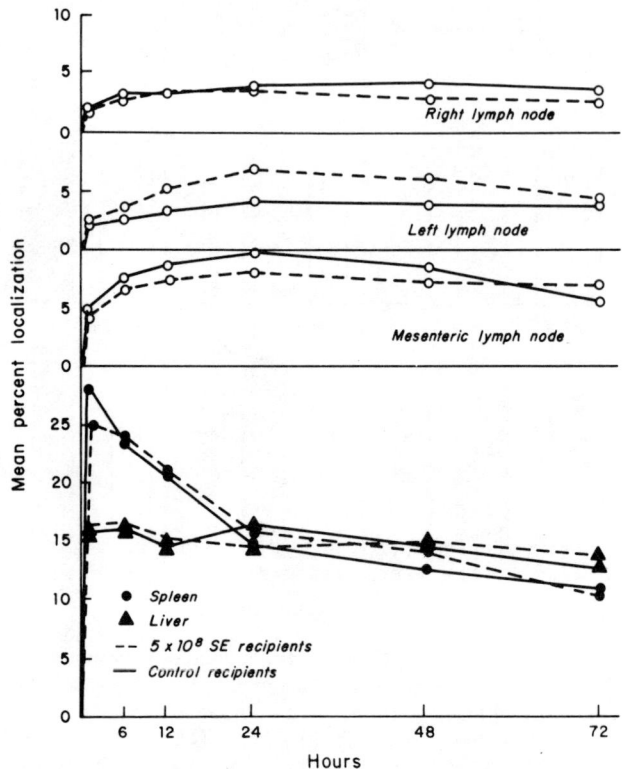

Figure 4.14 Kinetics of lymph node trapping after subcutaneous injection of antigen. Labelled lymph node cells were transferred into groups of three recipients 24 hr after subcutaneous injection of 5×10^8 SE, on the left flank, or into normal controls. Antigen-stimulated and control groups were sacrificed 1–72 hr after cell injection and the mean per cent of localization was determined in right, left, and mesenteric lymph nodes, spleen, and liver. Slightly modified from Zatz and Lance (1971)

(PPD), lipopolysaccharide (LPS), and horse red blood cells (Fig. 4.15). In response to some but not all antigens, a transient fall in lymphocyte output was observed immediately after stimulation (with LPS, bacteriophage φX174, allogeneic lymphocytes, and PPD, but not with HRBC and PWM). The decrease in cell output seems variable, whereas the later increase is the truly permanent feature of the response.

To investigate simultaneously the changes in lymphocyte input, ^{51}Cr-labelled autologous lymphocytes were infused intravenously either at the same time as or at varying intervals from antigen stimulation. The lymph nodes were removed 3 hr later and the radioactivity in them counted. When ^{51}Cr-labelled lymphocytes were infused intravenously at the same time as antigen was infused *via* the afferent

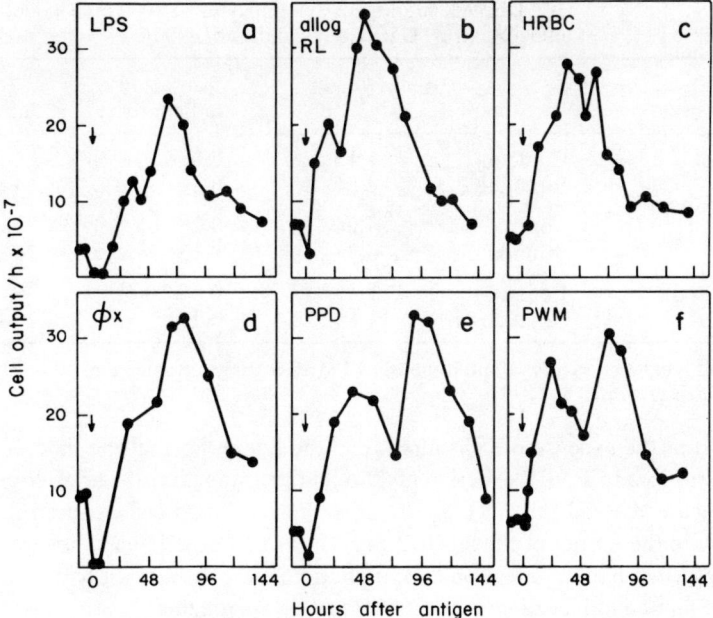

Figure 4.15 Each curve represents the total output of cells (●) after stimulation with antigen from the popliteal node of a different sheep. (a) LPS, 200 μg injected subcutaneously. (b) 4.5 x 10^8 irradiated allogeneic lymphocytes infused over 20 min *via* a cannulated afferent lymphatic. (c) HRBC, 0.5 ml packed cells infused over 20 min *via* a cannulated afferent lymphatic. (d) Bacteriophage φX174, 10^{12} PFU injected subcutaneously in a BCG-primed animal. (e) PPD, 100 μg injected subcutaneously in a BCG primed animal. (f) PWM, 15 μg injected subcutaneously. Slightly modified from Cahill *et al.* (1976)

lymphatic, more than four times as many ^{51}Cr-labelled lymphocytes entered the stimulated node as had entered the control unstimulated node. In spite of a 70% decrease in output, a 320% increase above the control was observed in cell input. The increase in lymphocyte input augmented with time, i.e. if antigen was given at time 0 and the labelled cells injected intravenously 13 hr later, the increase in input above the control was 611% (Table 4.9). The high input of labelled lymphocytes continues throughout the immune response but it takes some time before it influences the rate of cell output in the afferent lymph.

In these experiments the transit times through stimulated and unstimulated lymph nodes of labelled lymphocytes, injected simultaneously or 12 hr before the antigen infusion (human influenza virus), were also analysed. ^{51}Cr-labelled lymphocytes injected simultaneously with the antigen transited at the same time through stimulated and unstimulated nodes, in spite of a marked decrease in unlabelled cell output from the stimulated node. Labelled cells given 12 hr before antigen, however, were much delayed in appearing in the efferent lymph of the stimulated node. This delay was parallel to the decrease in cell output (Fig. 4.16). Thus, in these experiments it was clearly established that the drop in cell output

Table 4.9 Entry of ^{51}Cr-labelled autologous lymphocytes* into lymph nodes draining the site of injection of influenza virus. Data from Cahill et al. (1976)

Lymph node	Treatment	Weight (g)	% injected radioactivity	% increased input
Popliteal	Control	1.15	0.056	—
	Stimulated	2.65	0.40	611
Prescapular	Control	4.20	0.28	—
	Stimulated	6.71	1.13	298
Prefemoral	Control	1.49	0.09	—
	Stimulated	1.69	0.27	174

*Labelled lymphocytes infused intravenously 13 hr after antigen stimulation. Lymph nodes removed at 15 hr.

occurred at the expense of cells already in the lymph node at the time of antigen administration. In Ford's experiments too, antigen was given $1\frac{1}{2}$ hr after perfusion of labelled cells, and this, in the case of sheep red blood cells, caused a marked decrease in the output of the labelled cells. In Ford's experiments, however, swine influenza virus had no effect on tempo of circulation, in contrast with the marked effect of human influenza virus in Cahill et al.'s experiments.

In conclusion, administration of antigens causes a non-specific increase in

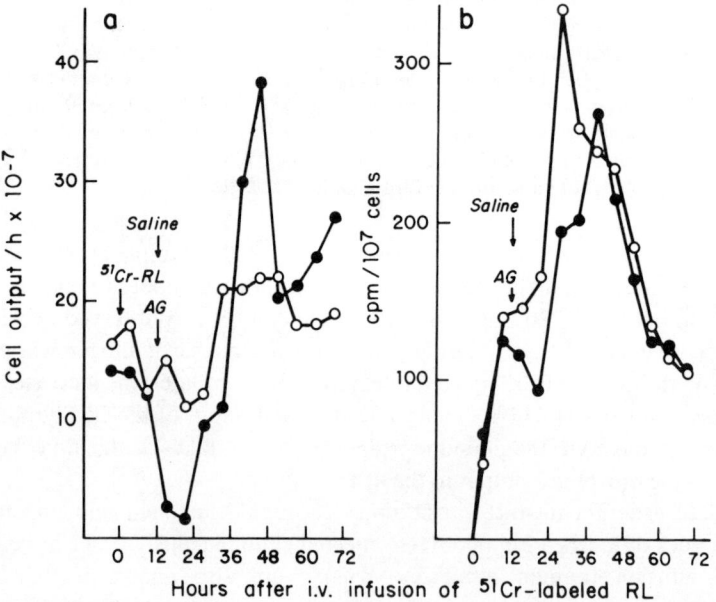

Figure 4.16 (a) Cell output from the right, influenza virus-stimulated (●) and the left, control (○) prescapular nodes. (b) Changes in concentration of ^{51}Cr-labelled autologous lymphocytes in the efferent lymph draining the stimulated and control nodes. Labelled cells given 12 hr before antigen. Note that the appearance of labelled cells in efferent lymph (b) parallels changes in cell output (a). Data from Cahill et al. (1976)

lymphocyte influx into the organ draining the site of injection of the antigen. The mechanism of this increase in influx is not clear, and one must compare experiments done in different experimental animals with different antigens with caution. It is plausible, however, that the observed increase in lymphocyte influx in the sheep is related to the reported increases in vascularity and blood flow occurring during the immune response (Herman *et al.*, 1972; Hay and Hobbs, 1977; Herman *et al.*, 1979; see Chapter 1). The possibility that an antigen-stimulated organ contains chemotactic factors (Dresser *et al.*, 1970), which positively attract circulating lymphocytes into it, must await further experimental evidence.

Lymphocytes entering a lymph node at the time of or shortly after administration of antigen are clearly not 'trapped' in it but simply transiting at the normal transit time in much higher numbers than through resting lymph nodes. The decrease in cell output often observed after the administration of most (but not all) antigens is related to the failure of cells which were already in it to leave a node.

Finally, increased cellularity in an antigen-draining lymphoid organ occurs 'at the cost' of a concomitant decrease elsewhere in the recirculatory pathway. An illustration of the functional consequence of this latter event is presented in Fig. 4.17: the response of mouse lymph nodes draining the site of a subcutaneous injection of antigen is reduced by the previous or simultaneous injection of the same antigen in the peritoneal cavity (O'Toole and Davies, 1971); this phenomenon has been termed 'preemption'.

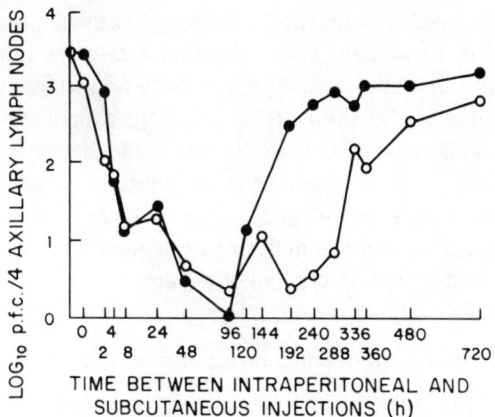

Figure 4.17 Preemption in immunity. Geometric means (expressed as log to the base ten) of the numbers of indirect plaque-forming cells per four draining lymph nodes of CBA mice 5 days after receiving a subcutaneous injection of SRBC at various times after an intraperitoneal injection of either SRBC (O———O) or HRBC (●———●). Abscissa plotted on a square root scale for convenience of presentation. Slightly modified from O'Toole and Davies (1971)

A number of other immunological phenomena fall in the borderline of the non-specific and specific influence of antigen on lymphocyte recruitment and function. Schlossman *et al.* (1971), in an elegant study of the compartmentalization of antigen-reactive lymphocytes in guinea pigs desensitized by the intravenous administration of antigen, demonstrated that persistence of antigen-responsive cells in the lymphoid organs coincided with their depletion from the blood and failure of the response of peritoneal exudate cells to the same antigen (DNP-polylysine) as measured by DNA synthesis and production of macrophage migration inhibition factor.

Antigen competition, the non-specific depression of immune responsiveness to one antigen following the administration of another non-reacting antigen (Adler, 1964), has also been attributed to a similar mechanism.

Augmentation of the response to weak immunogens by the simultaneous injection of a strong immunogen (antigenic 'promotion') has also been interpreted as the result of non-specific retention induced by one antigen, making cells more easily available to stimulation by the weak immunogen (Frost and Lance, 1974; Simic *et al.*, 1965; Wu and Cinader, 1971).

Immune deviation, a phenomenon basically similar to that described above in desensitized guinea pigs (Schlossman *et al.*, 1971), goes one step further insofar as depression of delayed hypersensitivity induced by pretreatment with the specific antigen occurs simultaneously with some enhancement of the production of certain classes of antibody (Asherson, 1966; Axelrod and Rowley, 1968).

The relevance of T lymphocyte maldistribution to the understanding of abnormalities of immunological function associated with disease will be discussed in Chapter 6. We have today the knowledge that T cells are indispensable both to the development of normal cell-mediated immunity and to the regulation of antibody production by B cells (Gershon, 1974). In all the experiments referred to so far in this chapter, no effort was made to determine the identity of the non-specifically retained populations. The experiments on immune deviation indicate, however, that in this case T cells are the ones predominantly 'redistributed', their absence from one site resulting in the simultaneous depression of cell-mediated immunity and enhanced antibody production in other sites.

4.4.2 Specific recruitment of antigen-responsive cells

One of the obvious advantages of the non-specific effects of antigen administration described above is to create the opportunity for the small minority of specific antigen-responsive cells (1 cell in 10^5 or 10^6) 'to see' the antigen. Evidence that cells do 'see' the antigen, and respond by transforming and dividing, derives from the increase in the output of large blast cells from a lymph node draining the site of antigen stimulation. In Cahill *et al.*'s experiments, for 100 hr after antigen stimulation, the output of blast cells in the efferent lymphatic was 50×10^6/hr (Cahill *et al.*, 1976). In earlier experiments in the sheep (Hall *et al.*, 1967), repeated injections of cells collected between 48 and 170 hr after cannulation from the efferent lymphatic of a popliteal lymph node which was infused *via* the afferent lymphatic with *S. typhi* 'O' organisms into a recipient twin resulted in a marked change in antibody titre against the same antigen in the recipient, starting one day after the first injection of cells (Fig. 4.18). This demonstrated that cells selectively stimulated in the donor lymph node left *via* the efferent lymphatic and, on transfer, induced the production of antibody against the same antigen in the recipient.

Other experiments in mice (Sprent *et al.*, 1971; Sprent and Miller, 1974) and rats (Rowley *et al.*, 1972) have shown that at early times (1–2 days) after immunization with heterologous erythrocytes or hapten–protein conjugates, a selective depletion of lymphocytes reactive to the injected antigen is observed in the thoracic duct lymph.

At the same time, normal or increased numbers of specifically reactive cells are present in the spleen (Sprent and Miller, 1974; Sprent and Lefkovits, 1976). Testing the GVH potential of thoracic duct lymphocytes from irradiated F_1 hybrid recipient rats of parental strain lymphocytes against the same F_1 hybrid type or a 'third party' F_1 hybrid, Atkins and Ford (1975) observed that the lymphocytes from the first 36 hr/lymph collections had a reduced GVH activity which was specific, i.e. no change was observed in the GVH potential against the third party F_1 hybrid.

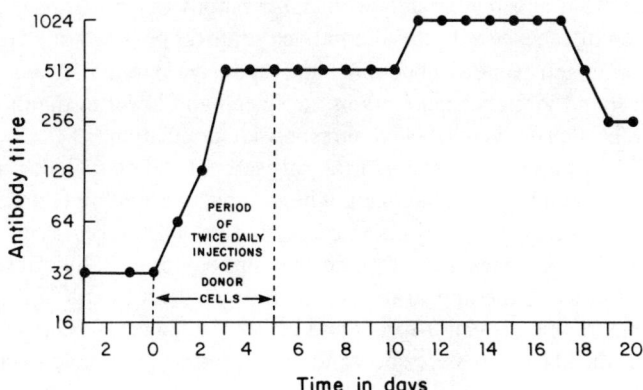

Figure 4.18 Data from the experiments of Hall *et al.* (1967), demonstrating that cells recirculating through an antigen-stimulated regional lymph node contain the pool of antigen-specific responding cells capable of specific antibody production to the antigen in question. Cells were collected from bilateral fistulae in the efferent lymphatics of the prefemoral lymph nodes after these nodes had been stimulated with killed *S. typhi* organisms, washed and injected daily for a period of 5 days into the jugular vein of the donor's chimaeric twin. The graph represents the changes in titre of antibody occurring in the blood plasma of the recipient animal following cell transfer. Slightly modified from Hall *et al.* (1967)

Earlier experiments in mice (Sprent et al., 1971) and rats (Rowley et al., 1972) had also shown that the capacity of thoracic duct lymphocytes from parental strain mice and rats to induce GVH reactions was specifically reduced or abolished 1 or 2 days after the injection of F_1 hybrid cells. Sprent and Miller (1976) have reported the observation of a dichotomy between selective depletion of TD cells with GVH potential, participating in allograft rejection and cell-mediated lympholysis, and only a negligible depletion of cells active in the MLR against the determinants of the stimulating semiallogeneic cells. This is in contrast with the findings of Hay et al. (1972) in the sheep and those of Howard and Wilson (1974) and Larner (1973) in the rat. In sheep, it was found that within 2–3 days of injecting allogeneic lymphocytes into the draining area of the popliteal lymph node, cells collected from the efferent lymphatics of the injected node and also from the contralateral node were devoid of reactive cells in the MLR to the injected determinants (Hay et al., 1975); in the rat, depletion of MLR reactive cells was observed in the peripheral blood shortly after the intravenous injection of low doses of allogeneic cells (3×10^7). In the peripheral blood of the injected rats, however, the failure to respond in the MLR was in part due to the presence of blocking factors.

In double labelling experiments, Atkins and Ford (1975) and Ford and Atkins (1973) provided a more direct demonstration of the transient selective recruitment of parental strain lymphocytes in the spleen of F_1 hybrid recipients. Parental strain lymphocytes were labelled with either [^{3}H]- or [^{14}C]-uridine and injected into F_1 hybrid recipient mixed intimately with an unresponsive population (F_1 hybrid or tolerant parental) labelled with the alternative radioisotope ([^{14}C] or [^{3}H]). Twenty-four hours after intravenous injection, the responsive parental strain population was always found in higher amounts in the spleen and lower in the thoracic duct lymph than the alternatively labelled unresponsive population.

The results of these experiments in the rat were attributed to T cell recruitment because of the quality of the labelling with radioactive uridine (Ford, 1975; see Section 4.3). In the mouse, the finding of responsive cells in the spleen and lymph nodes at 1–2 days after transfer of parental lymphocytes in F_1 hybrid recipients is followed at 4 days by the appearance in the thoracic duct lymph of the recipients of large numbers of blast cells (Sprent and Miller, 1972a,b,c; Cheers et al., 1974). Nearly all of the blast cells were shown to be of thymus origin and to carry Thy-1 antigen on their surfaces.

Thus all the examples of antigen-specific recruitment of recirculating lymphocytes reviewed so far are examples of T cell recruitment. They are also descriptions of events occurring during primary immune responses to antigens for the most part thymus-dependent. It has been argued that in primary immune responses the recruitment of B cells from the recirculating pool has not been shown, probably because it does not occur (Ford, 1975).

This view must await further experiments, in which the action of antigens known to be thymus-independent on the make-up of the recirculating pool of animals depleted of their thymus-derived population will be studied.

4.4.3 Role in the initiation, propagation, and persistence (memory) of immunity

4.4.3.1 Initiation

The contribution of circulating lymphocytes to the initiation of immune responses was first demonstrated in the allograft and graft *versus* host reactions (Gowans, 1962; Billingham *et al.*, 1954; Billingham *et al.*, 1962, 1963; Gowans *et al.*, 1963) and in the primary haemolysin response to sheep erythrocytes (McGregor and Gowans, 1963; McGregor *et al.*, 1967), at a time when the full implications of the existence of thymus-derived and non-thymus-derived populations of lymphocytes had not been fully realized, although contemporary work indicated that all the above immune responses were thymus-dependent (Humphrey *et al.*, 1964).

The first indication that both circulating and non-circulating lymphocytes are required for the development of a primary immune response, depending on the nature of the antigen studied, derived from a study by Strober (1968), in which the response to three different antigens, i.e. sheep red blood cells, bovine serum albumin, and alum precipitated tetanus toxoid, was investigated in the rat.

In experiments of design essentially similar to those of McGregor and Gowans (1963), the primary immune response was abolished by sublethal irradiation (500 r) and the ability of 2.5×10^8 first, second, third or fourth day thoracic duct lymphocytes to restore it was investigated. The response of rats subjected to prolonged thoracic duct cannulation was also investigated.

The primary immune responses to sheep erythrocytes and bovine serum albumin were indeed reduced in rats drained for long periods of time, and abolished in sublethally irradiated animals and restored by the injection of first day cannulated circulating lymphocytes (Fig. 4.19a). The response to alum precipitated tetanus toxoid, however, remained unaltered by prolonged thoracic duct drainage, and was not restored in sublethally irradiated animals by the injection of first day cannulated lymphocytes (Fig. 4.19b). The response to alum precipitated tetanus toxoid was restored, however, by normal rat spleen cells, or by second, third or fourth day lymphocytes. At the time of Strober's experiments the differences in tempo of migration of T and B cells (see Section 4.2) had not been discovered. Reading the original papers in the light of this knowledge, one is tempted to interpret the results as reflecting different contributions of circulating T and B lymphocytes to the initiation of primary responses with the different antigens tested.

Other less direct demonstrations of the contribution of circulating lymphocytes to the initiation of primary immune responses derive from the effect of single organ irradiation on the development of the primary immune response within the irradiated organ (Simic *et al.*, 1965, 1970; Hall and Morris, 1964). High doses of irradiation given selectively to a spleen or a lymph node have little effect on the antibody response evoked in the irradiated organ.

Ford (1969), comparing the restorative capacity in lymphocyte-free blood and thoracic duct lymphocytes of the haemolysin response to sheep red blood cells in

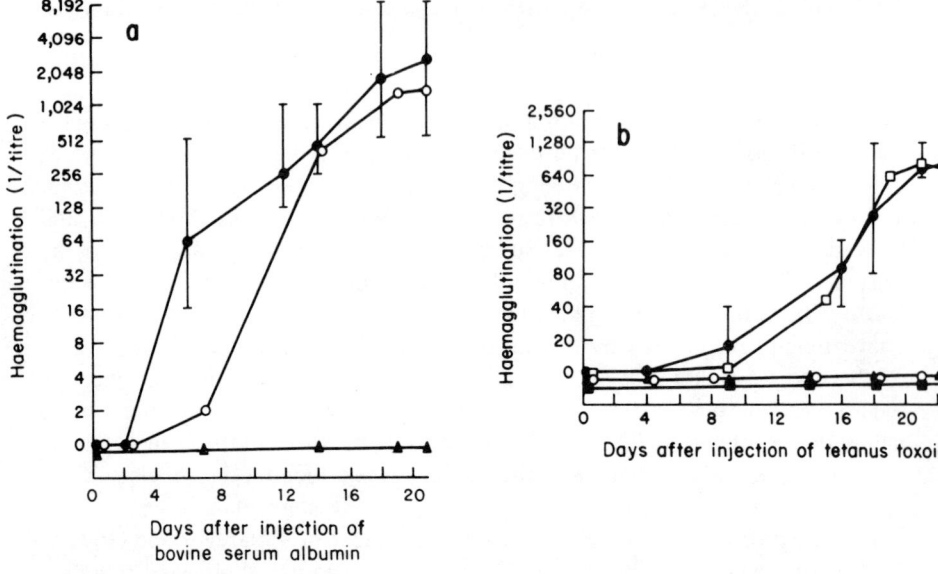

Figure 4.19 Demonstration from the experiments of Strober (1968) that recirculating lymphocytes are indispensable for the development of the immune response to some (a) but not all (b) antigens. (a) Tanned red cell haemagglutination response to a single subcutaneous injection of 0.8 mg of bovine serum albumin in complete Freund's adjuvant. ● Mean response of seven normal rats. ▲ Mean response of six rats exposed to whole body irradiation 24 hr before injection of bovine serum albumin. ○ Mean response of six rats given an intravenous injection of 2.5×10^8 first day thoracic duct cells 2 hr after irradiation; bovine serum albumin was injected 24 hr after irradiation. (b) Tanned cell haemagglutination response to a single intraperitoneal and subcutaneous injection of 15 Lf (total) alum precipitated tetanus toxoid. ● Mean response of eight normal rats. ▲ Mean response of eight rats exposed to 500 r whole body irradiation 24 hr before injection of tetanus toxoid. ○ Mean response of 13 rats given an intravenous injection of 2.5×10^8 first day thoracic duct cells 2 hr after irradiation; tetanus toxoid was injected 24 hr after irradiation. ■ Mean response of three rats given an intravenous injection of 1×10^9 first day thoracic duct cells 2 hr after irradiation; tetanus toxoid was injected 24 hr after irradiation. □ Mean response of five rats depleted of thoracic duct cells by 5 days of thoracic duct drainage; tetanus toxoid was injected immediately after drainage was stopped. Slightly modified from Strober (1968)

perfused spleens depleted of lymphocytes by X-irridiation and chronic thoracic duct drainage, demonstrated that the response was only restored to normal when the spleen was repopulated by adding thoracic duct lymphocytes to the initial perfusate. When lymphocyte-free blood was added to the perfusate traversing normal spleens, the haemolysin response was reduced by a factor of 8.

From all that is known today about the contribution of T and B cells to a normal response to sheep red blood cells (Greaves *et al.*, 1975), one can say retrospectively that most likely it was the T lymphocyte component in the perfusate that markedly influenced the development of the response in the isolated organ.

4.4.3.2 Propagation

The usefulness of having a physiological system sufficiently flexible to enable such drastic changes in cell flow in the draining node as those described earlier (Table 4.9) is obvious for the recruitment of antigen-specific responsive cells, but does it contribute to the propagation of the 'knowledge' that an antigen has arrived to such remote sites as the afferent lymphatic duct of a popliteal node?

Indeed it does.

Hall et al. (1967) were the first to demonstrate the role of the population leaving the efferent lymphatic of a node receiving S. typhi 'O' via the afferent lymphatic in the development of systemic antibody titre against the immunizing antigen.

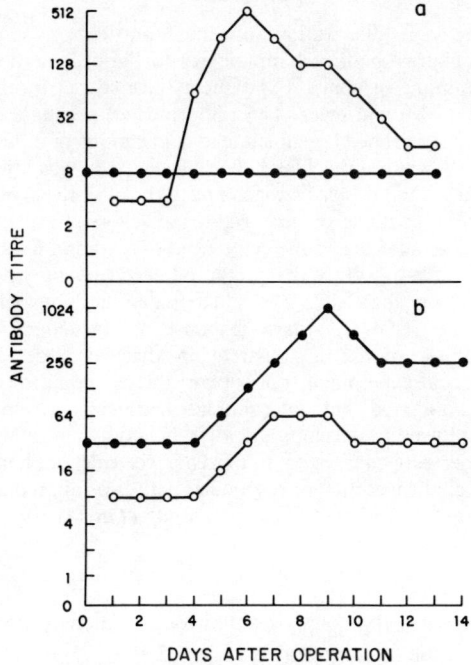

Figure 4.20 Changes in the antibody titre of the systemic blood plasma and the lymph from the prefemoral nodes of clun Forest sheep following the infusion of a suspension of killed S. typhi 'O' organisms into an afferent prefemoral lymphatic. In the test animals (a), the efferent duct of the stimulated node was cannulated. In the control animals (b), the efferent duct of the stimulated node was left intact and the efferent duct of the unstimulated node in the other flank was cannulated. ●———● titre of antibody in the blood plasma; ○———○ titre of antibody in lymph. Slightly modified from Hall et al. (1967)

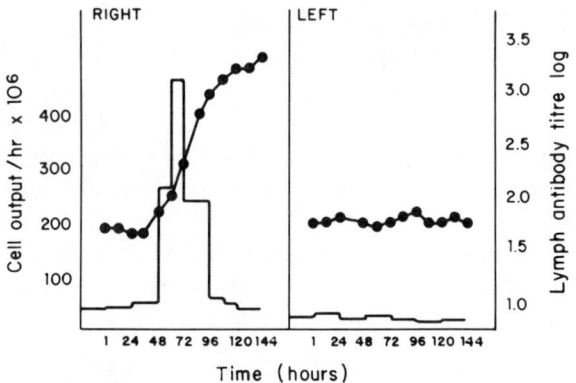

Figure 4.21 Illustration of the contribution of the recirculatory pool of lymphocytes to the propagation of the immune response. Experiments carried out by Smith et al. in Merino ewes. The right and left popliteal node were both primed by subcutaneous injections of influenza virus. Seventeen days later the right leg only was injected with a second dose of antigen and 12 hr after the injection the efferent ducts of both right and left popliteal nodes were cannulated and the cell output (———) and antibody content (●———●) of the lymph followed over the next 14 days. Note that while the right popliteal node responded with a typical secondary response, no evidence of an immune response is apparent in the left node. In a reciprocal experiment (not shown) the left popliteal node was stimulated, but not cannulated, a primary response was allowed to develop, and after 17 days both right and left legs were challenged. In this case, the side that had not been challenged before responded with typical secondary response. Slightly modified from Smith et al. (1970)

Animals whose efferent lymph was drained away failed to produce antibody, in marked contrast with the intact controls (Fig. 4.20).

Smith et al. (1970), studying the influence of draining the efferent lymph from a popliteal node receiving swine influenza virus *via* the afferent lymphatic on the development of the secondary immune response, verified that, after second challenge in the contralateral lymph node, the animals that had been drained gave an immune response with the characteristics of a primary immune response, whereas the controls (non-drained) gave a clearcut secondary response (Fig. 4.21). For further details see legend to Fig. 4.21.

4.4.3.3 Memory

In the remote English village, where the First World War dissipated a generation of men that today would be in their eighties, who remembers the War best? Little boys running around between village greens and sweet shops, or old men sitting still by bay windows? The latter, no doubt.

Thus, 'remembering' is an attribute linked fundamentally to long lifespan. Mammalian lymphocytes, however, combine two attributes which in human life belong to two clearly separate age groups – remembering and running around effortlessly.

Evidence for the linkage between lymphocyte recirculation between blood and lymph, long lifespan and memory has accumulated since the early seventies, mainly from the work of Strober (Strober, 1969, 1970, 1972) and Strober and Dilley (1973), and more recently from the work of Sprent and Miller (1976).

Thoracic duct lymphocytes from immunized rats were first shown by Strober (1969) to be less susceptible to *in vitro* treatment with vinblastine than TDL from non-immunized rats. On transfer to irradiated recipients immunized with *S. typhi* flagella or horse spleen ferritin, the restorative capacity of the response of immunized donor lymphocytes was unaltered by vinblastine treatment, in contrast with the deleting effect of similar treatment of TDL from non-immunized recipients. More recently, Strober and Dilley (1973), utilizing the experimental model illustrated in Fig. 4.22, demonstrated that the anti-DNP response in sublethally irradiated recipients of carrier-primed spleen cells and hapten-primed spleen cells, passaged or not through an intermediate irradiated host (collected from the thoracic duct lymph of the intermediate recipient), was 2.5 fold greater in the recipients of the passaged hapten-primed spleen cells.

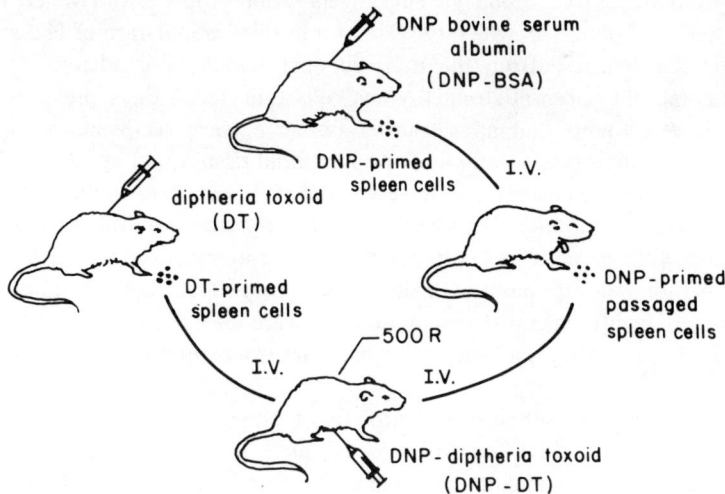

Figure 4.22 Experimental design of Strober and Dilley's experiments demonstrating the contribution of the recirculatory pool to immunological memory. Lewis rats are immunized with DNP–BSA or DT. DNP-primed spleen cells are injected intravenously into an irradiated intermediate host and recovered in the thoracic duct lymph. The passaged DNP-primed cells and non-passaged DT-primed cells are injected into an irradiated final host. Cell recipients are subsequently challenged with DNP–DT. Slightly modified from Strober and Dilley (1973)

Further experiments showed that hapten-primed thoracic duct cells, as well as passaged hapten-primed spleen cells, are more efficient in restoring the anti-DNP response than non-passaged spleen cells. Virtually all the memory spleen cell pool could be accounted for as belonging to the recirculatory pool. Spleen cells from hapten-primed donors which had been thoracic duct drained for 5 days failed to restore the response of irradiated recipients of carrier-primed cells; indeed, after challenge with DNP–DT, the response was reduced at least 25 fold, compared with the response of recipients of carrier-primed and hapten-primed spleen cells from non-drained donors.

Injection of 'suicidal' doses of [^{3}H]-thymidine (3.5 mCi every 8 hr for 48 hr before removal of the spleen), which normally produce a 20–100 fold decrease in the ability of thoracic duct cells from unimmunized rats to restore the adoptive *primary* response to horse spleen ferritin (Strober, 1972), injection of such suicidal doses of [^{3}H]-thymidine to the donors of the hapten-primed or the carrier-primed spleen cells caused only a minor reduction (2 fold) of the anti-DNP response, thus indicating that the majority of T and B memory cells are turning over at a considerably slower rate than B lymphocytes involved in the adoptive primary response. Moreover, these cells circulate poorly to the lymph (Strober, 1972). In essence, Strober's experiments can be summarized as indicating that in the rat, the thoracic duct lymph is a compartment enriched for long-lived memory cells. The same conclusion can be drawn from analysis of the more recent series of elegant experiments of Howard and Wilson (1974) in the rat and of Sprent in mice on the fate of H2-activated T lymphocytes in syngeneic hosts (Sprent and Miller, 1976).

In a series of papers in which the fate of a purified population of H2-activated blast T cells collected from the thoracic duct lymph of irradiated F_1 hybrid recipient mice of parental strain thymus cells (injected 4 days previously) was traced, it was found that after transfer into syngeneic recipients most of the activated cells disappeared rapidly from lymphoid tissues and intestines. A small proportion of the cells survived, however, and these persisted in the recirculating pool for several months (designated T.TDL, Sprent and Miller, 1976). The behaviour of these cells in GVH reaction, allograft reaction and in MLR was studied before and after passage through syngeneic B hosts. On the whole, T.TDL tested before or after passage through B mice were far more reactive to the determinants to which they had originally been activated than to third party determinants.

Their capacity to suppress the growth of allogeneic tumour cells was far superior to that of TDL control injected mice (Table 4.10), indicating good memory for the determinants of allograft reaction. Cells from T.TDL injected mice, however, unlike T.TDL injected rats (Howard and Wilson, 1974), were no more effective at producing GVH reactions and MLR than cells from mice injected with TDL alone. In the rat, Howard and Wilson, studying the fate of blast cells generated from rat TDL during MLR against AgB determinants *in vitro*, transferred into syngeneic B rats, observed that the thoracic duct lymphocytes harvested from the recipients weeks later gave high and specific MLR and GVH reactions against the sensitizing determinants (Howard and Wilson, 1974).

Table 4.10 Suppression of growth of DBA/2 tumour allografts by CBA T.TDL. Data from Sprent and Miller (1976)

CBA cells transferred subcutaneously to irradiated CBA mice together with 10^5 DBA/2 mastocytoma cells*	Lymphocyte : tumour cell ratio	No. of mice	% suppression of tumour growth in irradiated CBA mice
Spleen	200 : 1	5	40
	20 : 1	5	0
	2 : 1	5	0
Lymph node	200 : 1	5	60
	20 : 1	5	0
	2 : 1	5	0
TDL	20 : 1	5	0
	2 : 1	5	0
DBA/2-activated T.TDL	200 : 1	6	100
	20 : 1	6	100
	2 : 1	6	50
C57BL-activated T.TDL	200 : 1	6	100
	20 : 1	6	50
	2 : 1	6	16

*In 0.2 ml *via* 30 gauge needle.
T.TDL H2-activated blast T cells collected from thoracic duct lymph of irradiated F_1 hybrid mice which received parental strain thymus cells passaged further through syngeneic recipients.

As Sprent and Miller (1976) point out, to account for the discrepancy between the two sets of findings is clearly difficult, since the two populations were generated with different systems in different species.

4.5 FACTORS OTHER THAN ANTIGEN INFLUENCING LYMPHOCYTE CIRCULATION

4.5.1 Phenotype

In one of the early views presented to explain the ecotaxis of lymphocytes it was suggested that as a cell differentiates and acquires the surface components that define its phenotype, it acquires at the same time the surface make-up that will determine its ultimate destination and positioning in the peripheral lymphoid organs (de Sousa, 1973).

This view of the development of the circulation and specific positioning of lymphocytes has only recently been tested experimentally (de Sousa *et al.*, 1979). This has become possible with the recognition that different functionally distinct subpopulations of T lymphocytes can be distinguished and actually separated according to their Ly phenotype (see Chapter 2.4).

Experiments comparing the fate of ^{51}Cr-labelled Lyt-1 and Lyt-23 cells in syngeneic recipients demonstrated that the Lyt-1 cells behave like unselected T lymphocytes, i.e. after an early transit through the lungs and liver, the largest proportion of labelled cells is recovered from the spleen and lymph nodes (Fig. 4.23). Labelled Lyt-23 cells, however, differ from T and Lyt-1 cells in that only a small percentage (0.34%) reached the lymph nodes at 24 hr after injection (Fig. 4.23). At 24 hr, the majority of the radioactivity in the mice that had been given Lyt-23 cells was still recovered from the liver (19.1% ± 1.5) and spleen (24.9% ± 2.2). The different recoveries of ^{51}Cr-labelled Lyt-23 and Lyt-1 cells from the liver were not the result of cell death, but possibly the reflection of differences in surface carbohydrate composition of the two subsets of T cells. Similar transient increases in numbers of viable labelled lymphocytes in the liver are seen when the cells have been asialated by treatment *in vitro* with neuroaminidase (see Section 4.5.4). The possible binding of the anti-Lyt-1 antiserum used in the elimination of Lyt-1 positive cells to Lyt-23 cells without killing them may also have contributed to the finding of high numbers of these cells in the liver.

The poor circulation of Lyt-23 cells to the spleen and lymph nodes is also apparent from a study of the distribution of the two cell subsets in the spleen lymph nodes and thoracic duct lymph of B6 mice (Beverley, 1977). Lyt-1 cells constitute 30–40% of the spleen T cell population, 35–45% of the T cell population of the lymph node, and 40–60% of the T cells in the thoracic duct lymph (Table 2.4). Lyt-23 cells are found in small percentages in the spleen (10–20%), lymph node (5–10%), and thoracic duct lymph (2–10%).

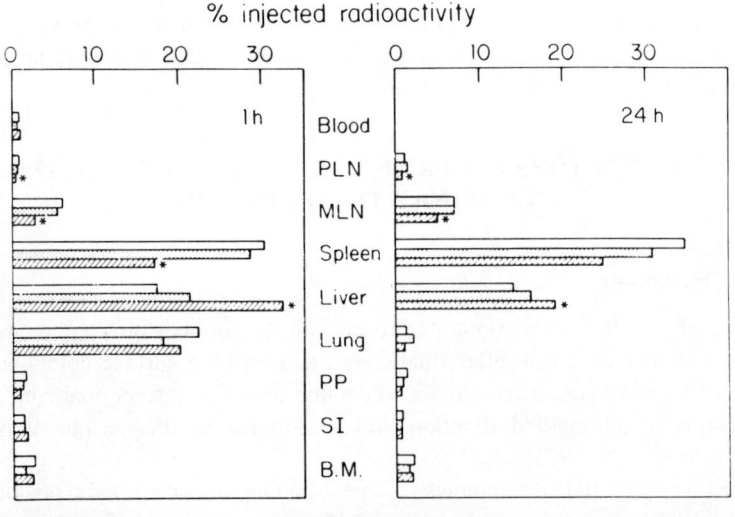

Figure 4.23 Migratory patterns of purified ^{51}Cr-labelled mouse T, Lyt-1 and Lyt-23 lymphocytes at 1 and 24 hr after intravenous injection in syngeneic recipients

Furthermore, in an autoradiographic study of the distribution of ^{3}H-adenosine-labelled Lyt-1 and Lyt-23 cells, the latter were found mostly in B cell areas of the mouse spleen and lymph nodes, in contrast with the migration of Lyt-1 cells to the T cell areas. Although very small numbers of Lyt-23 cells were seen in the lymph nodes, they seemed to 'prefer' the intermediate zone between the cortex and medulla. Another interesting feature of the distribution of Lyt-23 cells was their frequent association with polymorphonuclear cells. This finding was interpreted as indicating either that Lyt-23 cell migration is influenced by the release of products by polymorphs or that Lyt-23 cells and polymorphs are motivated to migrate to the same areas by the same chemotactic stimuli.

With the recent expansion in the field of immunogenetics and the delineation and the possibility of further separation of T as well as B cell subpopulations with monoclonal antibodies, we can envisage a time when the exact 'environmental' preferences of each cell type will be mapped rigorously in tissue sections.

4.5.2 Age

A few groups of workers have looked at the question of influence of age on the distribution of labelled cells from donors of different ages. Unfortunately, the experimental conditions are not comparable and therefore no general conclusions can be drawn from the slightly different groups of results. Zatz *et al.* (1971) conducted a study of the distribution of ^{51}Cr-labelled lymph node, spleen and thymus cells from CBA and NZB mice of different ages (ranging from 8 days to 12 months) in 2–3 months old CBA and 8–10 week old NZB recipients.

Failure of NZB mouse lymph node cells to reach the lymph nodes of syngeneic recipients was observed when the cells were obtained from 3 month old and 12 month old donors. The reduction in recovered radioactivity from the lymph nodes concurred with increased recoveries from the spleen and liver.

It is difficult to draw any clear conclusions from such experiments when we have no indication of the lymphocyte subpopulations included in the inoculum. As mentioned earlier, T and B lymphocytes have different tempos of circulation, and the failure of older NZB mice cells to reach the lymph nodes could be a reflection of the progressive B cell expansion that is known to occur in the peripheral lymph nodes of NZB mice with age (East *et al.*, 1965).

In the same study, Zatz and co-workers analysed the distribution of ^{51}Cr-labelled CBA lymph node cells in syngeneic recipients of different ages (1–12 months old). A trend towards decreasing lymph node localization and increasing spleen localization was observed.

In a study of the influence of donor age on the migration of [^{3}H]-adenosine-labelled bursa cells in 8-day irradiated chickens, De Kruyff *et al.* (1975) found that the age of the donors had no effect on the degree of migration to bursa or thymus. Differences were found in amount of recovered radioactivity in the spleen. When bursa cells from donors 3–8 days of age were transferred, recipient spleens contained only 4.6–9.7% of injected radioactivity per gramme of tissue. In

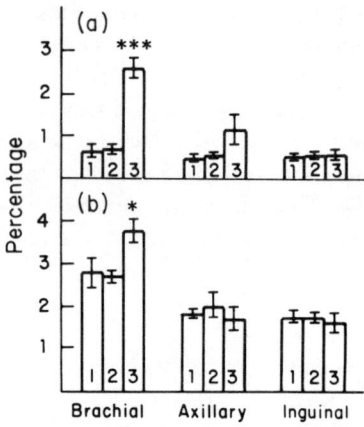

Figure 4.24 Data from Inchley et al. (1976) illustrating the failure of old recipients to recruit significant numbers of circulating lymphocytes to the regional lymph node draining an antigen injection of SRBC: 24 hr distribution of intravenously injected ^{51}Cr-labelled lymph node cells from 25 month old donors in the lymph nodes of young ((a), 3–4 months old) and old ((b), 24–26 months old) recipients, and the influence of local stimulation with SRBC. 1, mean of right and left lymph nodes of non-immunized control mice; 2, contralateral lymph nodes of immunized mice; 3, ipsilateral lymph nodes of immunized mice. Mean of five mice per group. Asterisks denote statistical comparison with next column to left. *$P < 0.05$; ***$P < 0.001$

contrast, when donors of bursa cells were 28–90 days old, the radioactivity per gramme of tissue associated with recipient spleens increased to a range of 9.00–17.6%.

Inchley et al. (1976), in studies of ^{51}Cr- or ^{75}Se-L-seleno-methionine-labelled young and old CBA lymph node cells, observed increased peripheral lymph node localization in recipients older than those studied by Zatz, i.e. 15 and 17 months old. Splenic localization in this case either declined slightly with age or, like the liver, showed no significant change.

One interesting observation in Inchley's study was the finding that 24–30 month old mice failed to respond to local injection of sheep erythrocytes with the expected increase in lymphocyte recruitment to the draining lymph node which occurs in younger animals (Fig. 4.24). Although the nature of the changes underlying this age-related decline in antigen-induced lymphocyte recruitment is not clear, it is probable that they are related to the defective immune responsiveness of older mice.

Another interesting aspect of this study is that the differences observed in lymph node cell migration, unlike bursa cells (De Kruyff et al., 1975), were not related to the age of the cells, but to the age of the recipients. This illustrates well the point that the host environment plays a crucial role in the control of lymphocyte circulation. Additional examples of the influence of host manipulation in lymphocyte circulation will be reviewed in Sections 4.5.6–4.5.8.

4.5.3 Antibody

The action of antibody on the migration of lymphocytes *in vivo* has been investigated in a limited number of studies (Martin, 1969; Durkin et al., 1975). This contrasts markedly with the numerous studies of the action of antibody on red cell traffic, and illustrates well how prevailing interests in one experimental subject dominate the choice of experiments done in that subject. The repercussion of these choices does not stay within the experimental field. Clinicians today are well aware of the effect of antibody on red cell sequestration, but seldom consider that antilymphocyte antibodies may have marked disturbing effects on peripheral blood lymphocyte counts and cause lymphocyte sequestrations similar to the known sequestration of sensitized red cells (see also Chapter 6.2).

Evidence of the induction by antibody of abnormal sequestration of ^{51}Cr-labelled lymphocytes in the liver was presented by Martin in a study of the distribution of ^{51}Cr-labelled lymphocytes treated *in vitro* with antilymphocyte antiserum (Martin, 1969).

More recently, Durkin *et al.* (1975) demonstrated that exposure of rabbit [^{3}H]-adenosine-labelled appendix cells *in vitro* to anti-immunoglobulin for 1 hr at 4°C caused alterations of their subsequent migration in the lymphoid organs of recipients killed at 5 hr after intravenous injection of the labelled cells. These alterations were transient and by 24 hr the numbers and distribution of labelled anti-Ig treated cells were identical to those of labelled control untreated cells.

4.5.4 Enzymes

4.5.4.1 Neuraminidase

Neuraminidase is a mucopolysaccharide, *N*-acetylneuraminylhydrolase, which cleaves the 2,3 and 2,6 glycosidic linkages between terminal *N*-acetylneuraminic acids and mucopolysaccharides. The discovery of its action on sialic acid moieties stemmed originally from the observation that filtrates from *Vibrio cholera* and *Clostridium perfringens* (*C. Welchii*) destroyed the receptor sites for influenza viruses at the surface of human erythrocytes (Burnet *et al.*, 1946). This observation led to the demonstration that the enzyme reduced the net surface negativity of human erythrocytes and that acidic groups were cleaved from the surface of enzyme-treated cells. It is now well established that the reduction in the net surface negativity of human erythrocytes induced by highly purified preparations of the enzyme is associated with cleavage of free sialic acid moieties which are resistant to release from glycolipids by neuraminidase (Winzler, 1970).

In the first study of the action of neuraminidase on the traffic of lymphocytes, a crude preparation of glycosidases, obtained from a culture of *C. perfringens*, was used (Gesner and Ginsburg, 1964). Subsequent studies with highly purified preparations of the enzyme (Woodruff and Gesner, 1969; Freitas and de Sousa, 1976a; Ford *et al.*, 1976; Kolb, Kriese, Kolb-Bachofen and Kolb, 1978; Kolb and Kolb-Bachofen, 1978; Kolb-Bachofen and Kolb, 1979) have yielded essentially the same results.

After the intravenous injection of *in vitro* labelled neuraminidase-treated lymphocytes, obtained from the thoracic duct lymph in rats or from mouse lymph node cell suspensions, at the early times after injection (up to 1 hr) most radioactivity is recovered from the liver. This increase in recovery of the labelled cells from the liver occurs concomitantly with significantly lower recoveries from the lymph nodes and slightly lower recoveries from the lungs and spleen. This effect can be directly related to the dose and time of exposure to the enzyme *in vitro* and is abolished by heating of the enzyme at 65°C for 19 min (Woodruff and Gesner, 1969). The effect has been directly related to action of the enzyme on the cell surface, in experiments in which it was found that the simultaneous *in vivo* administration of the enzyme and of labelled cells had no effect on the cells' distribution.

Evidence that the maldistribution induced by enzyme treatment is not related to cell death stems from the finding that at 24 and 48 hr after intravenous injection no differences are observed in the amounts of radioactivity recovered from the lymph nodes of recipients of treated or untreated lymphocytes (Woodruff and Gesner, 1969; Freitas and de Sousa, 1976a). Moreover, Woodruff and Gesner (1969), following up recovery of labelled neuraminidase-treated and untreated labelled autologous lymphocytes in the thoracic duct lymph, observed a delay in the peak recovery of radioactivity associated with cells in the recipients of the enzyme-treated cells.

Thus, these experiments indicate that failure of circulating lymphocytes to reach the lymph nodes at the early times after injection was related to their temporary sequestration in the liver (Fig. 4.25). Partial hepatectomy did not

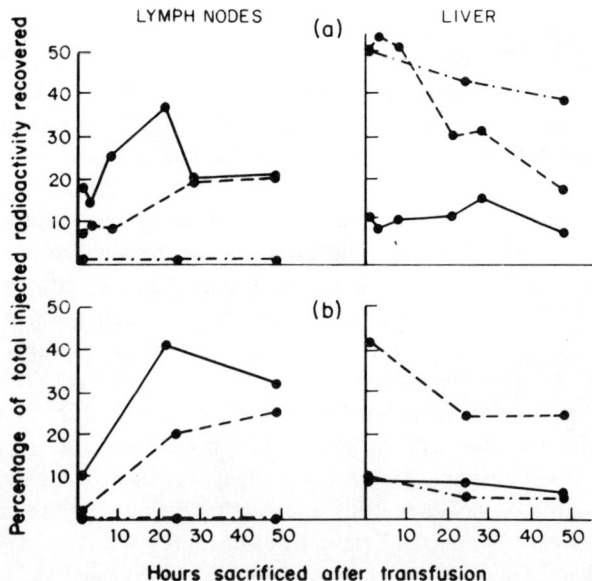

Figure 4.25 Effect of neuraminidase treatment (-----) and heat killing (-·-·-) on the distribution of ^{51}Cr-labelled rat lymphocytes to lymph nodes and liver. (a) Allogeneic lymphocytes. (b) Syngeneic lymphocytes. Distribution of ^{51}Cr-labelled untreated lymphocytes (●——●). Note that neuraminidase treatment reduced significantly migration to lymph nodes as the result of lymphocyte sequestration in liver. Slightly modified from Woodruff and Gesner (1969)

modify decreased lymph node entry in the rat experiments (Woodruff and Gesner, 1969), but ligature of the hepatic artery has been shown by Freitas (1976) to result in normal lymph node entry of the treated cells shortly after intravenous injection.

A more direct demonstration of the fact that neuraminidase treatment did not influence lymph node entry of circulating lymphocytes, however, derives from the experiments of Ford et al. (1976) in the rat. Studying the kinetics of direct entry of labelled thoracic duct lymphocytes in the perfused rat mesenteric lymph node, it was found that neuraminidase treatment did not influence entry, although there was some indication that transit through the node was slightly delayed (Table 4.11).

More recently, Kolb and co-workers (Kolb and Kolb-Bachofen, 1978; Kolb, Kriese, Kolb-Bachofen, and Kolb, 1978; Kolb-Bachofen and Kolb, 1979) have examined the molecular and ultrastructural aspects of the liver localization of neuraminidase-treated mouse spleen cells and found that although the majority of asialolymphocytes do not remain sequestered in the liver and regain their normal migratory pattern within 2 days, a small subpopulation persists in the liver, which adheres both to Kupffer cells and hepatocytes. The binding also takes place *in*

Table 4.11 Effect of neuraminidase and trypsin treatment on migration of perfused radiolabelled lymphocytes through the isolated mesenteric lymph node*

Enzyme	Ratio† of $\dfrac{\text{radioactivity associated with treated cells}}{\text{radioactivity associated with untreated cells}}$		
	Perfused lymph node	Extranodal tissue	Effluent perfusate
Neuraminidase	1.22	0.96	0.98
	1.46	1.31	0.98
	1.03	0.98	1.02
	1.44	1.28	0.93
	1.15	1.00	0.98
Median	1.22	1.00	0.98
Trypsin	0.44	0.91	1.09
	0.53	0.80	0.92
	0.45	–‡	0.93
	0.76	1.28	1.07
	0.83	1.09	1.04
	0.89	1.10	1.06
Median	0.64	1.09	1.05

*Data from Ford et al. (1976). Each set of results from one individual experiment rat thoracic duct lymphocytes was labelled with uridine-5-^{3}H or with uridine-^{14}C and treated or not with the enzyme under study mixed and perfused. The results are expressed as the ratio of the radioactivity associated with treated cells with the radioactivity associated with untreated internal control cells.
†Ratio standardized so that ratio in initial perfusate = 1.00.
‡Radioactivity too low to measure accurately.

vitro and is due to stereo-specific interactions between a D-galactose recognizing lectin-like receptor in liver cells (Ashwell and Morell, 1974) and β-D-galactosyl residues uncovered by neuraminidase (Kolb, Schudt, Kolb-Bachofen, and Kolb, 1978; Kolb and Kolb-Bachofen 1978).

In addition, auto-immune-like lesions were induced in the liver by repeated injections of asialolymphocytes (Kolb-Bachofen and Kolb, 1979). The mechanism of induction of these lesions will be discussed in detail later (Chapter 6.1).

4.5.4.2 Trypsin

In vitro treatment of rat thoracic duct lymphocytes (Woodruff and Gesner, 1968; Woodruff, 1974; Ford *et al.*, 1976; Ford, Smith, and Andrews, 1978) and of mouse lymph node cells (Freitas and de Sousa, 1976a) with trypsin results also in their maldistribution following intravenous injection.

Like neuraminidase-treated cells, the numbers of trypsin-treated lymphocytes entering lymph nodes are considerably reduced (Table 4.12a). With trypsin treatment, however, reduction in the per cent of injected radioactivity recovered from lymph nodes occurs with variable concomitant increases in the amount of radioactivity recovered from the spleen rather than the liver. This effect can be related to time of incubation of the cells with the enzyme (Freitas and de Sousa, 1976a), and trypsin-treated cells recover their capacity to migrate normally when incubated at 37°C in the absence of the enzyme for 12 hr (Woodruff, 1974). This has led to the suggestion that trypsin cleaves some component of the lymphocyte surface which is necessary for normal entry into the lymph nodes. Trypsin-treated lymphocytes incubated either at 17°C in the absence of the enzyme or in cultures to which puromycin was added failed to recover their normal circulation properties (Woodruff, 1974). This suggests that active synthesis of surface components is required for restoration of the ability of lymphocytes to circulate normally.

In an attempt to determine whether failure of trypsin-treated lymphocytes to enter lymph nodes is a 'genuine' effect or simply the reflection of their slower migration through the spleen, Freitas and de Sousa (1976a) have analysed the fate of trypsin-treated lymphocytes in splenectomized recipients (Table 4.12b). Under these circumstances, the amount of radioactivity recovered in the blood following intravenous injection is still much higher in the recipients of the treated cells than in the recipients of the untreated cells. In addition, Ford *et al.* (1976) have observed that trypsin-treated labelled thoracic duct lymphocytes fail to enter normally perfused mesenteric lymph nodes.

4.5.4.3 Phospholipases

Both the work on the action of neuraminidase treatment and the work on the action of trypsin on lymphocyte migration were prompted by interest in the role played by surface glycoproteins in the control of lymphocyte circulation (Gesner,

Table 4.12a Effect of pretreatment of ^{51}Cr-labelled lymphocytes with neuraminidase, trypsin, and phospholipase A (PL-A) on their distribution after i.v. injection. Data from Freitas and de Sousa (1976a)

	Control/treated						
	1 hr				24 hr		
	Neuraminidase	Trypsin$_{15'}$	Trypsin$_{5'}$	PL-A	Neuraminidase	Trypsin$_{15'}$	PL-A
Blood	0.3/0.2*	0.5/0.5	0.4/0.4	0.5/0.3	0.4/0.3	0.2/0.3	0.2/0.2
LN	10/4***	11/2***	8/5***	4/2***	15/7***	17/14*	13/8***
Spleen	23/10***	31/42***	31/31	30/30	16/13***	18/21*	22/26*
Liver	18/53***	13/16***	12/11	11/14**	19/36***	12/10	13/13
Lung	16/11***	13/12	11/10	14/24***	2/2	2/1	2/2

Table 4.12b Comparison between the fate of untreated and trypsin LPS on Con A treated labelled cells in splenectomized recipients. Data from Freitas and de Sousa (1976a)

	Control/treated				
	1 hr		24 hr		
	Trypsin$_{15'}$	Trypsin$_{5'}$	Con A	LPS	
Blood	0.7/0.9**	0.4/0.4	—	—	
LN	14/7***	18/16*	15/15	21/22	
Liver	21/20	15/13	14/15	18/17	
Lung	16/16	3/2*	3/3	2/2	

*$p < 0.05$
**$p < 0.01$
***$p < 0.001$

1966). The possibility that the results of the experiments with trypsin-treated cells could be due to the general action of trypsin on cell adhesiveness and knowledge of the effect of phospholipases on cell adhesion (Curtis et al., 1975) led Freitas and de Sousa to investigate the action of three phospholipases on lymphocyte migration (Freitas and de Sousa, 1976c).

Phospholipase A_2 (PL-A_2) lyses the phosphatidyl compounds in the plasmalemna to lyso compounds and a fatty acid (Fischer et al., 1967). Phospholipase C (PL-C) splits phospholipids at an O–P bond, i.e. acts on lecithin producing a diglyceride and phosphorylcholine (Bernheimer, 1970). Sphingomyelinase C (SMC) is a phospholipase C with a specific affinity for sphingomyelins, which are hydrolysed to acetylsphingosine and phosphorylcoline (Dorey et al., 1965).

Of the three studied, i.e. PL-A_2, PL-C, and SMC, only the latter had no effect on lymphocyte migration.

After treatment with phospholipase A_2(PL-A_2), decreased lymph node recovery was observed at 1 hr after cell transfer. This decrease occurred simultaneously with an increase in the amount of radioactivity recovered from the lungs and could be related to the dose of enzyme used. At 6 hr there was still a decreased localization of the treated cells into the lymph nodes, but by this time increased recoveries were observed in the spleen and liver (Fig. 4.26). At 24 hr a partial but not complete recovery of localization of the cells treated with 50 ng/ml cells in the recipient nodes was observed, and by 72 hr after cell transfer the recovery of a normal pattern of cell localization was complete and the distribution of labelled treated cells similar to the pattern of distribution of the control cells. Recovery of a normal pattern of cell localization in the recipients of cells treated with a lower dose (25 ng/ml) of PL-A_2 was observed at 24 hr.

Splenectomy of the recipients of the treated cells led to a partial, but never complete, recovery of the cells from the lymph nodes. With the higher dose of PL-A_2

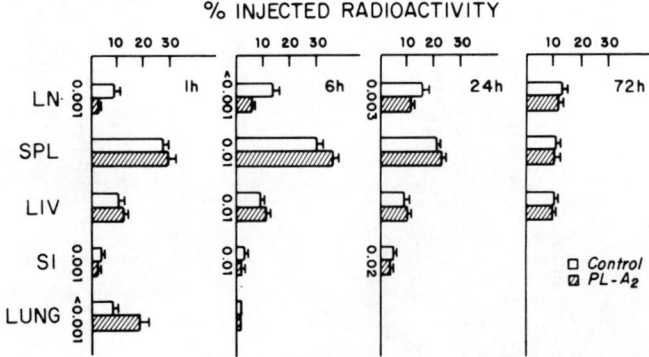

Figure 4.26 Distribution of normal and PL-A_2 (50 ng/ml)-treated ^{51}Cr-labelled lymph node cells, 1, 6, 24, and 72 hr after injection. Each bar represents the mean and 1 SD of the results obtained from 4–8 CBA mice expressed as a percentage of injected radioactivity. Data from Freitas and de Sousa (1976c)

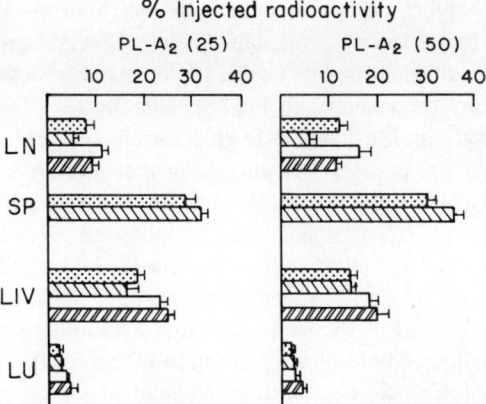

Figure 4.27 Comparison between the fate of ^{51}Cr-labelled lymph node cells exposed or not exposed to PL-A$_2$ (50 ng/ml right and 25 ng/ml left) in intact and splenectomized mice. Each bar represents the mean of 3–8 mice plus 1 SD. Normal cells–normal recipients ▨; PL-A$_2$-treated cells–N recipients ▧; N cells–splenectomized recipients ☐; PL-A$_2$-treated cells–splx recipients ▨

used (50 ng/ml) a significant constant deficit in the numbers of labelled cells recovered from the lymph nodes was observed; concomitant increases in the amounts of radioactivity recovered from the lungs and liver were observed (Fig. 4.27).

Phospholipase C treatment caused a transient increase at 1 hr after injection in the amount of radioactivity recovered from the blood, which was directly related to the dose of enzyme used. By 24 hr after cell transfer, there were no detectable differences between the migration of control and PL-C treated cells.

Investigating further the actual mechanisms of the effect of PL-A$_2$, whose treatment of the cell surface is known to lead to the accumulation of lysocompounds thus lowering cell adhesiveness (Curtis et al., 1975), Freitas and de Sousa (1976c) studied also the effect of incubation of ^{51}Cr-labelled lymph node cells with different dilutions of lysolecithin on their in vivo migration patterns. At a dilution of 1:100,000, lysolecithin induced significant differences in lymphocyte distribution at 1 hr after injection essentially similar to those induced by PL-A$_2$, namely decreased lymph node entry and increased lung recovery.

4.5.5 Non-specific mitogens

4.5.5.1 Plant lectins

Plant lectins are known to have an affinity for sugar residues on cell surfaces (Kornfeld and Kornfeld, 1974) which has been directly related to their blastogenic and mitogenic effect on lymphocytes (Lis and Sharon, 1973). Of the two most widely used plant lectins, concanavilin A (Con A) and phytohaemagglutinin (PHA), the binding characteristics of the former are best defined. *In vitro*, concanavilin A has been shown to bind specifically to α-D-mannopyranosyl, β-D-fructopyranosyl, and α- and β-D-glycopyranosyl groups on the lymphocyte surface. Thus, it is perhaps not surprising that Con A was the first plant lectin used in a study of lymphocyte traffic in the mouse (Gillette *et al.*, 1973).

Pretreatment of ^{51}Cr-labelled mouse lymph node cells with non-mitogenic doses of Con A *in vitro* (at 37°C for 1 hr) results in considerable changes of the lymphocyte distribution in syngeneic recipients. Migration to the lymph nodes is considerably reduced at the same time that accumulation of the radioactivity in the spleen is enhanced (24 hr after injection of the cells). This effect can be related to the dose of Con A used and is maximal at concentrations of 2–2.5 µg/ml (Gillette *et al.*, 1973; Freitas and de Sousa, 1975). Con A- and PHA-treated lymphocytes are found in the lungs at 1 hr after injection in significantly higher numbers than control untreated cells (Freitas and de Sousa, 1975); by 24 hr, however, the distribution of the radioactivity recovered in the recipients of PHA-treated lymphocytes is similar to that of the recipients of control untreated cells. Recovery from Con A treatment is observed later, at 72 hr after injection.

Proof that the Con A effect is directly related to the lectin's binding capacity to the cell surface is derived from the observation that simultaneous incubation with α-methyl-D-mannoside, a substance known to inhibit specifically binding of Con A to lymphocytes, completely reverses its effect on lymphocyte distribution (Table 4.13).

The finding of simultaneous reduced lymph node entry and increased spleen recovery after treatment with Con A was observed in four of the five studies (Gillette *et al.*, 1973; Freitas and de Sousa, 1975; Taub, 1974; Ford *et al.*, 1978; Schlesinger and Israel, 1974) reported to date on the effect of plant lectins on lymphocyte traffic.

Table 4.13 Influence of exposure time and αMM on the effect of Con A treatment on the distribution of ^{51}Cr-labelled lymph node cells at 24 hr (Data from Freitas and de Sousa, 1975)

Dose (µg/ml)	Time	αMM	LN	Distribution[a] (control/treated) Spleen	Liver	Lung
1	24 hr	–	13/3***	18/26**	10/19**	2/1
2.5	15 min	–	14/12	20/23	13/12	2/2
2.5	60 min	–	11/4***	20/37***	20/14**	2/1
2.5	60 min	+	11/13	20/23	20/19	2/2
–	60 min	+	11/11	20/21	20/20	2/2

[a]Expressed as % of injected radioactivity, each value represents the mean of the results of 3–10 mice per group.
*$p < 0.05$; **$p < 0.01$; ***$p < 0.001$; p values obtained from the statistical analysis of experimental and control groups within single experiments.

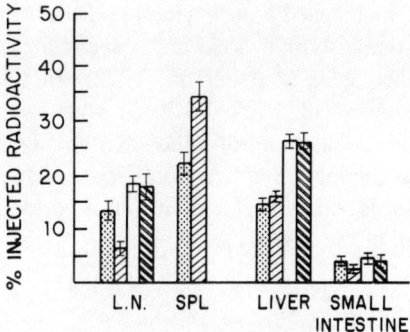

Figure 4.28 Comparison between the fate of ^{51}Cr-labelled lymph node cells treated or not with Con A in intact and splenectomized recipients. Note that removal of the spleen completely abolished any differences between the fate of Con A-treated and untreated cells. Con A-treated cells–normal recipients ▨; N cells–N recipients ▩; N cells–splx recipients ☐ ; Con A-treated cells–splx recipients ◩

In one study (Schlesinger and Israel, 1974), reduced lymph node entry of ^{51}Cr-labelled thymus and lymph node cells occurred concomitantly with reduced recovery of labelled cells from the spleen. Moreover, the effect on thymus cells was much more marked than on lymph node cells. The discrepancy between this study and the reproducibility of the results from the other studies is a little puzzling, and is perhaps related to the different manipulation of the cells utilized by Schlesinger and Israel (1974). In their study, the cells were incubated in normal saline, not washed after incubation, and injected in a suspension of 5% syngeneic normal mouse serum. In all other studies, the cells were incubated in routine culture media, washed, and resuspended in the media before injection.

The simultaneous increase in spleen recovery and decrease in lymph node entry observed in all other studies suggests that the reduced lymph node entry is simply a reflection of the fact that Con A-treated cells are sequestered in the spleen longer than untreated cells. The fact that recovery of treated and untreated cells is similar in splenectomized recipients (Fig. 4.28) strengthens this view.

4.5.5.2 Sodium periodate oxidation

Sodium periodate is an oxidizing agent which has been shown to induce blastogenesis of lymphocytes comparable to that observed with PHA (Novogrodsky and Katchalski, 1971; Parker *et al.*, 1972; Zatz *et al.*, 1972). Mild oxidation removes the terminal two carbon atoms from sialic acid and converts the alcohol group of carbon 7 to the aldehyde form (Van Lenten and Ashwell, 1971).

Mild oxidation of ^{51}Cr-labelled mouse lymph node cells *in vitro* with NaIO$_4$ was found to reduce drastically lymph node and spleen entry following intravenous injection of the labelled cells (Zatz *et al.*, 1972). In this study, reduction in lymphoid organ recovery of radioactivity could be accounted for by a simultaneous increase in the amount of radioactivity recovered from the liver. It is unlikely, however, that the increased liver recovery was due to cell death, for mild oxidation followed by reduction with sodium borohydride resulted in a return to the normal distribution of the oxidized cells.

4.5.5.3 *Lipopolysaccharide (LPS)*

LPS is a potent B cell mitogen in mice without affinity for glycoproteins which binds equally to B and T lymphocytes (Anderson *et al.*, 1972). To investigate the possibility that surface components other than glycoproteins were of importance in the control of lymphocyte circulation, Freitas and de Sousa (1976b) studied the action of treatment with LPS on the distribution of ^{51}Cr-labelled mouse T and B lymphocytes.

LPS-treated T lymphocytes were found in significantly higher numbers in the spleen at 24 hr after intravenous injection. This occurred with concomitant decreases in the amount of recovered radioactivity from the lymph nodes. Treated B cells were also found in significantly lower numbers in the lymph nodes but this did not occur with a simultaneous increase in the spleen. It is of interest to note that no differences were observed at 1 hr or 72 hr after injection, thus indicating that the action of LPS on the cell had a latent period. The nature of the changes induced by the LPS was not clarified. The possibility that the administration of LPS-treated cells was modifying the host was excluded in experiments where LPS-treated unlabelled cells were injected simultaneously with ^{51}Cr-labelled LPS-untreated control cells. The injection of the LPS-treated cells did not alter the migration of the untreated labelled cells.

4.5.5.4 *Sulphated polysaccharides*

Sulphated polysaccharides have striking effects on the distribution of lymphocytes *in vivo*. Injection of heparin, heparinoids, and synthetic polyanions causes a marked blood lymphocytosis which has been related to the number of sugar units in the sulphated carbohydrates, the sulphate groups, and the molecular size of the polyanion (Jansen *et al.*, 1962; Paluska and Hamilton, 1963; Sasaki, 1967; Bradfield and Born, 1974; Ormai *et al.*, 1973). Sulphated carbohydrates interact directly with cells, changing their net surface charge (Mehrishi, 1973) and adhesion (Curtis, 1973; Taylor and Culling, 1966; Vachek and Kölskh, 1975). Exposure of lymphoid cells to sulphated polysaccharides *in vitro* enhances their *in vitro* response to SRBC (Diamanstein, Meinhold, and Wagner, 1971; Battisto and Pappas, 1974) and they interact directly with B cells causing activation (Diamanstein *et al.*, 1973; Coutinho *et al.*, 1974).

In a study of the effect of exposure of ^{51}Cr-labelled mouse lymph node cells to dextrans of ranging molecular weights (Dextran 500, Dextran 40: MW 40,000; Dextran 70: MW 70,000), dextran sulphate, (MW 500,000) and sulphate (MW 2,000), it was found that the neutral dextrans had no effect on lymphocyte distribution in recipients killed at 1 and 24 hr after intravenous injection (Freitas and de Sousa, 1977). Dextran sulphate, however, altered significantly the normal pattern of lymphocyte distribution. Dextran sulphate-treated cells remained in the blood much longer than untreated cells (Fig. 4.29), and this occurred with a concomitant decrease in numbers of labelled cells recovered from the lymph nodes and spleen and also increases in the amount of radioactivity from the lung and liver (Fig. 4.29).

A complementary autoradiographic analysis of the distribution of the dextran sulphate-treated [^{3}H]-adenosine-labelled cells in syngeneic recipients revealed the presence of significantly higher numbers of treated than untreated cells in the lungs and in the marginal zone of the spleen at 1 hr after intravenous injection (Fig. 4.30). These differences were no longer apparent by 24 hr.

These results were attributed in part to the effect of the treatment with the polysaccharide on the net negative charge of the cell surface. This seems unlikely, for a similarly negatively charged dextran, i.e. dextran phosphate, has no effect on peripheral blood lymphocyte counts (Bradfield and Born, 1974). A slight action on distribution of ^{51}Cr-labelled lymph node cells has also been observed with pentosan sulphate. It seems more likely therefore that the sulphate groups

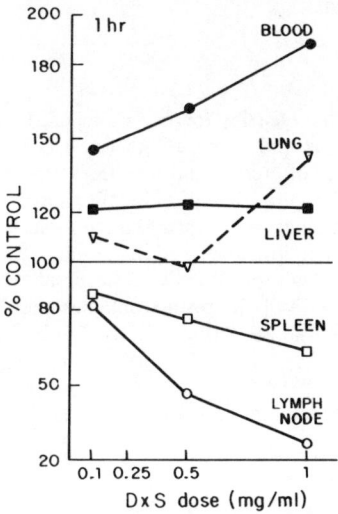

Figure 4.29 Effect of increasing doses of DxS *in vitro* on the distribution of ^{51}Cr-labelled cells in syngeneic recipients killed 1 hr after intravenous injection. Data from Freitas and de Sousa (1977)

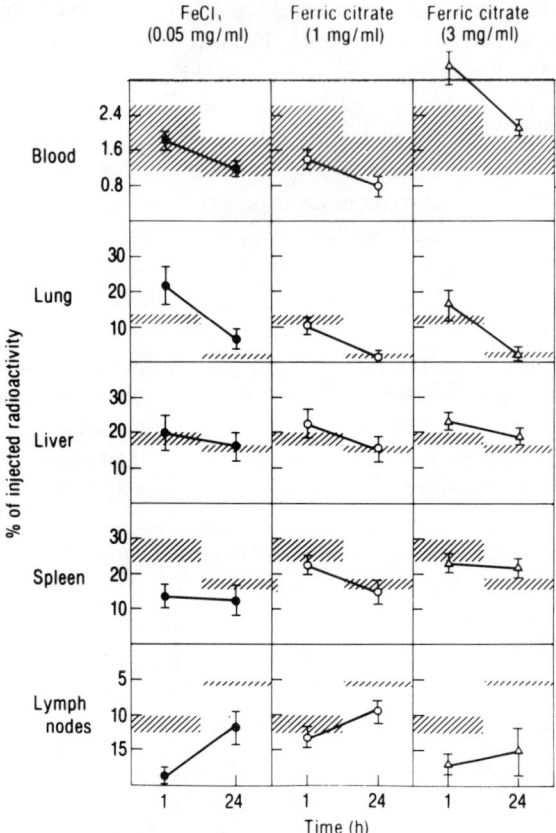

Figure 4.30 Distribution of ^{51}Cr-labelled mouse lymph node cells treated *in vitro* with ferric chloride (●) and two doses of ferric citrate, 0.3×10^{-5} M (○) and 1×10^{-5} M (△), at 1 and 24 hr after intravenous injection in syngeneic recipients. Shaded areas represent the control range (mean $\pm$ 1 SD), i.e. the distribution of ^{51}Cr-labelled untreated cells. Each point represents the mean ($\pm$1 SD) of the results obtained with 5–10 mice. From de Sousa (1978a)

themselves are playing a role in controlling the emigration of the labelled cells from the blood circuit.

4.5.6 Metal cations

The interaction of metal cations with lymphoid cell populations has been investigated only in a few experiments. Most of these have been concerned with the interaction of zinc with lymphocytes *in vitro*. Addition of zinc chloride to cultures of human peripheral blood lymphocytes stimulated by PHA enhances considerably their response to the antigen. In a detailed study of the possible mechanism of the binding of the metal to the cell. Phillips (1976) demonstrated that human peripheral blood cells bind zinc, and possibly iron, *via* a surface receptor for Zn-transferrin. In the same study, the existence of surface receptors for apotransferrin was also reported.

These observations, and the separate finding that increased numbers of T lymphocytes are found in spleens of patients with Hodgkin's disease in which large amounts of ferritin and ferritin-containing cells are found, led to the suggestion that iron and iron-binding proteins may play a role in directing lymphoid cell migration (de Sousa *et al.*, 1978). Experimental studies followed in which ^{51}Cr-labelled peripheral lymph node cells were exposed to ferric chloride or ferric citrate *in vitro* and their distribution followed in syngeneic recipients after intravenous injection.

The results shown in Fig. 4.30 are in many respects similar to those obtained with dextran sulphate. Ferric citrate-treated cells remain in the blood and fail to enter the lymph nodes and spleen.

The possible significance of these results and their relation to the physiology of the circulation of lymphocytes will be discussed in detail later (Chapter 8.2).

4.5.7 Agents that modify cell locomotion

4.5.7.1 Sodium azide

Treatment of lymphocytes *in vitro* with sodium azide alters their normal patterns of migration to lymph nodes (Ford, Andrews, and Smith, 1978; Freitas and Bognaki, 1979). Increased numbers of labelled cells were found in the blood, liver, and spleen at 1 hr after intravenous injection, but by 24 hr no significant differences were observed between the distribution of treated and untreated cells.

In splenectomized mice, the migration of sodium azide-treated cells was also found to differ from the migration of untreated cells (Freitas and Bognaki, 1979). At 1 hr after cell transfer significantly higher numbers of treated than untreated cells were present in the blood.

These results indicate that the azide treatment interferes with the selective interaction of lymphocytes with the endothelium of the postcapillary venules in the lymph nodes. In a more direct analysis of this interaction *in vitro*, Woodruff *et al.* (1978) confirmed that sodium azide-treated lymphocytes fail to adhere to HEV in lymph node frozen sections.

4.5.7.2 Cytochalisin A and cytochalisin B

Cytochalisin B treatment of ^{51}Cr-labelled lymphocytes only impaired partially the localization of the labelled cells into the lymph nodes in the mouse (Freitas and Bognaki, 1979). This effect was small, with a reduction of lymph node entry of only 15–20% of the control which was only observed at 15 min after cell transfer. Cytochalisin A treatment of rat thoracic duct lymphocytes, on the other hand, resulted in failure of the cells to enter the lymph nodes and reduced also splenic entry (Anderson et al., 1979).

4.5.7.3 Colchicine

Variable results have been observed in the migration of lymphocytes treated *in vitro* with colchicine (Anderson et al., 1979; Woodruff et al., 1978; Freitas and Bognaki, 1979). Rat thoracic duct lymphocytes treated with a concentration of 10^{-4} M colchicine showed depressed accumulation in lymph nodes which remained significantly reduced until 8 hr after infusion (Anderson et al., 1979). In contrast with these results, Freitas and Bognaki (1979) found that exposure of ^{51}Cr-labelled mouse lymph node cells to concentrations of 10^{-4} or 10^{-5} M did not influence their subsequent distribution *in vivo* at 15 min or 24 hr following transfer. Woodruff and co-workers (Woodruff et al., 1978) also found that treatment with colchicine had no effect on the adhesion of lymphocytes to HEV in frozen lymph node sections *in vitro*.

4.5.7.4 Cyclic AMP stimulators

Isoproterenol. Isoproterenol, an adenylate cyclase stimulator (Hadden et al., 1975), was found by Freitas and Bognaki (1979) to decrease the 1 hr localization of labelled mouse lymph node cells into the lymph nodes, with a concomitant increase in the amount of radioactivity recovered from the blood. An increased level of radioactivity was still recovered from the blood at 24 hr but the amount of radioactivity in the lymph nodes at this time was similar in the recipients of treated and untreated cells.

Theophyline. Exposure of mouse lymph node cells to theophyline caused a slight accumulation of the labelled cells in the blood which was only detectable at 1 hr after transfer. cGMP stimulators, in marked contrast with the effects of the cyclic AMP stimulators, had no effect on their *in vivo* migration.

4.5.8 Irradiation

Much of what is known of the participation of lymphocytes in the immune response has been learnt from experiments involving adoptive transfer of cells to irradiated animals. A prerequisite to the effective transfer of a memory cell response, for instance, is that the recipient should be irradiated. No response is elicited following transfer into unirradiated, immunocompetent hosts (Dresser, 1961; Mäkelä and Mitchison, 1965; Celada, 1966). Moreover, the level of antibody synthesis obtained from primed spleen cells adoptively transferred to an irradiated host is directly proportional to increasing doses of irradiation (Celada, 1966).

While we all have used these facts to the advantage of our experiments, few experiments examined the actual effect of radiation on lymphocytes (Anderson et al., 1974) or on the circulation of lymphocytes in irradiated animals (Sprent et al., 1974; Bell and Shand, 1975).

The cell output from the thoracic duct lymph of mice measured at 4 days after 800 r total body irradiation is reduced by more than 50 fold (Sprent et al., 1974). Of the remaining cells, 96% are T cells and only 1% B cells. This reflects the greater radiosensitivity of B cells, a fact which was demonstrated by the same authors after irradiation of T and B lymphocytes *in vitro* (Anderson et al., 1974). These experiments were done at a time when T lymphocytes were thought of as a major class of cells and no distinction was made between the radiosensitivity of cell subsets. More recently, Campbell and Cooper (1975) have demonstrated that after irradiation primed T cells retain helper function but fail to migrate normally.

Studies of the effect of irradiation *in vitro* on human lymphocyte subpopulations (Siegal and Siegal, 1977), have indicated that the suppressor T cell (Tγ) population is more radiosensitive than the T helper (Tμ) cell set. Marked decreases in the proportion of Tγ cells in a suspension of peripheral blood cells were observed after irradiation *in vitro* with a dose of 500 r. This seems a singularly high dose, when compared with the striking changes in thoracic duct lymphocyte output elicited by irradiating a whole mouse with 800 r, or a whole rat with 900 r (Bell and Shand, 1975).

Be it as it may, irradiating a whole rat with 900 r modifies the host environment considerably and affects significantly the circulation of transferred cells from blood to lymph through that modified host environment.

Bell and Shand (1975), in a most elegant study of the adoptive memory response in irradiated rats, demonstrated the effect of host irradiation on the circulation of transferred lymphocytes and related it to the effectiveness of the adoptive transfer.

Irradiated recipients were transferred with primed thoracic duct lymphocytes

Table 4.14 Effect of whole body irradiation on tissue distribution of [^{14}C]-leucine-labelled TDL. Data from Bell and Shand (1975)

Tissue	Experiment 1 (input/rat, 4.2×10^5 cpm)		Experiment 2 (input/rat, 7.2×10^5 cpm)	
	900 r	Normal	900 r	Normal
LN*	0.78†	0.33	1.00	0.46
Spleen	1.26	0.56	1.25	0.61
Liver	5.62	5.23	6.91	3.16
Kidney	0.69	0.64	0.71	0.68

*Cervical and brachial lymph nodes.
†Expressed as percentage of cpm input. Rats were killed 84 hr (Expt. 1) and 64 hr (Expt. 2) after injection of labelled TDL.

Table 4.15 Effect of unlabelled TDL on the recirculation of 10^8 [^{14}C]-lecine-labelled TDL in the irradiated rat. Data from Bell and Shand (1975)

Collection interval (hr)	cpm		Percentage of input	
	900 r	900 r + Nor. TDL*	900 r	900 r + Nor. TDL*
0–5	35	566	0.03	0.27
17	1,035	3,604	0.49	1.71
29	620	3,706	0.29	1.76
41	244	1,293	0.12	0.61
53	194	236	0.09	0.11
65	258	197	0.12	0.09

*6×10^8 unlabelled TDL were injected 1.5 hr before labelled TDL.

('TDL) at 2 hr, 1 week, and 4 weeks post irradiation times and the antigen-binding capacity of the recipients' serum measured at 2, 4, and 6 weeks after challenge with the same antigen.

There was a decline in antibody synthesis by the transferred 'TDL which was inversely related to the return of host immunocompetence. The suppressive effect of the presence of non-immune TDL (TDL) on the adoptive transfer of the memory response could be reproduced by the transfer of 'TDL combined with increasing numbers of TDL.

Tracing the pattern of the blood to lymph circulation of ^{14}C-labelled TDL in irradiated and normal recipients, Bell and Shand demonstrated that the recirculation of the transferred cells was significantly impaired in the irradiated recipients (Table 4.14). A final important aspect of Bell and Shand's work was the observation that unlabelled, normal TDL 'helped' the establishment of a normal blood to lymph circulation of the transferred labelled cells in irradiated hosts (Table 4.15).

4.5.9 ACTH

Following the observation that a simple manipulation such as the intravenous injection of 2.5 ml of medium 199 in rats with a previously placed tail vein cannula caused a transient decrease in the output of lymphocytes from the thoracic duct, Spry (1972) investigated further the effect of stress and cortisone on lymphocyte output (Fig. 4.31). Reduction in lymphocyte output was observed after an intravenous injection of 1 unit of ACTH. A more marked reduction was observed after the continuous infusion of ACTH (100 mU/hr) which was reversed after the infusion was stopped.

In the continuous infusion experiments both output and total recovery were decreased, indicating that lymphocyte lysis as well as inhibition of blood to lymph recirculation had occurred. Spry argues that these observations could be significant in diseases and after operations which result in adrenal stimulation. He adds that 'it is also tempting to postulate that endogenous steroid levels have an

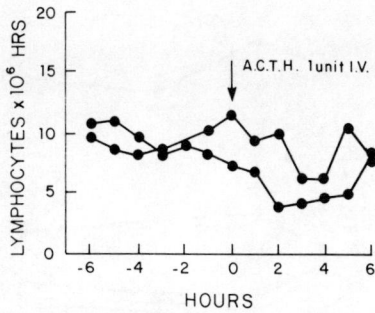

Figure 4.31 Change in output of thoracic duct lymphocytes in two rats injected intravenously with 1 u of corticotropin (ACTH). Note reduction in lymphocyte output. Slightly modified from Spry (1972)

effect on the dynamics of lymphocyte circulation under normal conditions'. The possible validity of such an attractive postulate remains untested.

4.5.10 *Bordetella pertussis*

One elegant series of experiments on modification of lymphocyte traffic *in vivo* is that of Morse's group on the effect of *B. pertussis* (Morse, 1964; Morse and Riester, 1967a,b; Morse and Bray, 1969; Morse and Barron, 1970; Taub *et al.*, 1972).

B. pertussis causes a striking blood lymphocytosis in mice. Morse demonstrated that the increase in numbers of lymphocytes was not due to newly formed cells but to the retention of long-lived cells in the blood (Morse and Riester, 1967a). Secondly, it was shown that the lymphocytosis was confined to the blood and that lymphocytes failed to circulate to lymph (Morse and Riester, 1967b). Finally, in a most thorough comparative study (Taub *et al.*, 1972) of the effect of the whole organism *versus* 'lymphocytosis promotor factor' obtained from supernatants of *B. pertussis* cultures on traffic of injected ^{51}Cr-labelled lymph node or thoracic duct cells *in vivo*, the following results were obtained.

1. Administration of the supernatant before or after the labelled cells resulted in a redistribution in the host: more radioactivity was recovered from the blood, less from the lymph nodes, and less from the spleen.
2. Administration of the whole organism provoked a similar decrease in lymph node entry and blood increase, but, in addition, increased numbers of cells were retained in the spleen (Fig. 4.32).
3. *In vitro* treatment of labelled cells with plasma from *B. pertussis* supernatant injected mice failed to alter their migration.
4. Unlabelled erythrocytes or lymphocytes which had bound *B. pertussis*

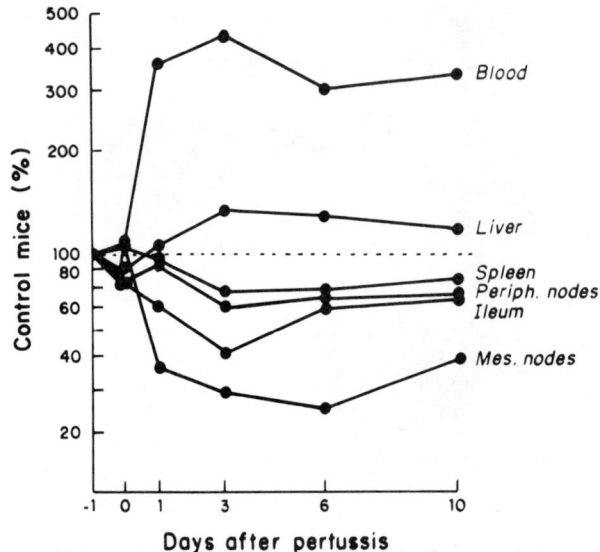

Figure 4.32 Changes with time in distribution of ^{51}Cr-labelled lymph node cells in mice injected intravenously with *B. pertussis* organisms 24 hr after labelled cells. The results are expressed as per cent of control values. Each point represents: mean radioactivity of *pertussis*-treated group of 3 mice x 100 radioactivity of normal untreated group for each organ. Slightly modified from Taub *et al.* (1972)

supernatant *in vitro*, when mixed with untreated cells, altered their migration (Table 4.16).

The implications of these observations are manifold. Two aspects in particular must be stressed: one, the fact that cells, not plasma, carried on their surface a factor that after elution could actively influence the migration of other cells, indicating that direct or short range cell interactions are at play in this system; secondly, the fact that after an intravenous injection, the whole organism, but not the supernatant, caused some degree of cell retention in the spleen.

4.5.11 Complement

C3 receptors are a well-known B cell marker in animals (Papamichail *et al.*, 1975); it has been shown that lowering the C3 level of blood before antigen administration affects markedly the localization of antigen in spleen follicles in mice and chickens (Papamichail *et al.*, 1975; White *et al.*, 1975), with resulting decreases in germinal centre formation in chickens (White *et al.*, 1975). Studies were designed, therefore, to determine whether lowering C3 levels in blood by injection of cobra venom (CVF) (Pepys, 1975) influences cell localization in mice

Table 4.16 Elution of *pertussis* from red blood cells or lymph node cells. Data from Taub et al. (1972)

^{51}Cr-labelled lymph node cells incubated with:	Blood	Lymph nodes†	Spleen	Liver
Medium only	0.19‡	10.36	17.02	9.39
	(0.01)	0.22	0.30	0.70
1/100 *pertussis* supernatant	0.40	2.76	22.35	15.28
	(0.07)	0.00	1.28	2.14
Supernatant after absorption by red	0.52	5.74	22.02	14.53
blood cells	(0.10)	0.58	1.58	1.74
Supernatant after absorption by	0.23	8.86	22.36	15.33
lymph node cells	(0.12)	0.86	2.33	0.66
Eluate from *pertussis*-treated red	0.46	1.88	21.61	13.77
blood cells	(0.01)	0.81	1.11	2.57
Eluate from *pertussis*-treated lymph	0.19	11.73	19.36	13.74
node cells	(0.03)	0.55	1.55	1.25
Pertussis-treated red blood cells	0.51	4.30	23.65	13.70
	(0.05)	0.00	1.42	1.46
Pertussis-treated lymph node cells	0.47	8.93	21.90	15.37
	(0.05)	1.00	0.76	3.02
Normal unlabelled lymph node cells	0.25	12.05	17.45	11.29
	(0.08)	1.34	2.18	1.48

*0.25 ml/mouse.
†Brachial, axillary, inguinal, mesenteric.
‡Mean ± SD of four animals.

Table 4.17 Lack of effect of C3 depletion of recipients on localization of ^{3}H-labelled lymphoid cells.* Data from De Kruyff et al. (1977)

Donor tissue	Recipient pretreatment	% injected radioactivity†				
		Spleen	LN‡	Liver	Lung	Blood
Expt. 1						
Mouse NW-adh.	PBS	10.9	3.2	1.9	2.3	2.1
spleen	CVF	10.0	3.7	1.5	1.7	2.1
Expt. 2						
Mouse NW-adh.	PBS	6.7	2.4	0.9	0.9	3.1
spleen	CVF	5.4	2.3	1.0	0.7	1.9
Expt. 3						
Chicken bursa	PBS	5.1	2.5	0.8	0.4	
	CVF	4.8	0.9	0.9	0.3	
Chicken thymus	PBS	15.0	1.9	0.5	0.3	
	CVF	15.8	2.1	0.5	0.3	

*[^{3}H] adenosine-labelled chicken bursa and thymus cells and [^{3}H] uridine-labelled SJL/J mouse nylon (NW)-adherent spleen cells.
†Average values for 3 recipients per group 24 hr after transfer. Expressed as % of injected radioactivity per 100 mg tissue (mice) or per g tissue (chickens).
‡Combined left and right brachial lymph nodes (LN).

Spry *et al.*, 1977 and chickens (De Kruyff *et al.*, 1975, 1977). In both species (Table 4.17) pretreatment of irradiated recipients with CVF 8 hr prior to transfer of labelled cells had no effect on the quantitative or qualitative distribution of cells within the spleen and other organs examined (De Kruyff *et al.*, 1977).

Chapter 5

Lymphocyte Circulation Outside the Lymphoid System

D. M. V. PARROTT

5.1 INTRODUCTION

Varying numbers and subpopulations of lymphocytes enter and leave various non-lymphoid tissues and organs, often in response to inflammatory and antigenic stimuli. They may be estimated by measuring the arrival in the tissue of labelled lymphocytes by gamma or scintillation counting or by autoradiography. In larger animals where it is possible to cannulate a lymphatic draining a tissue (the afferent lymphatic to a lymph node), a measurement can be made of the cells draining from or leaving a tissue. It should be appreciated, however, that there is not necessarily a direct correlation between these two measurements either in numbers or in type of cell. Some lymphocytes may differentiate further after entering a tissue, for example cells which enter as lymphoblasts may leave as small lymphocytes, or remain behind as sessile cells, e.g. plasma cells. The transit time through a tissue may vary according to whether an antigenic stimulus is present or not. Rannie and Donald (1977) have shown that the transit time through unstimulated skin is relatively rapid, but during primary sensitization to a contact sensitizer (Rose *et al.*, 1978: Ottaway and Parrott, 1979) or during delayed type reactions (Rannie, Smith, and Ford, 1977) cells may be retained for longer periods so that there is a lag period between peak entry and peak exit.

Most normal tissues contain very few lymphocytes. After the injection of labelled lymphocytes the amount of radioactivity in normal, non-lymphoid tissues is very small indeed when compared with lymphoid tissues (Asherson and Allwood, 1972; Rose *et al.*, 1976a, 1976b; Rannie and Donald, 1977), and corresponds with the low number of lymphocytes (200–800/mm^3) found in afferent lymph (often termed peripheral lymph) in man and sheep draining all tissues with the exception of liver and the gut mucosa (Smith, McIntosh, and Morris, 1970a; Hall *et al.*, 1976; Cahill *et al.*, 1976; Miller and Adams, 1977). The first response in the skin to the application of contact sensitizing agents or intradermal injections of antigen is usually an early appearance of polymorphs or macrophages (de Sousa and Parrott, 1969; Hall and Smith, 1971; Cahill et al., 1976), though lymphocytes both small or blast-like can be induced to extravasate 20–30 times above baseline levels and have been observed especially at sites of application of contact sensitizing agents (Asherson and Allwood, 1972; Ottaway and Parrott, 1979; Hall, 1980) and in adjuvant induced granulomas (Smith, McIntosh, and Morris, 1970b; Rannie, Smith, and Ford, 1977). These observations prompt several questions. What is known of the mechanisms which increase the traffic of lymphocytes and how does it differ from traffic through lymph nodes and spleen? Is the increase in numbers brought about by an increase in the proportion of lymphocytes leaving the bloodstream as they traverse the capillary bed, i.e. is the proportion of cells stimulated to locomote increased and does the increase apply to all lymphocytes indiscriminately or is there selection, i.e. are some lymphocyte populations 'persuaded' to locomote in preference to others?

Mucosal sites, especially the gut mucosa, are throughout life submitted to constant antigenic stimulation and as a consequence normally contain lymphoid cells which differ in number and type from other non-lymphoid sites such as the skin. Nevertheless, the actual process of extravasation of lymphocytes into the tissues is very similar regardless of site. It is the intention of this chapter to emphasize the common characteristics of this aspect of lymphocyte migration and to highlight the differences where they exist rather than to discuss mucosal lymphocyte traffic as if it were unrelated to that of non-mucosal sites.

5.2 MIGRATION OF LYMPHOCYTES TO NON-MUCOSAL SITES

5.2.1 Number and composition of cells in afferent lymph draining non-mucosal sites

The most extensive studies on the numbers of cells contained in afferent lymph are those of Smith et al. (1970a) (Table 5.1) and Miller and Adams (1977) who cannulated the lymphatics draining sites of skin, muscle, and other organs. With the exception of the afferent lymph draining the liver, all other sites under normal conditions contained very small numbers of lymphocytes (200–800 mm^3), i.e. only 5–10 per cent of those in afferent lymph from lymph nodes. The paucity of lymphocytes in afferent lymph has also been reported by other workers in the sheep (Hall, 1967; Hall et al., 1976; Cahill et al., 1976) and the rabbit (Kelly et al., 1972; Kelly et al., 1978).

One point that should not be overlooked is the effect of the surgical procedures following introduction of an indwelling cannula (Hall, 1980). However skilful the surgeon, some degree of inflammation must occur and persist throughout the period of experimentation and thus induce a traffic of cells which does not exist in normal undisturbed tissue. Hill (1969) demonstrated that the injection of distilled water would change cellular infiltration in the skin. We would expect, therefore, that the true baseline cellular content of afferent lymph is very small indeed.

This surprising conclusion is, however, confirmed by the numerous studies which have traced isotopically labelled cells after infusion into the bloodstream

Table 5.1 White cell content of normal peripheral lymph collected from various organs in the sheep. Figures for the numbers of cells present in efferent lymph draining various regional lymph nodes are given for comparison. Data from Smith et al., (1970a)

Source of lymph	Flow rate (ml/hr)	Cell count/mm^3	Lymphocytes	Macrophages	Others
					Differential
Afferent					
Hind limb	1.0–8.0 (10)	200–700	80–90	5–15	3–5
Fore limb	3.0–5.0 (5)	500–1,000	85–90	6–10	0–5
Prescapular	2.5–5.0 (4)	600–800	80–90	5–15	0–5
Prefemoral	1.5–3.0 (4)	500–800	78–85	7–20	0–6
Liver	1.0–3.0 (12)	2,000–6,000	70–85	5–20	5–10
Kidney	1.0–3.0 (9)	100–700	75–85	15–22	2–4
Ovary	1.0–9.5 (6)	200–700	90–95	5–10	<1
Testis	10.0–30.0 (5)	100–300	75–82	5–20	0–8
Thyroid	0.3–0.6 (4)	200–800	85–92	5–13	2–5
Efferent					
Popliteal node	1.0–9.0 (10)	3,000–10,000	95–100	<1	0–5
Prescapular node	4.5–8.0 (9)	8,000–12,000	92–100	<1	0–8
Prefemoral node	3.0–6.0 (5)	5,000–8,000	96–100	<1	0–4
Portal node (liver)	1.0–10.0 (10)	8,000–12,000	95–100	<1	0–5

( ) number of animals.

and measured their arrival in the tissues by gamma or scintillation counting or by autoradiography.

In the absence of antigenic or inflammatory stimuli, the amount of radioactivity found in, say, a measured area of skin is minimal and probably represents cells still confined to the bloodstream. Although this conclusion may be debated, there is little evidence to suggest that appreciable numbers of lymphocytes normally traffic through the skin or most other tissues and those that do so have a rapid transit time (Hall *et al.*, 1976; Rannie and Donald, 1977).

Despite the small numbers of lymphocytes present in the tissues there does appear to be some selection process at the level of the capillary bed, for in most non-mucosal sites the proportion of B lymphocytes which extravasate is much smaller than T cells. Scollay *et al.* (1976) showed in sheep that only 5–10% of cells in afferent lymph to popliteal lymph nodes were B lymphocytes. Miller and Adams (1977) extended these observations to other sources of afferent lymph. Even hepatic lymph, which normally has relatively high numbers of lymphocytes, contains relatively few B lymphocytes, and, after a kidney allograft, when the cell output increased 20–40 fold within 48 hr, only 6% were B cells (Miller and Adams, 1977). T cells also predominate in human peripheral lymph (Engeset *et al.*, 1974) and other extravascular fluids in man (Manconi *et al.*, 1978). The preference for T lymphocytes is also reflected by the greater 'enthusiasm' with which radiolabelled T lymphocytes, particularly activated T lymphoblasts, enter the skin (Asherson *et al.*, 1973; Rose *et al.*, 1976a). It is unlikely that the paucity of B lymphocytes in the skin is a result of some sort of exclusion mechanism and more likely that circumstances promote the extravasation of T lymphocytes, along with other blood leukocytes. Certainly the capillaries of the skin and other tissues do not exclude other blood leukocytes as vigorously as the HEV of lymph nodes; monocytes and macrocytes and so-called veiled or frilly cells are always present in afferent lymph as well as lymphocytes (Smith *et al.*, 1970; Hall *et al.*, 1976) and their proportion in sheep is 5–15% but can be as high as 50% in the rabbit (Kelly *et al.*, 1978).

The numbers of macrophages are far greater than in efferent lymph (Smith *et al.*, 1970). Cahill *et al.* (1976) have noted a possible relationship between these cells and monocytes in the blood, an interesting speculation in view of observations (Wilkinson *et al.*, 1976) on the close similarity of the *in vivo* locomotion behaviour of monocytes and lymphoblasts. Thus, as summarized in Table 5.1, afferent or peripheral lymph contains remarkably few lymphocytes, a considerable number of macrophages, and a different proportion of T:B cells (7.6:1) as compared with efferent lymph (2.5:1) or blood (2:1).

5.2.2 Alterations in afferent lymph following antigenic stimulation

Application of an antigenic stimulus usually results in changes in afferent lymph but the nature and size of the alterations varies enormously according to the stimulus. There is little approaching the reproducible and large increase in lymphocyte number and appearance of lymphoblasts which characterizes the efferent lymph from a lymph node after regional antigen stimulation.

Hall and Morris (1963) reported a slight but significant increase in numbers of lymphocytes and macrophages and the appearance of some blast cells in the afferent lymph draining the site of injection of antigen in sheep. Kelly *et al.* (1972) noted a 5 fold increase in lymphocytes, macrophage and blast cells at 3–6 days in the afferent lymph draining the rabbit hind footpad after injecting alum-precipitated diphtheria toxoid or bovine SRBC. When DNFB was applied to the rabbit hind paw, there was only a transient increase in polymorphs and no increase in lymphocytes or blast cells (Kelly *et al.*, 1972). Their results were thus similar to those of Hall (1967), who applied a skin allograft to the flank of sheep and found virtually no increase in lymphocytes; only the number of macrophages increased. But Soeberg *et al.* (1977) did find an increase in lymphocytes in the afferent lymph of the pig following DNFB. Recently, the veiled or frilly cells have been found to contain Birbeck granules and are almost certainly related to Langerhans cells (Hoefsmit *et al.*, 1979). Cahill *et al.* (1976) reported a transient increase in polymorphs, a slight increase in macrophages, and no change in lymphocytes whatsoever in afferent lymph draining the site of injection of swine influenza virus in sheep. However, following the injection of PPD (Hay *et al.*, 1973) and after a severe normal transfer reaction (Hay *et al.*, 1977), a 20–30 fold increase in all cells occurred, including lymphocytes and blast cells, over a period with a maximum at 4–8 days.

The largest and fastest increase in lymphocyte population in afferent lymph was observed by Pederson and Morris (1970) in sheep with a renal allograft. They observed a 20–30 fold increase in cell numbers, particularly blast cells, within 48 hr of transplantation. A similar increase, though evolving over a period of 20–40 days, occurred when a chronic granuloma developed after the injection of either swine influenza virus or chicken RBC in Freund's complete adjuvant in sheep (Smith *et al.*, 1970b).

In all these instances the most consistent cellular change in afferent lymph following antigenic stimulus was the early appearance of polymorphs followed by macrophages, a subsequent increase in lymphocytes or blast cells being much less consistent. Thus, deposition of antigen frequently produced reactions in afferent lymph comparable to simple inflammatory reactions, the only exception to this being the observation of Smith *et al.* (1970b), who after producing hydronephrosis in sheep by ligating the ureter noted that within 24–48 hr there was a considerable increase in lymphocyte numbers in the afferent renal lymph. Apparently, when the ureter was ligated large numbers of lymphocytes migrated from the blood into the kidney and infiltrated through the renal cortex. There was no evidence of an immune process, i.e. blast cells or multiplication of lymphocytes, and no evidence of inflammation since there were neither polymorphs nor eosinophils; so far this is an unexplained phenomenon.

5.2.3 Vascular permeability and composition of lymphoid cells in non-lymphoid tissues

An increase in vascular permeability with consequent leakage of protein occurs after antigen deposition (Hall and Smith 1971; Hay *et al.*, 1977; Rose and Parrott, 1977) and it has been postulated that this increase in vascular permeability is responsible for the increased extravasation of mononuclear cells during the delayed hyperpersensitivity reaction in the skin (Gershon *et al.*, 1975). It has been known for some time, however, that even in a tissue such as the ovary where there is a high rate of leakage of blood protein (1,500 mg/g ovary/day) (Morris and Sass, 1966) the cellular concentration in lymph from the ovary is nevertheless very low (Smith *et al.*, 1970). Moreover, we have shown that enhancing vascular permeability by injection of serotonin does not promote lymphoblast extravasation and although an increase in vascular permeability does occur during primary sensitization to oxazolone it is not related directly to increased lymphoblast migration (Rose and Parrott, 1977) (Table 5.2). It should be borne in mind, however, that serum albumin does act as a chemokinetic agent to lymphocytes *in vitro* (Wilkinson *et al.*, 1977) and could well accelerate locomotion of lymphocytes *in vivo*, especially when transudation has occurred.

5.2.4 Migration of inflammatory T blasts

Asherson and his co-workers (Asherson and Allwood, 1972; Asherson *et al.*, 1973) and more recently we (Parrott *et al.*, 1975; Rose *et al.*, 1978; Ottaway and Parrott, 1979) have shown that activated T blasts have a special ability to move into sites of inflammation. Cells taken from nodes draining the site of a contact sensitizer, for example oxazolone, 3 or 4 days after application and labelled with the thymidine analogue ^{125}Iododeoxyuridine accumulated non-specifically in sites

Table 5.2 Illustration of the fact that increased vascular permeability *per se* does not enhance lymphoblast migration to skin. From data published by Rose and Parrott (1977)

Treatment	^{125}I-labelled HSA† (cpm)	^{125}IUdR-labelled blast cells‡ (% of injected dose)
Oxazolone*	306 ± 110	1.9 ± 0.3
Serotonin	1,449 ± 252	0.0

*The mice received an application of 10 mg oxazolone on both ears 24 hr before being injected intradermally with 0.02–0.03 ml of 4×10^{-4} M serotonin.
†Immediately after serotonin ^{125}I-labelled HSA was injected intravenously and the ears removed 1 hr later.
‡Immediately after serotonin the mice received an intravenous injection of blast cells prepared from donor lymph nodes draining oxazolone-sensitized ears.
†‡Results from separate groups of mice.

Table 5.3 Effect of picryl chloride and oxazolone* on the 24 hr localization of ^{125}I UdR-labelled OX–PLN to the gut of infected mice.† Data from Rose et al. (1978)

Group recipients		Mean % injected dose ± SD				
	Ears	Auricular lymph nodes	Mesenteric lymph nodes	Small intestine	Spleen	Total‡
A Untreated	0.1 ± 0.0	0.2 ± 0.1	0.3 ± 0.1	1.9 ± 0.4	3.3 ± 0.6	8.5 ± 1.7
B Infected	0.1 ± 0.0	0.2 ± 0.1	0.8 ± 0.2	3.4 ± 0.5	3.0 ± 0.4	9.5 ± 0.8
C Infected plus picryl chloride	1.4 ± 0.2	0.9 ± 0.3	0.7 ± 0.1	2.9 ± 0.6	2.8 ± 0.5	10.5 ± 2.0
D Infected plus oxazolone	2.3 ± 0.7	0.9 ± 0.9	0.4 ± 0.0	1.9 ± 0.2	1.4 ± 0.2	8.5 ± 0.9

*10 mg of oxazolone or picryl chloride were painted on the ears 1 day before cell transfer.
†Mice were infected with T. spiralis 4 days before cell transfer.
‡Total amount of radioactivity recovered from all the excised organs expressed as percentage of the injected dose.

inflamed with turpentine or croton oil or an unrelated chemical sensitizer as well as into the site to which the priming chemical had been applied (Table 5.3). The use of the thymidine analogue ensured that only proliferating cells were followed; moreover, the cells were non-adherent to cotton wool, killed by anti-Thy-1 antiserum (Asherson *et al.*, 1973), and passed through a nylon wool column (Rose *et al.*, 1976a), thus proving that most if not all the cells were activated T blasts. Cells taken from unstimulated nodes are much less able to move into sites of inflammation and activated T blasts cannot move out into the tissues if they are not inflamed.

Although these cells are activated by antigenic stimuli applied to the skin, and they readily return to, indeed may have a preference for, sites thereon, nevertheless they will move into inflammatory sites elsewhere, for example the peritoneal cavity whether inflamed by liquid paraffin (Asherson and Allwood, 1972), *C. parvum* or thioglycollate (Rose *et al.*, 1978). Furthermore, Rose *et al.* (1976a) have shown that although the normal gut is impervious to T blasts from peripheral lymph nodes, whether activated by oxazolone or picryl chloride, after infection of mice with the nematode *T. spiralis* a large amount of injected radioactivity was recovered in the gut; peripheral T blasts will therefore enter the inflamed gut mucosa. If, however, the skin is also inflamed with a contact sensitizer or inflammatory agent in an animal with a parasitized gut, then the injection of T blasts from peripheral nodes to the gut is abrogated or inhibited and they revert to their 'first *choice*', namely the skin.

The capacity for T blasts to move into sites of inflammation is also well illustrated by the series of experiments of McGregor and his colleagues (Jungi and McGregor, 1978, 1979; McGregor and Logie, 1974). These workers showed that activated T blasts formed in the caudal lymph nodes after the injection of *Listeria monocytogenes* are delivered into the thoracic duct lymph and thence to the blood. They can then be drawn into the peritoneal cavity by the induction of an appropriate inflammatory stimulus, which is not immunologically specific. Thus, thoracic duct blast cells taken from donors immunized against BCG or *Listeria* and labelled *in vitro* with isotopically labelled thymidine accumulated well in peritoneal exudates induced by killed bacteria, whether *Listeria monocytogenes*, BCG or *S. typhi* (McGregor and Logie, 1974).

5.2.5 Lymphocyte traffic through the skin in CMI

The response to a second application of the same stimulus is very different. It has long been known that lymphocytes and the mononuclear cells appear primarily in the skin in delayed type reactions (Waksman, 1960; Uhr, 1966). For example, lymphocytes are already present in the skin at 4 hr after testing of oxazolone-sensitized mice although the numbers may not peak until 24 hr (de Sousa and Parrott, 1969).

In 1970 Smith and co-workers (Smith *et al.*, 1970b) described the evolution of a chronic granuloma in the skin of sheep injected with Freund's adjuvant and influenza virus. The lesion developed over a period of 20–40 days until the number of lymphocytes passing through became equivalent to that passing through a lymph node, and this increased flux was associated with the change in the appearance of the endothelium of small venules which came to resemble the morphologically distinct high-walled endothelium of lymph nodes. This is especially interesting because such structures although common in the lymph nodes of many species rarely occur in sheep lymph nodes (Fahy et al., 1980). Comparable observations on the increase in lymphocyte flux through granuloma have also been made in the rabbit (Hay et al., 1977) and the rat (Rannie et al., 1977). There is now evidence that the nature of lymphocyte traffic through CMI reactions is substantially different from that through non-immune and immune inflammation sites or through the sites of initial contact with antigen; thus small lymphocytes localize (and migrate) through such areas as well as lymphoblasts (Rannie et al., 1977; Ottaway, unpublished data).

5.2.6 The role of blood flow in the delivery of lymphocytes

Hay et al. (1977) have measured blood flow to the skin in three types of immune reactions: the reaction to allogenic lymphocytes, the evolution of a Freund's adjuvant induced chronic granuloma, and a delayed type of reaction to PPD. An increase in blood flow occurred in all three situations, up to 20–30 times after the injection of allogenic lymphocytes down to a more modest 2–3 times after PPD (see also Chapter 1, Table 1.4). Recently the changes in blood flow and cell traffic following initial reaction to the contact sensitizer oxazolone (Ottaway and Parrott, 1979) were measured simultaneously. The resultant increase in blood flow was directly connected to the concomitant increase of migration of lymphoblasts to the skin. There was also a much smaller increase in small lymphocyte migration to the skin but this was not connected with blood flow. At the same time, there was also an increase in blood flow to the draining lymph node (Chapter 1.5), but in contrast this was directly connected to small lymphocyte and not blast cell traffic. Preliminary observations indicate, however, that at recall to the same contact sensitizer the relationship changes and that increased blood flow to the skin is also related to increased small lymphocyte traffic (Ottaway, unpublished).

5.2.7 Antigen-specific migration

It is obviously of interest to determine whether or not the antigenic stimulus which promotes the activation of lymphocytes to lymphoblasts will subsequently modify their migration pathway or their net accumulation over time in the site of antigen deposition.

There is general agreement that S-phase T lymphoblasts have a ready capacity to leave the circulation at sites of non-immune inflammation, situations in which antigenic recognition can play little or no part. As already described, large numbers of lymphoblasts accumulate, after intravenous injection, in skin sites

Table 5.4 The effect of oxazolone* on the regional blood flow and 24 hr localization of [^{125}I]UdR-labelled OX–PLN or PC–PLN to the ears.† Data from Ottaway and Parrott (1979)

Treatment of recipients	Donor cells	C.O. (%)	Injected dose of cells (%)
Unsensitized	PC–PLN	0.29 ± 0.07	0.03 ± 0.01
Unsensitized	OX–PLN	0.34 ± 0.06	0.05 ± 0.01
Oxazolone on day of cell transfer	PC–PLN	0.64 ± 0.20	0.54 ± 0.11‡
Oxazolone on day of cell transfer	OX–PLN	0.55 ± 0.10	1.49 ± 0.30‡
Oxazolone 1 day before cell transfer	PC–PLN	0.49 ± 0.09	0.66 ± 0.12‡
Oxazolone 1 day before cell transfer	OX–PLN	0.60 ± 0.18	1.34 ± 0.46‡

*10 mg of oxazolone were painted on the ears at times shown.
†Responses are the mean ± SD for 5–6 mice per group.
‡$p < 0.01$. Significantly different response for the value found in the ears of animals receiving OX–PLN *vs.* PC–PLN at the same stage of oxazolone treatment.

inflamed by croton oil or turpentine (Asherson and Allwood, 1972; Moore and Hall, 1973; Parrott *et al.*, 1975) and in peritoneal exudates inflamed with various non-antigenic stimuli, e.g. glycogen or thioglycollate (McGregor and Logie, 1974; Love and Ogilvie, 1977; Rose *et al.*, 1978). Even when antigen is involved by using contact sensitizers or preparations of bacterial antigens, these also produce considerable non-immune inflammatory reactions as well as antigenic change and the inflammatory reactions induced promote sufficient lymphoblast migration to mask any element of antigen-induced migration.

Allwood (1975), however, compared the migration of cells primed against picryl chloride or oxazolone into mice that had been primed previously and subsequently challenged with either oxazolone or picryl chloride 24 hr before receipt of cells; by using a careful cross-over design he detected an element of specific blast cell accumulation. More recently Ottaway and Parrott (1979), also using the sensitizers oxazolone and picryl chloride but using recipients which had not been sensitized previously, also obtained a significant increment of increased localization due to antigen (Table 5.4) which was comparable to that obtained by Jungi and McGregor (1978, 1979) when they measured the differential accumulation of specific antigen-activated S-phase lymphocytes in peritoneal exudates containing either *L. monocytogenes* mitogen or *F. tularensis* antigen. For other situations such as skin grafting (Tilney and Ford, 1974; Emeson, 1978) a similar element of 'specific' accumulation was observed, but it should be emphasized, however, that a major element of 'non-specific' accumulation is always present and is probably obligatory.

5.2.8 Role of chemoattractants and complement in modifying lymphoblast migration *in vivo*

Jungi and McGregor (1978) reported a small degree of antigenic specificity in their experiments on lymphoblast assembly in induced peritoneal exudates.

However, the presence of specifically sensitized lymphoblasts could substantially increase the assembly of lymphoblasts primed to another antigen. Jungi and McGregor (1978) have postulated that the numbers of 'pioneer' lymphoblasts which make the initial contact with antigen can be quite small yet they attract substantial numbers of other lymphoblasts; the mechanism by which the lymphoblasts achieve this is not known but could be by the release of chemoattractive lymphokines. More recently, Jungi and McGregor (1979) have investigated whether complement-dependent factors are involved in lymphoblast migration by treating rats with cobra venom factor, which inactivates C3. This treatment did reduce the numbers of lymphoblasts appearing in exudates of specifically immunized donors but did not prevent it entirely. It did not reduce non-specific lymphoblast accumulation.

5.3 MIGRATION TO MUCOSAL SITES

5.3.1 Composition of lymphoid cells in the gut and other mucosal surfaces

Many mucosal surfaces and especially the gut and the lungs are subjected to large and continuous antigenic stimulation and as a consequence contain many lymphoid cells. Intensive study of the predominant immunoglobulin-secreting cell, which in most animals and man is IgA, has been the main springboard for the development of the concept of a 'local immunological system' in the gut and other mucosal surfaces (Tomasi and Bienenstock, 1968; Bienenstock, 1974).

Histological studies of the human gut have demonstrated that there are 10^5–10^6 cells/mm^3 (Crabbé and Heremans, 1966; Bazin, 1976). The major classes of IgA, IgM, and IgG appear in relative frequencies of approximately 40:3:1, smaller numbers of IgD and IgE also being present (Brandtzaeg and Baklien, 1976; Crabbé and Heremans, 1966; Skinner and Whitehead, 1974; Brown et al., 1975). In ruminant animals, however, the predominant immunoglobulin-producing cell is IgG (Newby and Bourne, 1976).

Identification of T cells in the gut mucosa has excited less attention than immunoglobulin-producing cells although they probably occur almost as frequently (Guy-Grand et al., 1974). In 1972, Ferguson and Parrott (1972a) reported that there were fewer intraepithelial lymphocytes in the gut of thymus-deprived than normal mice, and Parrott and de Sousa (1974) found virtually no intraepithelial lymphocytes in homozygote nude mice, although heterozygotes had normal numbers and after implantation of a thymus graft into nude mice intraepithelial lymphocytes appeared. From these observations it was deduced that most intraepithelial lymphocytes were T cells, a deduction which was confirmed by the identification of a T cell surface antigen on the surface of all intraepithelial lymphocytes as well as many cells in the lamina propria (Guy-Grand et al., 1974; Meuwissen et al., 1976). Rudzick et al. (1975) examined suspensions of intraepithelial lymphocytes separated from the gut mucosa of rabbits and found a low proportion of cells (11%) with T cell surface antigen, 17% with immunoglobulin in their surface, and a high proportion of null cells

(65–70%). Mowatt (1975) found a higher proportion of T cells (33%) in lymphocytes separated from the epithelial layer of mice, none with immunoglobulin, but the same number of 'null' cells. Various explanations as well as species differences may be proferred for these disparities. Most lymphocytes in the gut are in an 'activated' form and activated lymphocytes have less cell surface antigen on their surface than resting lymphocytes so that many 'null' cells could be T lymphocytes, but it should also be appreciated that extraction of lymphocytes from epithelium or mucosa is a traumatic procedure which may well remove or change cell surface properties.

Intraepithelial lymphocytes differ morphologically in several respects from normal circulating small T lymphocytes. At least half of them are medium to large in size and some are large and blast-like (Marsh, 1975a). They have dense nuclei, granular cytoplasm, some rough endoplasmic reticulum, and a well-developed Golgi apparatus. Many IE contain tiny metachromatic granules (Rudzick and Bienenstock, 1974; Guy-Grand et al., 1978).

Examination of the lymphocyte content of the lamina propria of biopsies of human colon has shown that these also are larger than circulating lymphocytes; many have prominent nucleoli and basophilic cytoplasm. Fifty-eight % of the total mononuclear cells were identified as T cells and 32% as B cells, the remaining 10% being monocytes or macrophages (Bull and Bockman, 1977).

In theory it should be possible to assess the constituents of gut mucosa by cannulation and measurement of the cellular content of afferent intestinal lymph, as has been achieved with non-mucosal tissues (see above). So far, however, there are no published estimates of the numbers of small B and T lymphocytes, but there are larger numbers of blast cells (8–15%) of which half are probably T blasts (Hall et al., 1977) than in other afferent lymph. Like other afferent lymph, intestinal lymph in both species studied, sheep (Hall et al., 1977) and rat (MacPherson and Steer, 1979), contains approximately 5% of mononuclear phagocytes.

The assumption, however, that counting the cellular content of intestinal afferent lymph mirrors the cellular content of the intestinal mucosa is open to several potential sources of error. Many cells, especially B cells, differentiate into end cells which do not leave the mucosa and other cells, especially during pathological changes and inflammation, may be lost through the mucosa (see below). There may also be difficulty in differentiating between cells coming from the mucosa alone and those derived from efferent lymphatics of Peyer's patch tissue. As long ago as 1933 Baker observed in cats that the lymph coming from Peyer's patches was much richer in lymphocytes than the lymph coming directly from lacteals; these observations have been confirmed recently in the rat (Steer and MacPherson, personal communication). But problems obviously arise in, for example, the adult sheep when macroscopic patches are not seen (Hall et al., 1977), especially since the absence of macroscopic patches does not preclude the presence of small yet clearly defined patches by histological examination (Keren et al., 1978).

The bronchial mucosa apparently contains a much higher proportion of monocytes and macrophages to lymphocytes than the gut mucosa. Thus in the guinea pig (Hunninghake and Fauci, 1976) 50–70% of the mononuclear cells are monocytes or macrophages and only 30–50% are lymphocytes; of these, 68% formed E-rosettes (T cells) and 20.5% EA C-rosettes (B cells). In estimates of lung lavage (Daniele et al., 1977) which presumably represent the cells which have been persuaded to move into the alveolar air space, the proportion of lymphocytes is lower still, namely 14%. Most other mucosal surfaces presumably contain few if any lymphocytes, but there are now several estimates of the number of lymphocytes secreted from the mammary glands into colostrum and milk. Human colostrum contains 7–8 million leukocytes per ml of which up to 90% are monocytes or macrophages. The proportion of lymphocytes is highest immediately after parturition, and at that time 55% of the lymphocytes are T and 35% (approx.) are B lymphocytes (Diaz-Jouanen and Williams, 1974). In milk the proportion of T lymphocytes decreases to some 30–35% (Ogra and Ogra, 1978).

5.3.2 Identification of mucosal lymphocytes as effector cells

The numbers of cells in the gut mucosa directly reflect the antigenic stimulation *via* the gut lumen, for in germ-free animals or in 'antigen-free' gut grafts (Ferguson and Parrott, 1972b) the numbers of cells, both B and T, are drastically reduced. On the other hand, in some forms of antigen challenge, for example in coeliac disease (Ferguson, 1977) and in the response to protozoal or nematode infection, the numbers of lymphoid cells increase (MacDonald and Ferguson, 1978). In our current understanding, most of the cells in mucosal surface are effector cells rather than affector or memory cells (Parrott, 1976b; Cebra et al., 1977). In the case of B cells this is obvious since most are differentiated into immunoglobulin-secreting cells, many in the form of plasma cells. Effector T cells have also been demonstrated in mucosal sites. Thus, cells capable of mediating cellular immune responses (Waldman and Henney, 1971) and non-specific cytotoxicity (Hunninghake and Fauci, 1976) have been recovered from the bronchiolar air space by lavage; there are cytotoxic T lymphocytes present in human colostrum (Parmely and Williams, 1979) and cells able to mediate spontaneous cell-mediated cytotoxicity, mitogen-induced cellular cytotoxicity as well as antibody-dependent cellular cytotoxicity in the gut mucosa of guinea pigs (Arnaud-Battandier et al., 1978). But quantitation of the proportions of effector T cells is a difficult proposition because of the problems involved in preparing cell suspensions from mucosal sites. Nevertheless, the balance of evidence is in favour of the theory that most cells in mucosal sites are effector cells which have entered from the circulating blood and that they or their antecedents were primed by exposure to antigen in the specialized lymphoepithelial organs which abound in the walls of the nasopharynx, the intestinal tract, and the lungs. The logical place to start any study of the traffic of lymphocytes to mucosal surfaces is, therefore, with the specialized lymphoepithelial organs.

5.3.2.1 The beginning of the journey

Interaction of antigen on mucosal surfaces with circulating small lymphocytes from the bloodstream takes place in those structures in which the epithelium is specifically adapted to enhance trapping and uptake of antigenic material and particulate material. The organized lymphoepithelial structures in the intestinal tract, collectively termed GALT or gut-associated lymphoid tissues, include tonsils, Peyer's patches, appendix, and caecal patch, which are common to several species including man, rabbit, rat, mouse, hamster, dogs, and monkeys (Owen and Nemanic, 1978). Some species have additional but comparable tissue such as the sacculus rotundus in the rabbit and the caecal tonsil in the bird. Similar lymphoepithelial structures in the respiratory tract include the adenoids (Owen and Nemanic, 1978) and the bronchus-associated lymphoid tissues (BALT) (Bienenstock and Johnston, 1976).

5.3.2.2 Structure of the gut-associated and bronchus-associated lymphoid tissues

In general terms both GALT and BALT have many features in common with other secondary or peripheral lymphoid tissues such as the spleen and lymph nodes. For example, Peyer's patches may be subdivided roughly into T and B areas in which either T or B lymphocytes predominate (Parrott, 1976; de Sousa and Good, 1978). The nodules and germinal centres are composed primarily of B cells and the corridors between the nodules are occupied by T cells. Prominent postcapillary high endothelial walled venules (HEV) similar to the ones present in normal lymph nodes (Plate 15) are located in the interfollicular zones through which circulating T and B lymphocytes enter. As would be expected, the T areas of Peyer's patches and appendix are selectively depleted in animals deprived of T cells by neonatal thymectomy, by thymectomy plus irradiation or in the congenitally athymic nude mouse (de Sousa et al., 1969; de Sousa et al., 1973; Parrott and Ferguson, 1974). When selectively enriched populations of T or B lymphocytes are injected they can then be shown to migrate to specific T or B areas (see Plate 11).

An anatomical feature common to all mucosal lymphoid tissues is the unusual nature of the epithelial layer covering them. There may be several layers of squamous epithelium as in the tonsil (Curran and Jones, 1977) or a single layer of cuboidal epithelium without goblet cells as in Peyer's patches and appendix (Faulk et al., 1971; Plate 16) and flattened epithelium without cilia or goblet and glandular cells as in BALT. But in all instances there are large numbers of lymphocytes infiltrating the epithelium and there are specialized cells with micropinocytic properties known as the M cell (Plates 17 and 18; Bockman and Cooper, 1973; Owen and Jones, 1974). Immediately beneath the epithelium is a mixture of T and B lymphocytes, macrophages, and plasma cells, an area of lymphocyte traffic (Parrott, 1976a) called the dome. Unlike lymph nodes, there are no afferent lymphatics conveying antigen into GALT or BALT but antigen appears to enter through the epithelium. Several authors have reported that soluble and particulate antigen, India ink, and even intact bacteria can pass into the dome areas of Peyer's patches and appendix, but it could well be that the vital process of antigen–lymphocyte interaction takes place within the epithelium itself. Recently Owen (1977) has reported that in mouse Peyer's patches epithelium cells take up the enzyme horseradish peroxidase and transfer it to adjacent lymphocytes (Plate 17). Owen and Jones (1974) and Curran and Jones (1977) have also suggested that the lymphocytes within the epithelium are sufficiently close to make direct contact with antigen in the lumen. Certainly neither GALT nor BALT seems to require the antigen-handling mechanisms by macrophages which characterize the perifollicular region of the spleen and the sinuses of lymph nodes.

5.3.2.3 Other routes of antigen entry and lymphocyte interaction

Experimental manipulations such as the application of antigen to isolated loops of small intestine with or without Peyer's patches and removal of the mesenteric lymph node chain have emphasized the importance of Peyer's patches in the production and supply of IgA precursors and specific antibody-forming cells to the lamina propria of the gut (i.e. local humoral immunity), for certain antigens. It may be that the importance of Peyer's patches declines with age; they are certainly reduced in number after puberty in man (Cornes, 1965) and apparently disappear altogether after 6 months of age in the sheep (Hall *et al.*, 1977). The relative importance of other routes of entry of antigen from the gut and other mucosa have yet to be assessed. For example, there is direct lymphatic drainage from the lacteal of the villi to the mesenteric nodes and there is also access *via* the portal system to the liver and from thence either to the portal nodes or to the spleen through the general circulation, and either of these routes could be more important than Peyer's patches in some manifestations of systemic immunity as distinct from local immunity. For discussion of these problems see Parrott (1976b) and Ottaway *et al.* (1979).

5.3.2.4 The ontogeny of lymphocytes in the mucosa

The age at which lymphocytes appear in the GALT and BALT varies according to species, well before birth in humans and sheep but at, or around, birth in most rodents. Their first appearance is a consequence of the development of the primary lymphoid tissues and not upon antigen stimulation. Pearson *et al.* (1976) demonstrated that lymphocyte recirculation through Peyer's patches takes place in the foetal lamb; grafts of foetal gut and foetal lung (Ferguson and Parrott, 1972b; Milne *et al.*, 1975) which are free of antigenic stimulus nevertheless develop recognizable Peyer's patches and bronchus-associated lymphoid tissue. T cells appear in the T areas of Peyer's patches and in mice within 3 days of birth (Joel *et al.*, 1972; Ferguson and Parrott, 1972a) and at the same time in the dome area and in the covering specialized layer of cuboidal epithelium (Joel *et al.*, 1972;

Waksman, 1973) of mouse Peyer's patches and rabbit appendix (Niewenhuis, 1971). The population of B areas follows a day or so later. By contrast, no lymphoid cells appear in the rest of the mucosa until 2 weeks of age and these are manifestly a response to antigen challenge from the lumen (Crabbé et al., 1970; Ferguson and Parrott, 1972a).

5.3.2.5 Peyer's patches – the source of effector cell precursors (Fig. 5.1) in the gut mucosa

As a result of their observations on the sequential appearance of IgA-producing cells, Crabbé et al. (1970) were the first to postulate that Peyer's patches might be the source of IgA-forming cells (Fig. 5.1). Subsequently, in a series of elegant cell transfer experiments, Cebra and his co-workers (Craig and Cebra, 1971, 1975; Cebra et al., 1977) have demonstrated that Peyer's patches are a much richer source of IgA precursors than spleen, peripheral lymph node or peripheral blood lymphocytes and that these precursors over a period of 10–14 days can repopulate the lamina propria of the intestine of irradiated allogeneic rabbits or congenic mice with IgA-producing cells. They have also shown in rabbits (Cebra et al., 1977) that by placing an antigen, keyhole limpet haemocyanin, into isolated ileal loops, with or without a Peyer's patch secretory antibody was produced in both loops without a detectable systemic response but local production of antibody was much greater when antigen was placed in a loop with a Peyer's

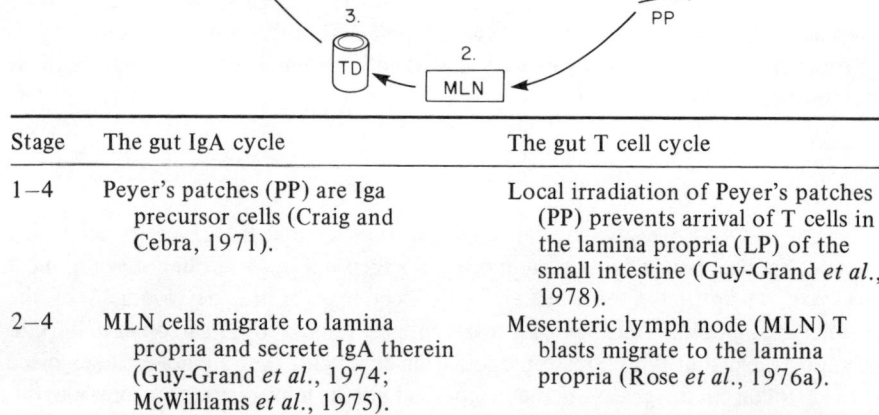

Stage	The gut IgA cycle	The gut T cell cycle
1–4	Peyer's patches (PP) are Iga precursor cells (Craig and Cebra, 1971).	Local irradiation of Peyer's patches (PP) prevents arrival of T cells in the lamina propria (LP) of the small intestine (Guy-Grand et al., 1978).
2–4	MLN cells migrate to lamina propria and secrete IgA therein (Guy-Grand et al., 1974; McWilliams et al., 1975).	Mesenteric lymph node (MLN) T blasts migrate to the lamina propria (Rose et al., 1976a).
3–4	Thoracic duct (TD) IgA blasts migrate to LP (Guy-Grand et al., 1974).	TD blasts migrate to LP (Freitas et al., 1980).

Figure 5.1 Schematic representation of evidence leading to the definition of accepted stages in the populating of the gut mucosa by T cells and B cells

patch than without. These experiments do not, however, show how the cells producing antibody travel from the Peyer's patch of one loop to the mucosa of the other loop or indeed to the rest of the gut. This has been achieved by monitoring the arrival of specific antibody- and Ig-producing cells in thoracic duct lymph (Husband *et al.*, 1977) and by tracing isotopically labelled mesenteric and thoracic duct lymphoblasts to the lamina propria of the intestine (Hall *et al.*, 1972; Parrott and Ferguson, 1974; Guy-Grand *et al.*, 1974), for it has not been possible to demonstrate directly by means of isotopic labelling that Peyer's patch cells migrate to the lamina propria, since they are retained in the spleen (Guy-Grand *et al.*, 1974). Using a system of isolated ileal loops similar to that of Cebra *et al.* (1977) but in rats instead of rabbits, Husband *et al.* (1977) showed that antibody-producing cells appeared. And Pierce and Gowans (1975) had earlier shown the importance of the thoracic duct in the circuit from Peyer's patch to lamina propria, for introduction of a thoracic duct fistula drastically reduced the number of specific antibody-containing cells in jejunum and ileum after intraduodenal challenge with cholera toxin.

It would seem proven, therefore, that IgA precursor cells in Peyer's patches, having responded to the challenge of antigen entering through the specialized dome epithelium, migrate *via* the mesenteric node and mesenteric lymphatics to the thoracic duct and bloodstream to the mucosa (Fig. 5.1). These observations do not, however, exclude the participation of other organized lymphoid tissues in supplying IgA precursors, indeed there is evidence that both appendix (Craig and Cebra, 1975) and BALT do so (Rudzig *et al.*, 1975). In primed animals the route from GALT *via* the thoracic duct may be less important as cells already present in the mucosa may respond to antigenic stimulation (Husband and Gowans, 1978; Husband *et al.*, 1979). Conversely, it cannot be assumed that Peyer's patches only supply IgA precursors, for T cells of mesenteric origin also accumulate selectively in the gut mucosa (Rose *et al.*, 1976b; Guy-Grand *et al.*, 1978) and local irradiation of Peyer's patches reduces the numbers of T cells in the gut mucosa (Guy-Grand *et al.*, 1978).

5.3.2.6 *The nature of the lymphoid cell which enters mucosal sites*

In their now classical experiments, Gowans and Knight (1964) demonstrated by means of autoradiography that only large lymphocytes from thoracic duct lymph would localize in the lamina propria of the villi after intravenous injection, although small lymphocytes from the same source were found in Peyer's patches, as well as in lymph nodes and spleen.

These basic findings have been confirmed in a succession of papers (Griscelli *et al.*, 1969; Hall *et al.*, 1972; Parrott and Ferguson, 1974). Only cells which are in large blast-like form and are undergoing DNA synthesis or have recently synthesized DNA as manifest by their capacity to take up DNA precursors or analogues during *in vitro* incubation will enter the mucosal villi, the only exception to this rule being those villi which are immediately adjacent to the nodules of Peyer's patches and which are accessible to small lymphocytes presumably entering *via* the Peyer's patches; there are both lymphatic (Parrott and Ferguson, 1974) and venous extensions from Peyer's patches (Anderson *et al.*, 1976; Plate 15) to these villi. In these earlier studies most emphasis was placed on the fact that the blast cells entering the lamina propria were IgA-containing cells, but it has been shown that activated T blasts from mesenteric lymph node (Rose *et al.*, 1976b) or thoracic duct lymph (Sprent, 1976; Guy-Grand *et al.*, 1978) also enter selectively the lamina propria, whilst mesenteric lymph node T cells deprived of their blast cell component have a reduced capacity to enter the lamina propria (Freitas *et al.*, 1977). Very recently, Freitas, Rose, and Rocha (1980) have further clarified the difference in the capacity of blast cells and small lymphocytes to enter the gut mucosa. They separated mouse thoracic duct T cells on a nylon wool column and then selectively enriched the proportion of blast cells in the cell suspension by velocity sedimentation on a discontinuous gradient of BSA. After labelling with ^{51}Cr they found that the proportion of cells which after 24 hr localized in the mucosa of the small intestine increased directly with the proportion of blast cells in the inoculum, whilst the radioactivity found in Peyer's patches and all other lymphoid tissues decreased with the increase in blast cells.

It is important to realize that although the thoracic duct drains principally the intestine, it does nevertheless drain other viscera including the caudal lymph nodes in rodents; thus, after recent antigenic stimulation it will contain mixtures of blast cells from both peripheral and mesenteric sources although in unstimulated animals only mesenteric blasts are present (Hopkins and Hall, 1976). Thus, peripheral blasts taken from the thoracic duct lymph after antigen injection into the flank can be persuaded to extravasate into the skin or peritoneal cavity as the experiments of Moore and Hall (1973) and McGregor and his colleagues (McGregor and Logie, 1974, Jungi and McGregor, 1978, 1979) have shown, but mesenteric blasts will not do so (Rose *et al.*, 1976a). In contrast, blast cells taken from peripheral sites will not enter the gut mucosa (Rose *et al.*, 1976a; Hall *et al.*, 1977) unless the gut has been inflamed by infection with *T. spiralis* (Table 5.3; and even so the peak accumulation of peripheral blasts is less than that of mesenteric blast cells (Rose *et al.*, 1976a, 1978). It has been suggested that the capacity of lymphocytes to differentiate between mesenteric and peripheral sites is possessed by small lymphocytes as well as blast cells in sheep (Cahill *et al.*, 1977), although this suggestion was not confirmed by later observations in mice (Freitas *et al.*, 1977, 1980). More recently, however, Cahill *et al.* (1979) have shown that separate migration pathways do not exist in the sheep foetus and appear only after birth. It is obvious, therefore, that the capacity to differentiate between sites is only acquired by lymphocytes after they have responded to antigen in a particular location.

5.3.2.7 Factors which control the numbers of effector cells in the gut mucosa

The lifespan of most of the cells which enter the lamina propria is comparatively short (see below) and their numbers are sustained by the cells which continually

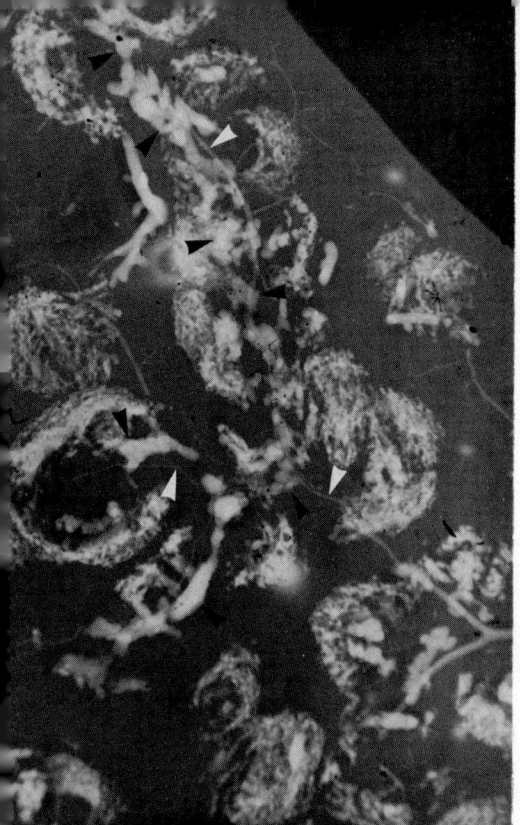

Plate 1: Spleen microcirculation. Microradiograph of a 400 μm cross-section (×14). Note the short interconnecting irregular channels forming the marginal sinus. White arrows, central artery; black arrows, lymphatic channels. Data from Dubreuil et al. (1975), courtesy P. G. Herman

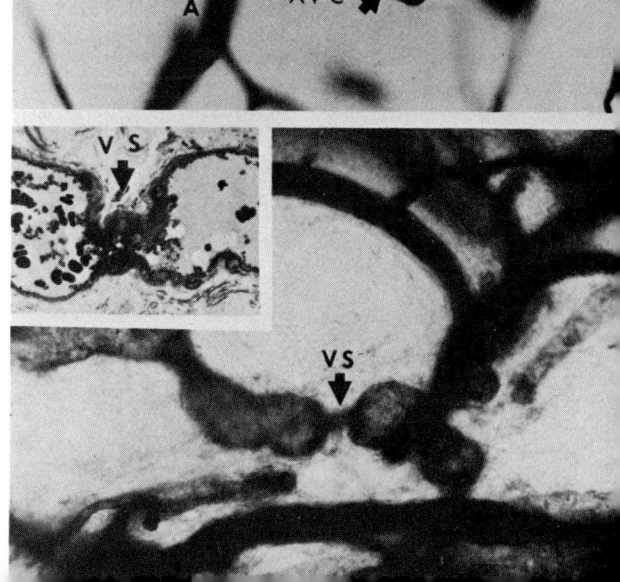

Plate 2: (a) Arteriovenous communication (AVC) between artery (A) and a high endothelial venule (HEV) in a cleared section from an alcian blue perfused rat node. (b) A local constriction is shown near the terminal end of a segmental vein in this cleared section (×135). Serial 1 μm sections through this site demonstrated a sphincter (VS) composed of circumferential smooth muscle bundles (see inset). For further evidence for the existence of arteriovenous shunting, see Table 1.1 Microphotograph courtesy A. Anderson, from Anderson and Anderson (1975)

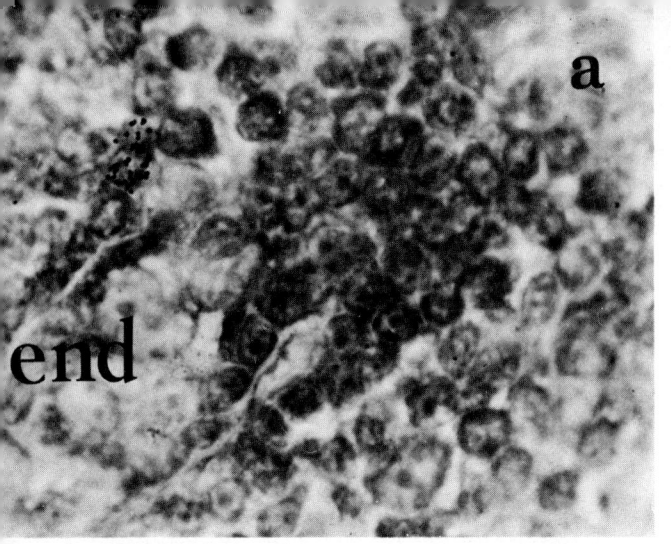
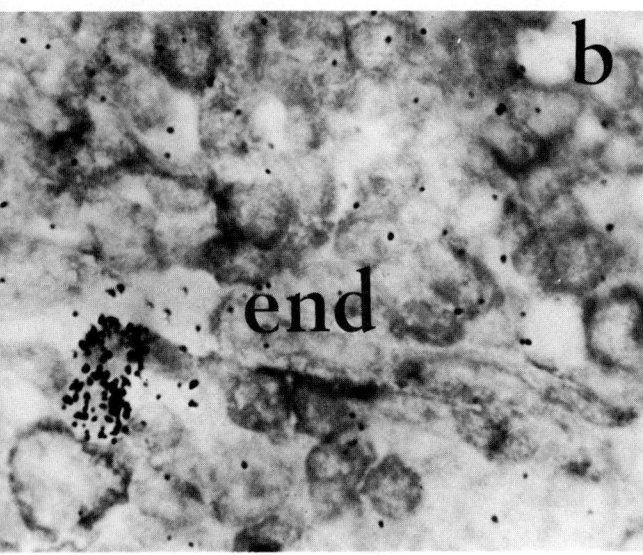

Plate 3: Recirculating rodent lymphocytes enter the lymph circuit through postcapillary venules located in the mid-cortex of lymph nodes. In normal animals (a) the venules, at the point of lymphocyte crossing, have a characteristic and remarkable high endothelium, which has led to the generalized designation of HEV. In animals depleted of circulating lymphocytes, however, the endothelial cells appear flat and unremarkable (b). Endothelium morphology *per se* does not appear to influence lymphocyte entry into the lymph node. Following the intravenous injection of labelled lymphocytes the labelled cells are found closely associated with the venules in both instances (a, b). Autoradiographs of lymph nodes removed from intact (a) and neonatally thymectomized (b) mice killed at 24 hr after the intravenous injection of ^{3}H adenosine-labelled lymphocytes

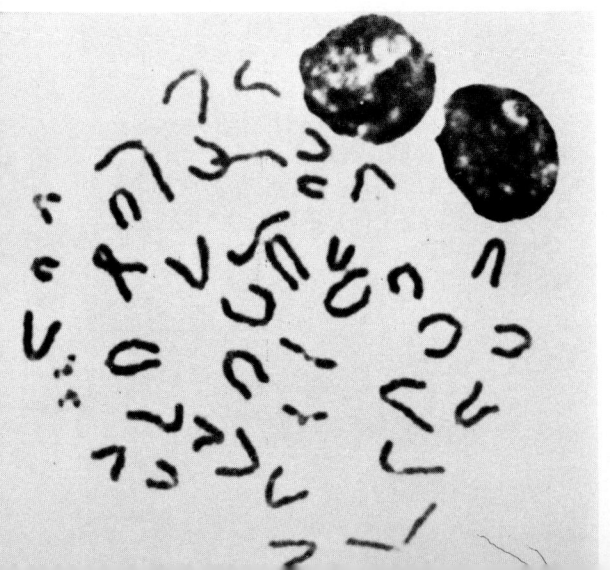

Plate 4: The T6 chromosome marker (see page 15 for description). Courtesy H. S. Micklem.

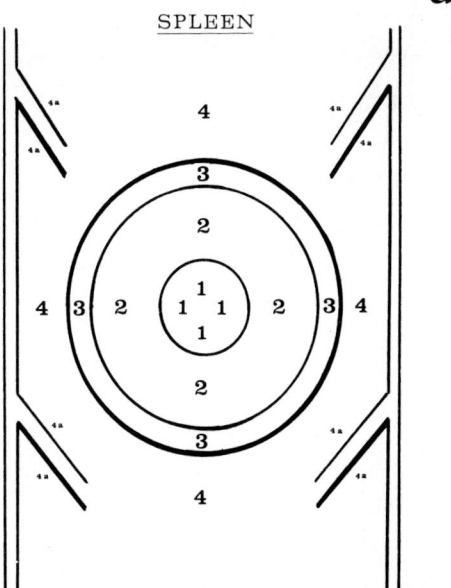

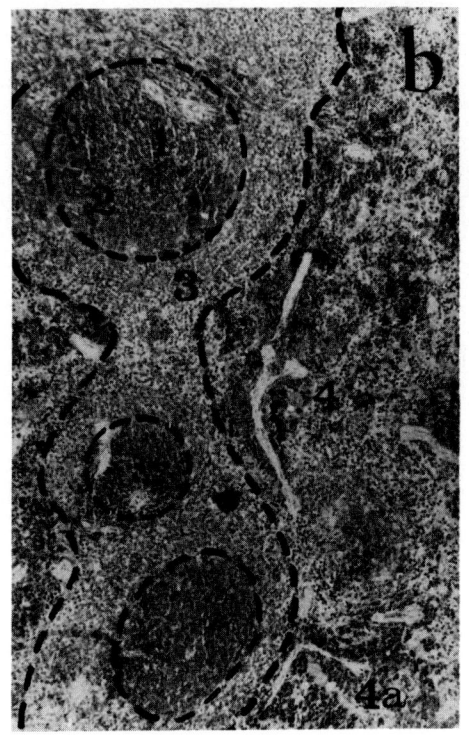

Plate 5: Diagrammatic representation (a) of the main areas of the mammalian spleen, also shown in microphotographs of the mouse spleen (b, c). 1, thymus-dependent or T cell area, consisting mostly of cells of thymus origin and occupying the zone immediately surrounding the central arteriole; 2, thymus-independent or B cell area, occupying the outer zone of the Malpighian follicle; 3, marginal zone, at the interface of white and red pulp; 4, within seconds of an intravenous injection, labelled cells or dyes (India ink) are found in the marginal zone (3c); 4a, peritrabecular aggregates of lymphoid cells and plasma cells are also seen in the red pulp (4)

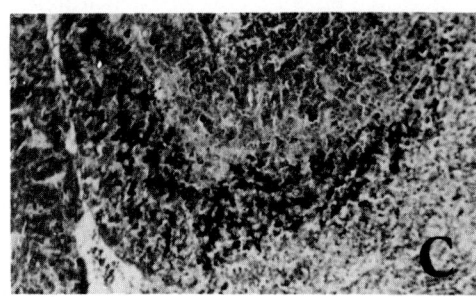

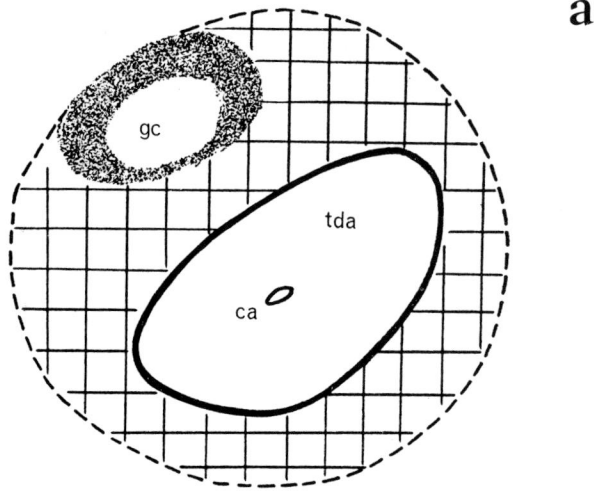

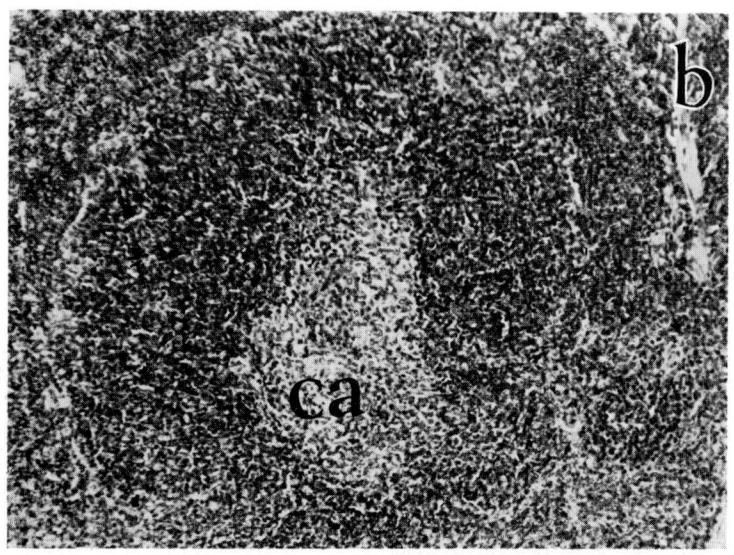

Plate 6: Diagrammatic representation (a) and microphotograph (b) illustrating the lymphoid cell depletion observed in the thymus-dependent area (tda) located round the central arteriole (ca) in the spleen of neonatally thymectomized mice. gc, germinal centre. In mice born without a thymus, germinal centre formation is impaired. Diagram from Parrott *et al.* (1966)

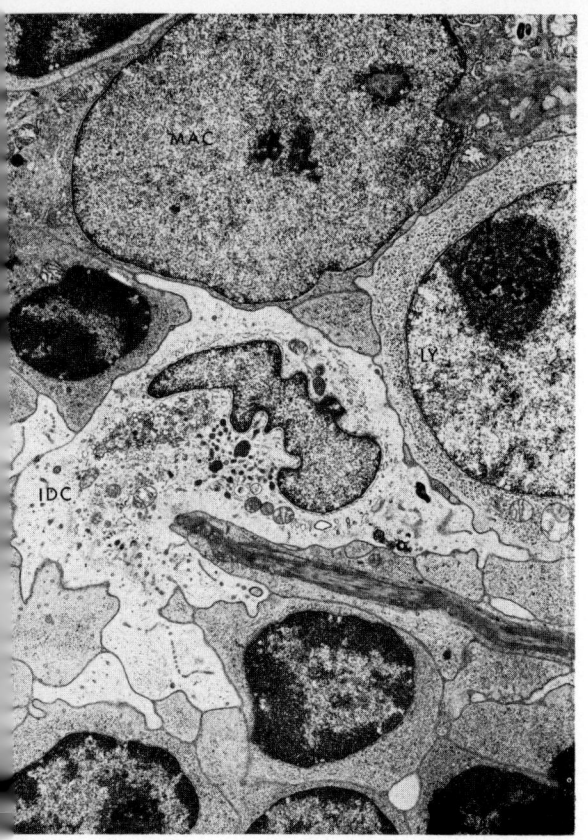

Plate 7: Electronmicrograph illustrating an interdigitating cell (IDC) in thymus-dependent area of mouse lymph node. Courtesy Dr. A. Anderson (from Anderson, 1980)

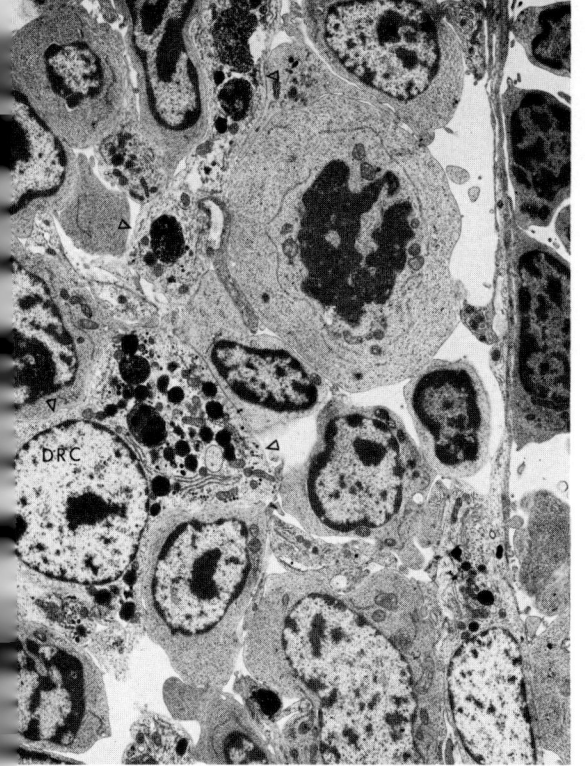

Plate 8: Electronmicrograph illustrating a dendritic reticulum cell (DRC) found in the follicular, B cell area, of lymph node. Edge of follicle indicated by line between asterisks. Outlines of cytoplasmic ramifications of cell indicated by triangles. Courtesy Dr. A. Anderson (from Anderson, 1980)

LYMPH NODE

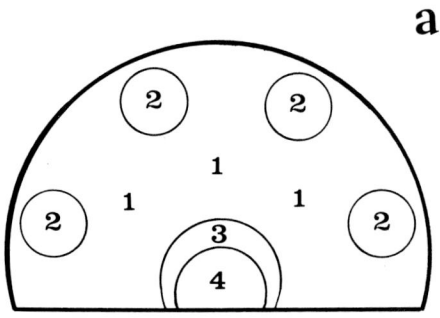

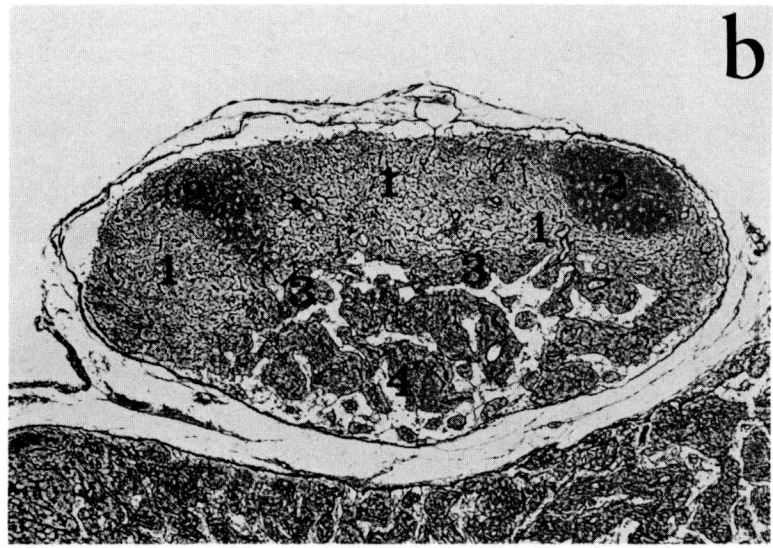

Plate 9: Diagrammatic representation (a) of the four major lymph node areas, also shown in the microphotograph of a mouse lymph node section stained for reticulin (b). 1, thymus-dependent or T cell area, also designated paracortex; 2, thymus-independent, B cell areas, sometimes incorrectly designated cortex; 3, cortico-medullary junction or deep cortex; 4, medulla (see also Plate 10).

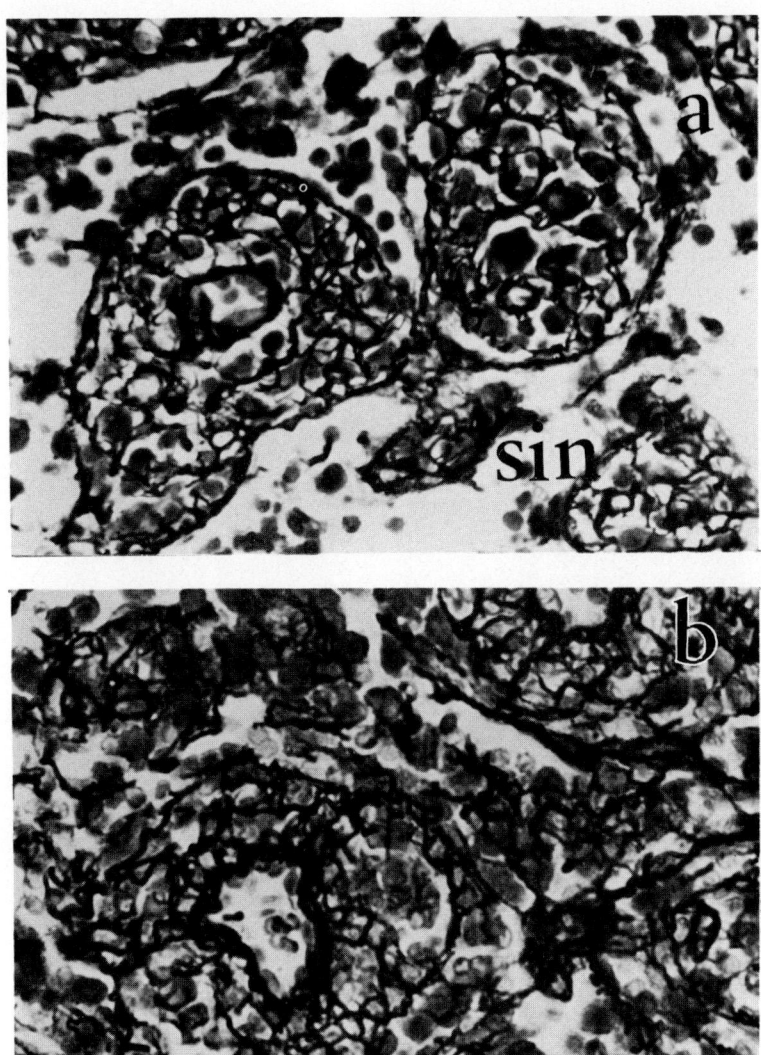

Plate 10: Microphotographs of mouse lymph nodes illustrating the reticulin framework of the medullary cords and the changes in cellularity of the sinuses (sin) observed in situations of continuous antigen stimulation (b). Note that the comparatively empty sinuses observed in a normal lymph node (a) become 'choked' with mononuclear cells in an animal which has received repeated injections of antigen from birth (b). From data published in de Sousa *et al.* (1971)

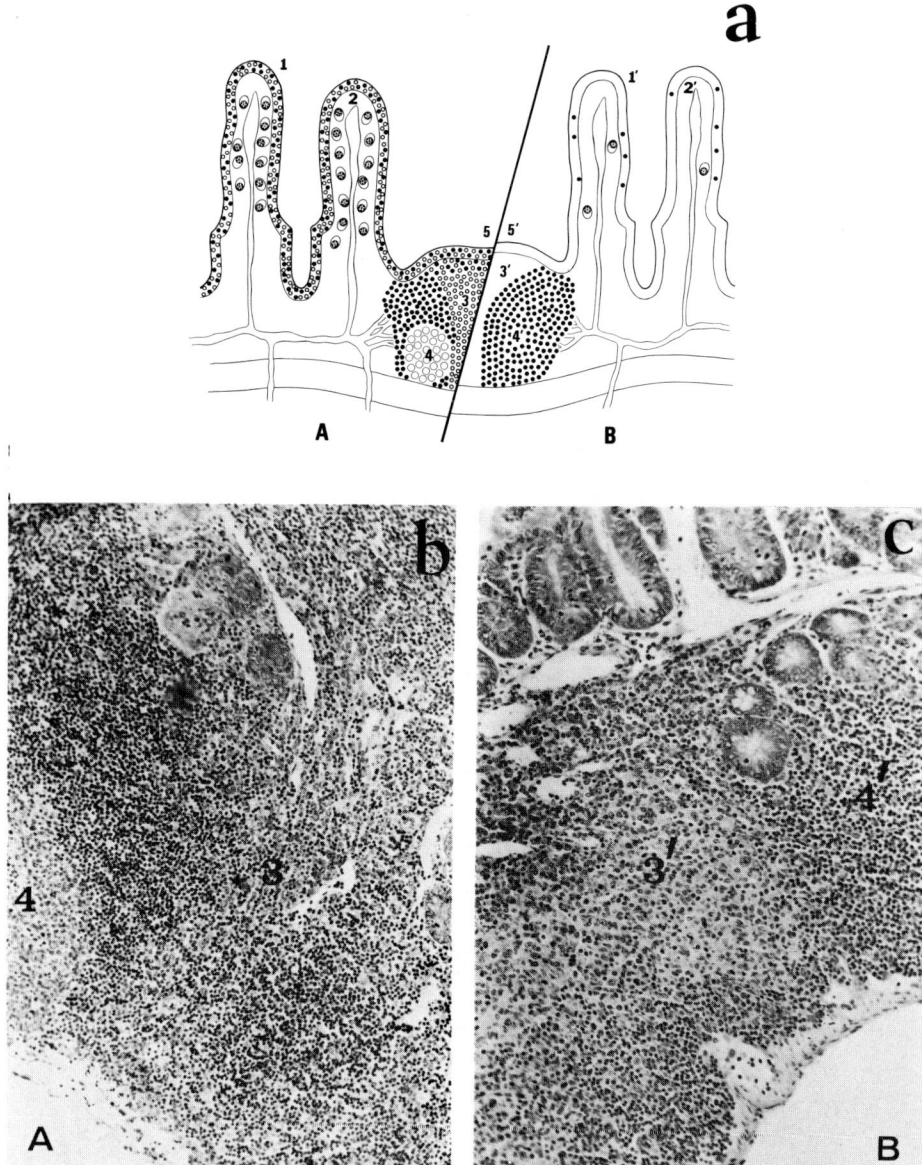

Plate 11: Schematic representation (a) and microphotographs of intact (b, A) and *nu nu* (c, B) Peyer's patches illustrating the distribution of T(○, 3) and B(●, 4') lymphocytes, plasma cells, and germinal centres (○, 4) in the gut. Numerous T lymphocytes and variable numbers of B lymphocytes have been observed in the gut epithelium (1). The numbers of intraepithelial lymphocytes are markedly reduced in thymus-deprived animals (1'). Numerous IgA-containing plasma cells are normally present in the lamina propria (2). In the absence of T cells, the numbers of IgA-containing cells are reduced (2'). Thymus-dependent (3, 3') and B cell areas (4, 4') have been delineated in Peyer's patches. In thymus-deprived animals (B: a and c) germinal centre development is impaired. Interaction between antigen and immunologically competent cells occurs in the dome area of the Peyer's patches (5, 5'). For further details of the ultrastructure of this area, see Plate 16. Diagram from de Sousa and Good (1978). Photomicrographs from de Sousa *et al.* (1969).

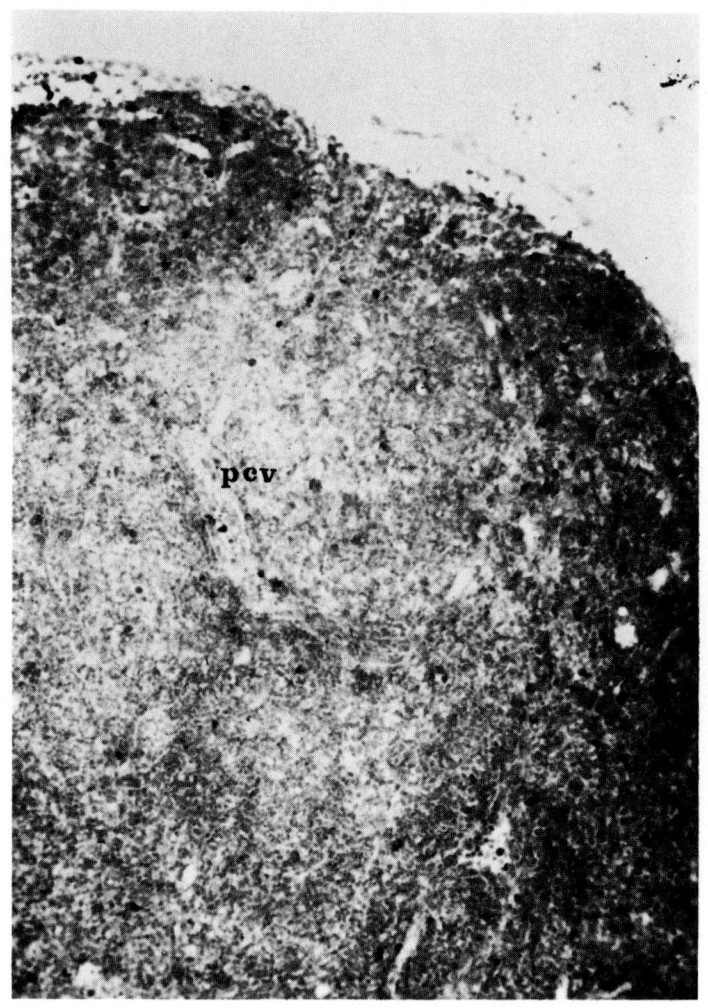

Plate 12: Autoradiograph of mouse lymph node. [^{3}H]-5-uridine-labelled B lymphocytes over B areas of the lymph node cortex. Note a few labelled cells close to postcapillary venules (pcv)

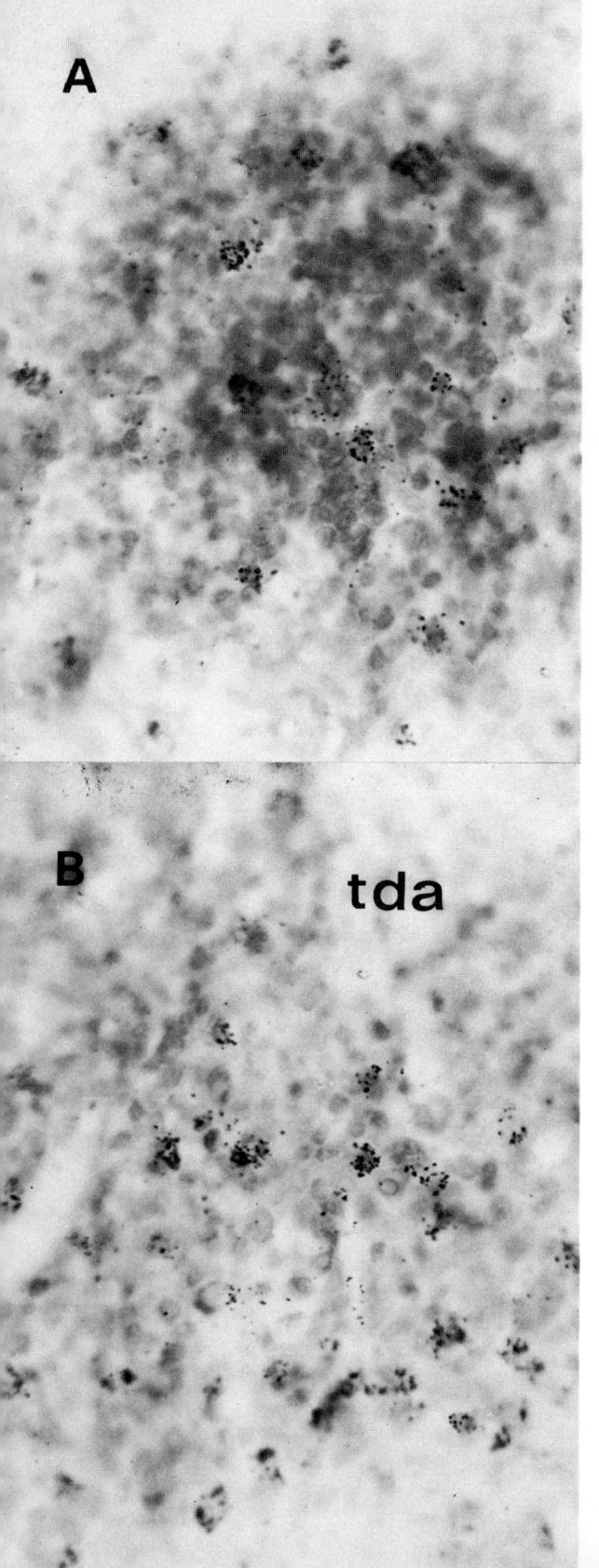

Plate 13: Lymph node. Illustration of the selective migration of radio-labelled B (A) and T (B) lymphocytes to the primary nodule (A) and thymus-dependent area (tda) (B) of the lymph node. Autoradiographs of mouse lymph nodes removed at 24 hr after the injection of [^{3}H]-adenosine-labelled cells

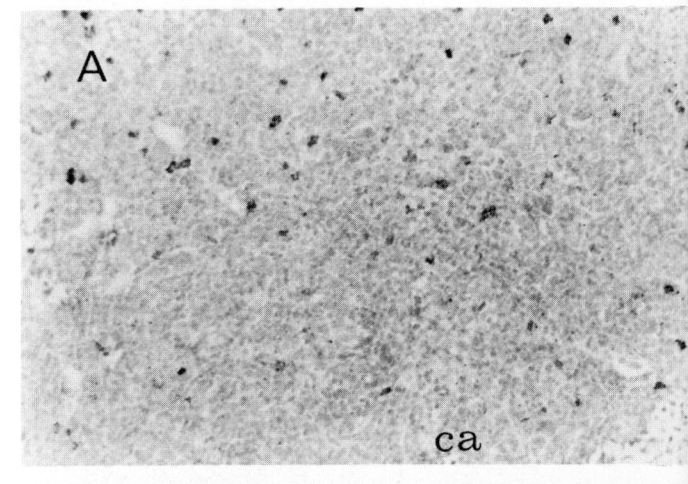

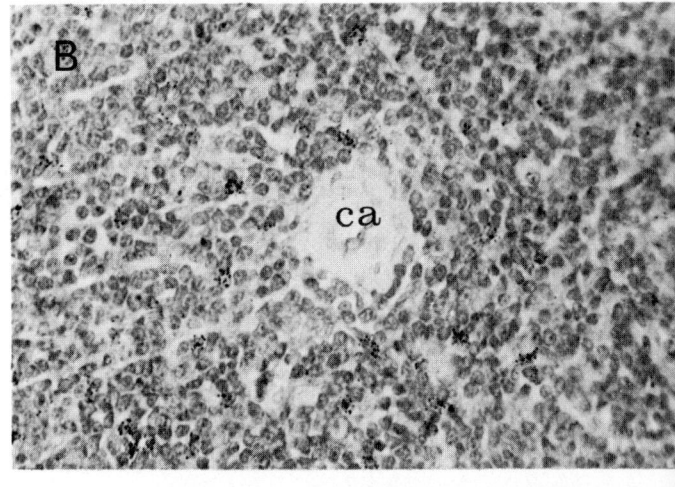

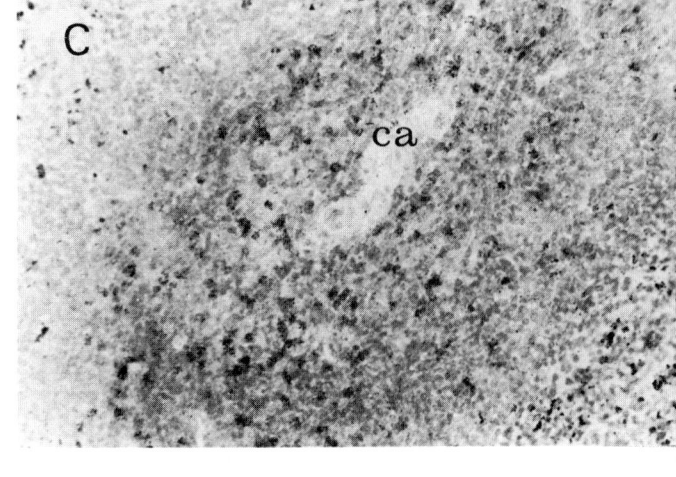

Plate 14: Spleen. Illustration of the selective migration of B (A) and T (B) lymphocytes to the outer follicular area of the Malpighian body (A) and the periarteriolar, thymus-dependent area (B). Following the injection of labelled spleen cells, containing both B and T lymphocytes (C), labelled cells are found in both areas of the white pulp nodules. Studies using specific anti-T or anti-B antisera have also demonstrated the selective distribution of the two cell types in the two separate regions of the spleen and lymph node. Autoradiographs of mouse spleens removed at 24 hr after the intravenous injection of [³H]-adenosine-labelled cells

Plate 15: High endothelium venules (HEV) in Peyer's patch: HEV form a freely anastomosing network in the interfollicular region (see also Plate 2). Venus plexuses situated near the muscularis propria (MP) and muscular mucosa and merge with capillary beds at the base of intestinal crypts. Relatively few blood vessels are seen in the adjacent nodule (N). (Magnification ×51,450 from section of cleared Peyer's patch.) Courtesy Anderson *et al.* (1976). Reproduced with permission of the author

Plate 16: Scanning electronmicrograph of single Peyer's patch lymphoid nodules protruding among finger-shaped villi in mouse ileum (R. G. Bruce) Courtesy Dr. R. G. Bruce

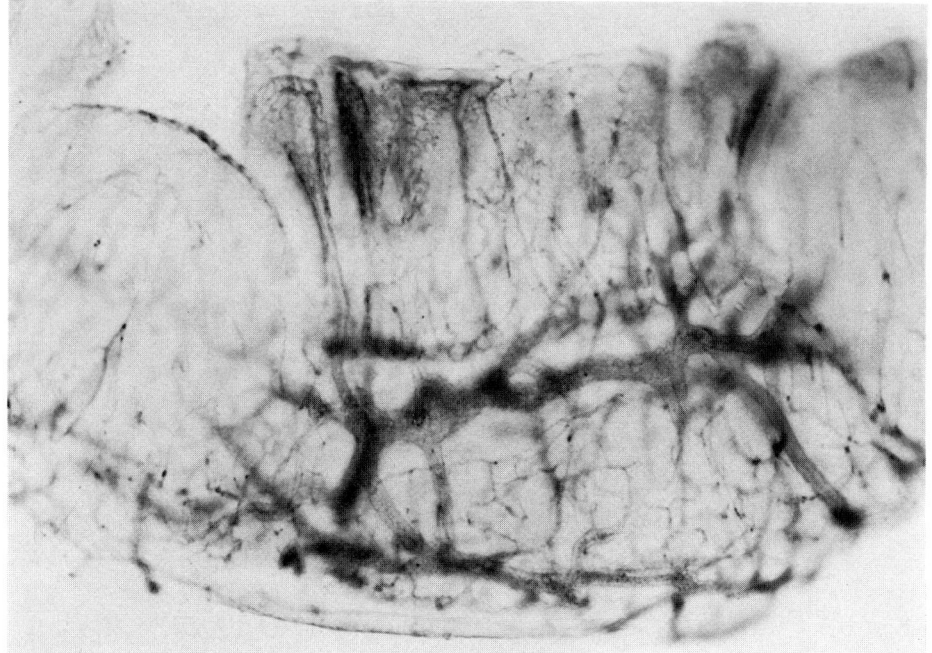

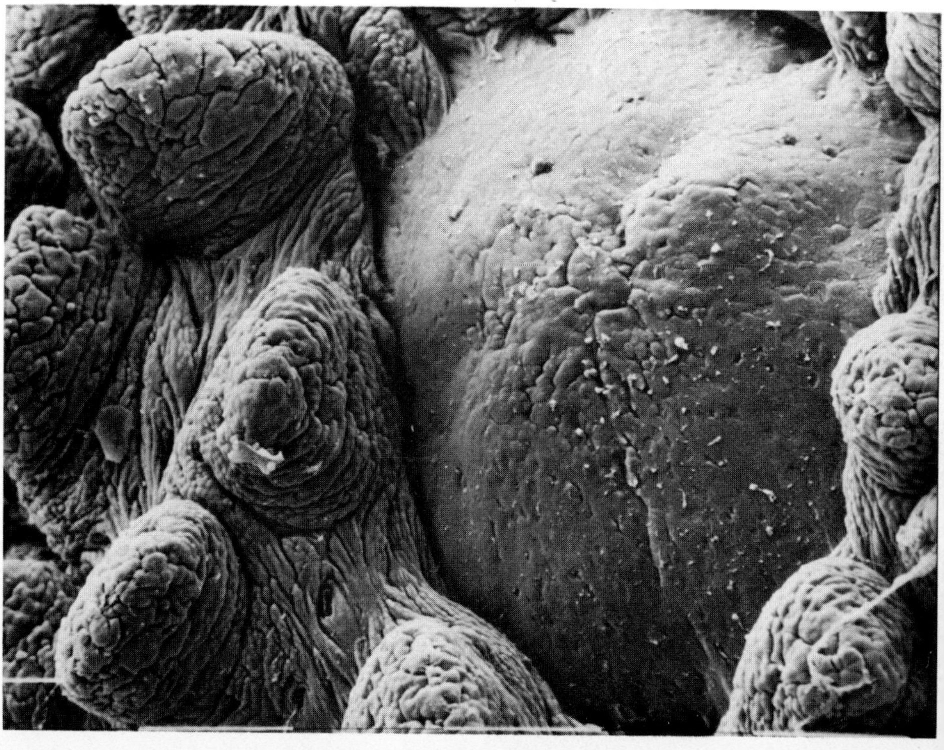

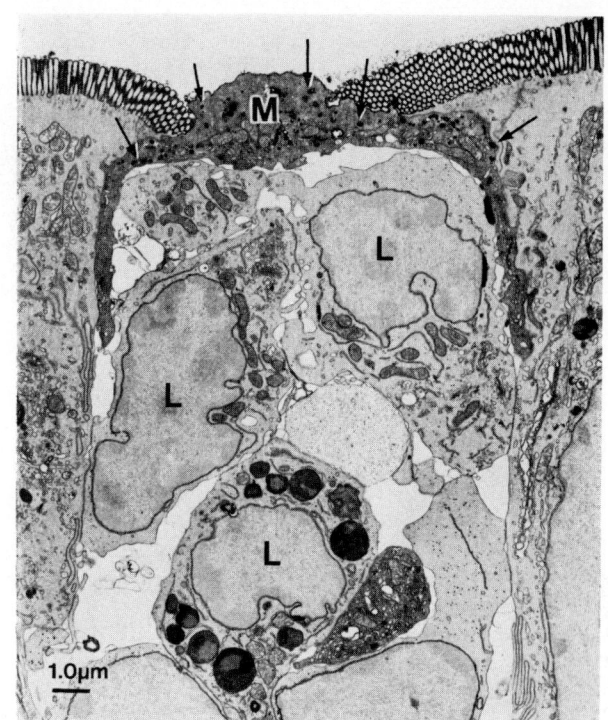

Plate 17: Mouse Peyer's patch: M cell (M) surrounding several lymphocytes (L). Arrows mark vesicles transporting exogenously administered horseradish peroxidase. Courtesy Owen and Nemanic (1978). Reproduced with permission of the authors

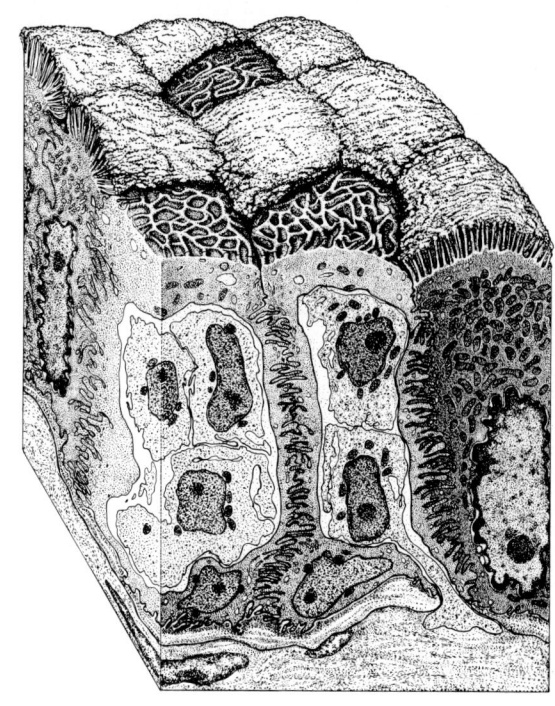

Plate 18: Artist's view of human Peyer's patch epithelium. Note migrating lymphocytes enfolded by M cells, extending from the basal lamina and interdigitating with adjacent columnar cells. Courtesy Owen and Nemanic (1978). Reproduced with permission of the authors

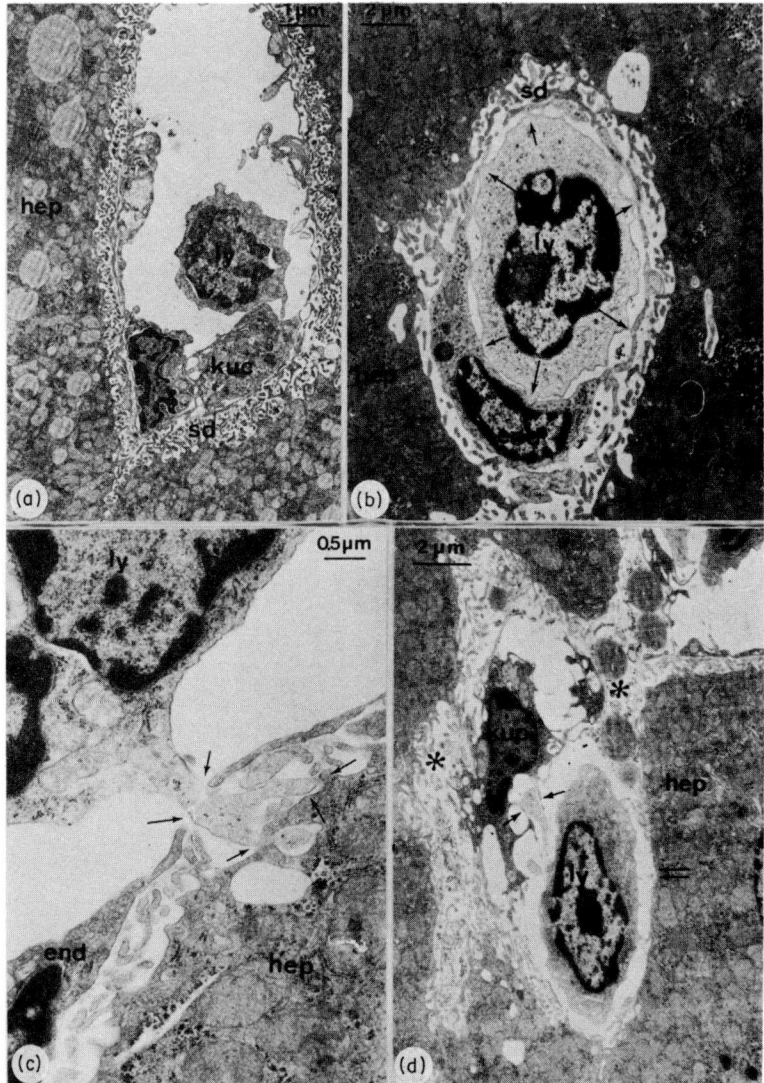

Plate 19: Autoimmune reactions against liver cells 7 days after a single injection of asialosplenocytes. a, lymphocytes (ly) persisting in the capillary lumen are found adhering (arrow) to Kupfer cells (kuc); b, or to endothelial cells (end, arrows); hep, hepatocyte; sd, space of Disse. c, infiltration starts with the lymphocyte (ly) extending microvilli through endothelial (end) fenestrations and establishing contact (arrows) with hepatocellular (hep) microvilli in the space of Disse (sd). d, infiltrating lymphocyte (ly) in contact (arrow) with Kupfer cell (kuc). The endothelial cell is already lysed.* double lysed fat-storing cells; hep, hepatocyte. Courtesy of Kolb-Bachofen and Kolb (1979)

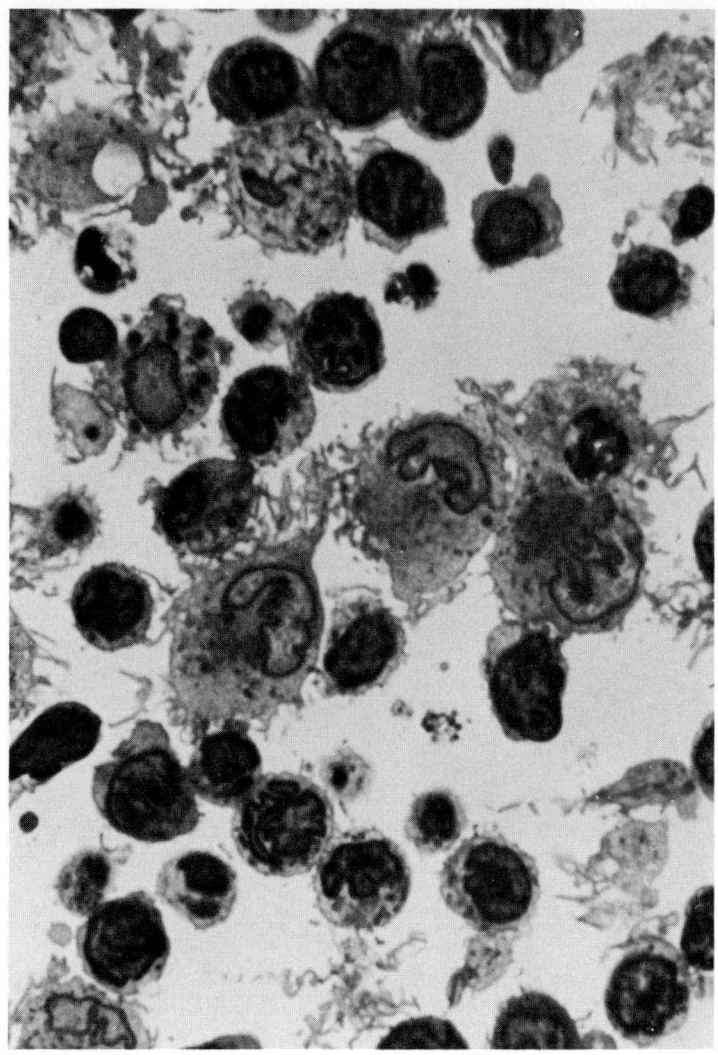

Plate 20: Interdigitating dendritic cells (light cells) and malignant T lymphocytes (dark cells) in lymph node cell suspension from patient with mycosis fungoides. A similar close interaction between the two cell types is seen in the skin of patients with mycosis fungoides or Sezary syndrome. Courtesy D. H. Wright

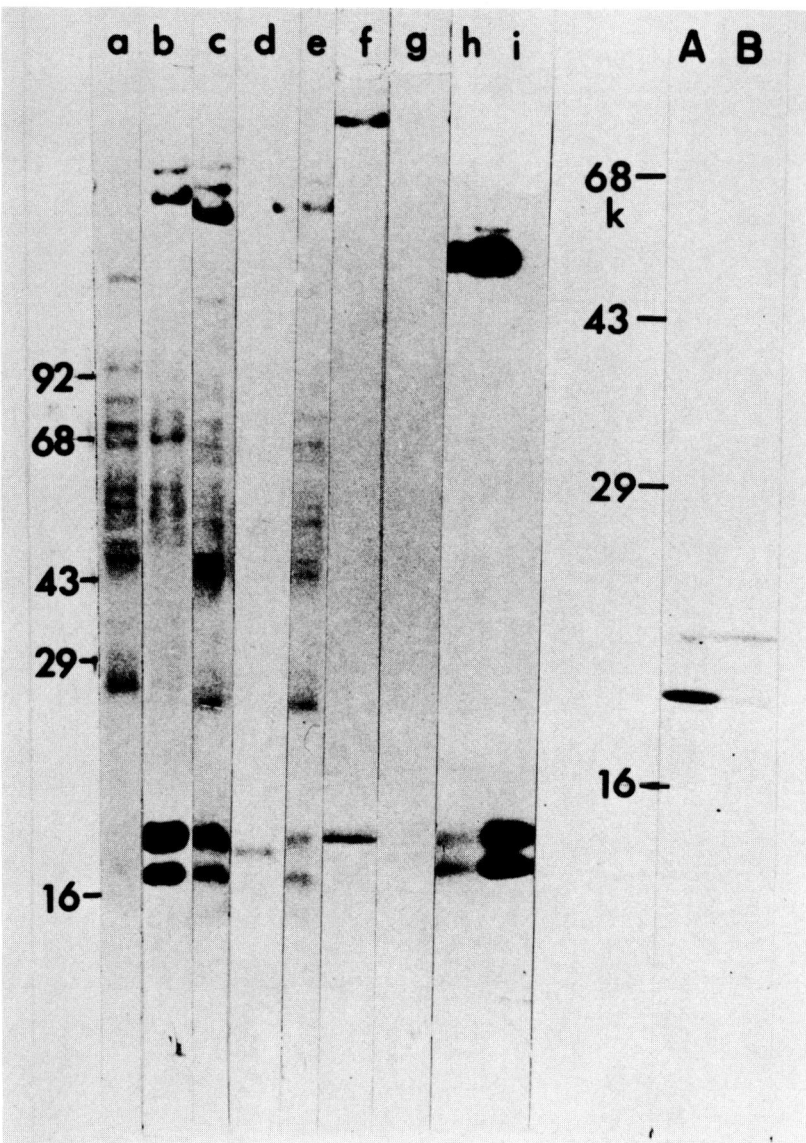

Plate 21: Evidence of synthesis and secretion of ferritin by human lymphoid cells. SDS-PAGE analysis of metabolically labelled (^{3}H-leucine) cell extracts and supernatants from selected Hodgkin's disease spleen cells. a, T cell lysate precipitated with normal rabbit serum (7.8×10^5 cpm). b, identical lysate precipitated with antiferrin antiserum (AFS). c, T cell supernatant precipitated with AFS (10^6 cpm). d, B cell lysate precipitated with AFS (7.8×10^5 cpm). e, B cell supernatant lysate precipitated with AFS (10^6 cpm). f, g, ^{3}H-leucine-labelled cell lysate from fractionated peripheral blood mononuclear cells. f, T-cell lysate precipitated with AFS. g, identical sample precipitated with AFS previously absorbed with human spleen ferritin. h, i, iodinated human spleen ferritin. h, unreduced sample (no 2-mercaptoethanol in sample buffer). i, reduced sample. A, B, photographs of Coomassie blue stained proteins in SDS-PAGE analysis of purified ferritin. A, human spleen ferritin. B, human heart ferritin (from Dörner et al., 1980)

enter from the bloodstream. Therefore, the efficacy of immune responses is dependent upon the efficiency with which the effector cells, whether T or B, are transported from the GALT tissues to the mucosa by a route which, as we have seen, is somewhat circuitous. So far, it has not proved possible to determine what proportion of cells within Peyer's patches reach the gut mucosa. This has, however, been achieved with cell preparations from 'further along the route', namely mesenteric lymph node cells and thoracic duct lymphocytes. Isotopically labelled lymphoblasts from either of these sources arrive in significant numbers at the mucosa within an hour of injection (Hall *et al.*, 1972; Rose *et al.*, 1976b), and the numbers peak within 12 hr of injection. Significantly, the highest proportion of labelled cells (60%) is present in the small intestine. Far less is found in the large intestine, caecum, or mesenteric node. Lymphoblasts are both fragile and short-lived and after injection much of the radioactive label is recovered in the urine (Sprent, 1976). By 72 hr after injection only a small percentage (5–6%) of the injected radioactivity is recoverable yet 70% of it is in the small intestine (Rose *et al.*, 1978). It would seem, therefore, that the small intestine is the preferred site of localization of lymphoblasts from the GALT and if the cells do not arrive there, they do not survive beyond a few hours.

One important factor which affects the delivery of lymphoblasts to the gut is blood flow (Ottaway and Parrott, unpublished). Measurement of cardiac output by ^{86}Rb Cl method in normal mice showed that the proportion of blood flow received by the duodenum and jejunum is much greater than that to the ileum and that differences in blood flow are also present at different levels of the small intestine. A mirror image of this distribution pattern has been reported already for mesenteric lymphoblasts (Parrott and Rose, 1978) and has also been found with separated T mesenteric blasts (Manson-Smith *et al.*, 1979). Recently it has been found that the proportional distribution of mesenteric T and B lymphoblasts to the gut was directly related to blood flow, an additional aspect in which migration to a mucosal site resembles migration to the peripheral site (Ottaway and Parrott, unpublished).

It is interesting that the relative distribution of IgA-producing cells resembles the distribution of blast cells and the blood flow to the gut in that it is highest at the proximal section of the small intestine rather than in the distal section, the caecum or the large intestine in mice (Crabbé *et al.*, 1970), in calves (Porter *et al.*, 1972) and humans (Crabbé and Heremans, 1966). There is also some indication that the numbers of intraepithelial (T) lymphocytes are higher in the proximal section of the intestines than elsewhere. Nevertheless, it is obvious that factors other than blood flow must be involved in the delivery of lymphoblasts to the intestine or as many lymphoblasts of peripheral origin would appear in the mucosa as those of mesenteric origin and this is not the case (see above).

Many factors could affect the total number of either immunoglobulin-producing (B) or effector (T) cells present in the mucosa. These include the ability to adhere to and migrate through the vascular endothelium, the presence of substances, e.g. antigen, to attract and/or retain the cells once they have entered, the

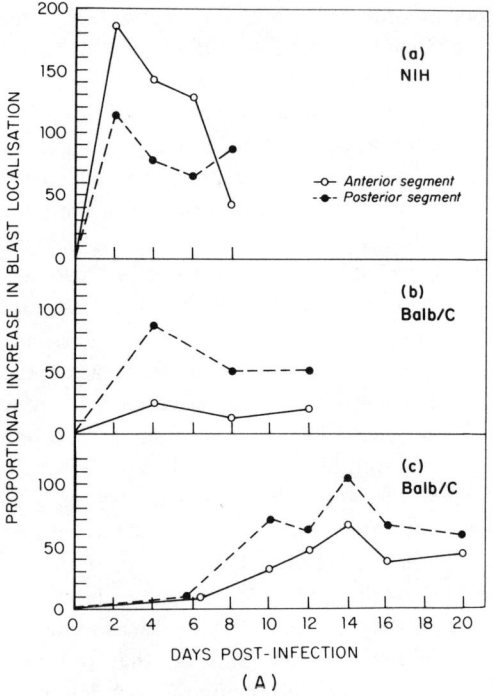

Figure 5.2 (A) Proportional increases in the 24 hr localization of ^{125}IUdR-labelled mesenteric lymphoblasts in the anterior and posterior halves of the small intestine during *T. spiralis* infection. (a) NIH strain recipients of cells from donors infected 4 days previously; (b) Balb/c strain recipients of cells from donors infected 4 days previously; (c) Balb/c strain recipients of cells from donors infected 12 days previously

lifespan of the cells and their ability to multiply whilst in the mucosa, and whether they stay in or migrate out of mucosa. The *in vitro* locomotor behaviour of lymphoblasts and the possible relevance of these studies to *in vivo* locomotor behaviour is presently under investigation. Suffice it to say here that there is nothing to suggest that blasts of mesenteric origin are not as equally motile as peripheral blast cells (Parrott and Wilkinson, 1980).

The much smaller number of IgA-producing cells and intraepithelial lymphocytes in germ-free and 'antigen-free' gut grafts testifies that antigen in the gut lumen does affect significantly the lymphoid population of the mucosa but does not demonstrate how. Thoracic duct or mesenteric lymphoblasts taken from primed donors (Pierce and Gowans, 1975: Rose *et al.*, 1976b) not only migrate to the intestine of non-primed recipients, but also to gut grafts which contain no antigen (Moore and Hall, 1972; Parrott and Ferguson, 1974). However, lymphoblasts are also found in larger numbers in regions of gut which are

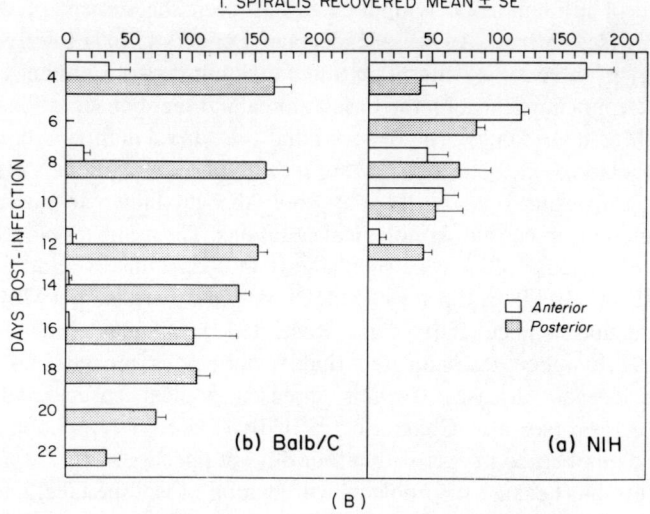

Figure 5.2 (B) Recovery of adult *T. spiralis* from the small intestine of infected mice. Distribution between the anterior and posterior halves in (a) NIH strain and (b) Balb/c strain mice

stimulated than in those which are not, as is shown by the 'segmental' distribution of ^{125}IUdR-labelled mesenteric lymphoblasts to different segments of the intestine during the course of infection with *T. spiralis* (Fig. 5.2). This segmental increase occurs rapidly, i.e. within 2–4 hr of injection of cells and apparently involves a non-specific facilitation of lymphoblast accumulation. Another separate and slower antigen-dependent mechanism for increasing effector cell representation has also been described (Husband and Gowans, 1978). More specific antibody-forming cells appear in gut regions or gut loops of rats in which antigen is placed than in non-stimulated regions or loops (Pierce and Gowans, 1975; Husband and Gowans, 1978). This increase takes place over a period of several days and is considered to be the result of retention and cell division rather than the attraction of more cells into the mucosa. Certainly, IgA-forming cells in the mucosa are capable of further division (Cebra *et al.*, 1977; Husband and Gowans, 1978).

5.3.2.8 *The fate of B and T lymphoblasts in the gut mucosa*

The fate of B and T lymphoblasts once in the mucosa is different. The B blasts do not recirculate (Hall *et al.*, 1972; Husband and Gowans 1978) but die *in situ* after a short half life of 4–7 days (Mattioli and Tomasi, 1973; Cebra *et al.*, 1977). T cells also have a short lifespan as shown by autoradiography (Parrott *et al.*, 1975; Marsh, 1975a,b) and by cell traffic studies (Sprent, 1976; Rose *et al.*, 1978). There is a rapid fall in isotopes recovered from the intestine and colon within 3 days after the injection of T blasts and complete disappearance at 7–14 days, though a very small minority continue to recirculate as small lymphocytes (Sprent, 1976).

The fate of intraepithelial lymphocytes has been the subject of debate over many years (see Parrott, 1976). Meader and Landers (1967) inferred from the morphology of direction of migration that equal numbers of lymphocytes entered and left the epithelium through the basal lamina and these observations were confirmed by Marsh (1975a,b), who deduced that substantial numbers returned to the general circulation *via* the lacteals. More recently, however, there is evidence that lymphocytes (presumed to be T) may enter the gut lumen in pursuit of their effector functions in certain pathological situations. The numbers of intraepithelial lymphocytes increase often very significantly in coeliac disease and giardiasis in man (Ferguson, 1977) and in mice (MacDonald and Ferguson, 1978), and in *T. spiralis* infection in mice (Parrott and Rose, 1978). Douglas *et al.* (1976) using ^{51}Cr-labelled lymphocytes indicated that lymphocytes moved into the faecal stream in coeliac disease, Crohn's disease, tropical sprue, and intestinal lymphangiectasia (see also Chapter 6). ^{125}IUdR-labelled T lymphoblasts migrate in increased numbers to the gut within four days of infection with *T. spiralis* (Rose *et al.*, 1976b; but because of problems with elution of isotope label and excretion of label from dead cells into the stomach it was not valid to conclude that any increase in label in gut contents was due to migrating cells (Sprent, 1976). Recently, however, in scanning electronmicrograph studies of Peyer's patches, clusters of lymphocytes were found in the crypts, close to Peyer's patches, in mice infected with *T. spiralis* and some were found attached to the nematode (Bruce and Parrott, unpublished observations). Owen *et al.* (1979) have found similar clusters of lymphocytes also in scanning electronmicrograph studies in mice infected with *Giardia muris* often attached to the trophozoites. To date, there is little evidence of the extent of this migration in uninfected animals or whether any lymphocytes are retrieved from the faecal stream. It may be that lymphocytes do migrate normally into the gut lumen as they do into the alveolar air space and into colostrum and milk (Smith and Goldman, 1968; Diaz-Jounanen and Williams, 1974), but only in detectable numbers when the appropriate antigenic stimulus is present.

5.3.2.9 The source of effector cells at sites other than the small intestine – a common mucosal traffic system

The extensive studies on cell traffic from Peyer's patches *via* mesenteric node and thoracic duct lymph to the lamina propria of the small intestine are in marked contrast to the comparative lack of interest which cell 'traffickers' have taken in the mechanisms by which the lamina propria of the rest of the gastrointestinal tract is populated, despite the obvious clinical importance of such studies, for example, to the understanding of the immunology of dental caries, the pathological processes of inflammatory bowel disease, the response to parasitic infections of the stomach, liver, large bowel, and caecum, and the incidence of carcinoma of the stomach and colon (for a discussion of this latter problem see de Sousa and Good, 1978). There is circumstantial evidence from studies on the reduced response to Salk vaccine in subjects after tonsillectomy (Ogra, 1971) that the tonsils may serve to populate the upper gastrointestinal tract with immunoglobulin-producing cells. There are indications that cells from the mesenteric nodes can be 'persuaded' to enter the colon in secondary infections with *T. spiralis* (Parrott and Rose, 1978). There are hints from the experiments of Pierce and Gowans (1975) showing that chronic thoracic duct drainage, although substantially reducing the numbers of antibody-forming cells in jejunum and ileum, nevertheless does not affect the numbers in the colon, indicating that cells *en route* to the colon must travel by a different route than those bound for the small intestine. But these casual observations merely highlight our general ignorance. Our comparative lack of 'hard' evidence is obvious when one faces the problem of the sources of other cellular populations in other mucosal surfaces. Rudzik *et al.* (1975) made the important observation that cells from BALT (bronchus associated epithelial tissue), after transfer into irradiated rabbits, would repopulate after an interval of 6 days not only the lungs with IgA-producing cells, but also the lamina propria of the gut; and that the Peyer's patch tissue would, as was shown earlier by Craig and Cebra (1971), not only populate the lamina propria of the intestine, but also contribute IgA-producing cells to the bronchial tree. As a consequence of these experiments they suggested that there might be a 'common mucosal immunologic system' (Bienenstock *et al.*, 1978). Several studies have shown that either oral or inhalation immunization has given rise to antibody at remote sites, suggesting that the cells have migrated, either from the small bowel or the lungs, into the glandular tissue concerned. Montgomery *et al.* (1978) showed that secretory IgA antibodies appear in saliva and milk as well as in bronchial and intestinal fluids of rabbits immunized by an endotrachial or gastric intubation with DNP–BGG or DNP–KLH. Mestecky *et al.* (1978) found S-IgA antibody in the saliva and lacrimal secretions of humans fed with *S. mutans* antigen. Specific IgA antibodies were demonstrated in the milk of humans infected with *S. typhimurium* (Allardyce *et al.*, 1974) and, more significantly, IgA antibody-producing cells were detected in the colostrum and milk of lactating women orally immunized with *E. coli* (Goldblum *et al.*, 1975). The experiments of Lamm and co-workers using radiolabelled mesenteric lymph node cells and combined immunofluorescent and autoradiographic analysis in mice showed that radiolabelled IgA-containing cells appeared in breast tissues in increasing numbers after parturition, confirming the gut–mammary gland association; similar autoradiographic studies in mice (Bienenstock *et al.*, 1978) using [^{3}H]-thymidine-labelled mesenteric node cells, which were found in significant numbers in lungs, cervix, vagina, and uterus, as well as in the small intestine and mammary glands, emphasize the possibility of cell seeding as the method whereby a common mucosal system could probably function. Attractive as this theory is, some degree of reservation and caution should be exercised. However, one of the most valuable functions of an attractive theory is that it should promote further experimentation as this has done – if only to prove it false.

The observation that IgA is selectively transported from plasma into biliary secretions at a rapid rate (Lemaitre-Coelho et al., 1978) has disturbed the original concept since it provides a ready explanation for those experiments which did not look for the presence of antibody. It may be that the ability to transport secretory immunoglobulin from the blood to the luminal side of mucosa is a general property of all mucosal surfaces. Montgomery et al. (1977) have already shown that there is selective transport of dimeric IgA into the saliva in dogs. Such a mechanism would readily explain the presence of antibody in, for example, lachrymal and salivary glands and the uterus in the absence of more than a trivial number of immunoglobulin-secreting cells.

Moreover, most cell traffic studies do not provide evidence which supports the common mucosal theory. Thus the amount of radioactivity in lungs, salivary glands, lachrymal gland, and uterus after the injection of ^{125}IUdR-labelled gut-destined blasts is normally very small in comparison with that in the intestine even when allowances are made for the differences in size and weight of tissue (Sprent, 1967; Hall et al., 1977; Rannie and Donald, 1977) and is not significantly higher than other extralymphoidal tissue. Quantitative assessment by means of autoradiography is especially open to error when the numbers of labelled cells found are small relative to the numbers and areas of sections to be scanned. Guy-Grand et al. (1974) found no [^{3}H]-thymidine-labelled mesenteric lymph node or TDL cells in tracheal, bronchial mucosa or salivary glands of mice; it should be noted, however, that they did not find any significant numbers of recipient IgA-forming cells in these locations. Rannie and Donald (1977) found variable numbers of [^{3}H]- or [^{14}C]-thymidine-labelled TD cells in all tissues of rats examined including non-lymphoid and non-mucosal, indicating that following injection of a bolus of blast cells, most of which have little capacity for recirculation but considerable capacity for extravasation, small proportions of them will lodge wherever they happen to be when they have differentiated beyond their blast-like and mobile form. All these findings contrast with those of Bienenstock et al. (1978) and Bienenstock et al. (1979) who, after transfer of [^{3}H]-thymidine-labelled mesenteric blast cells, found significant numbers in lungs, bronchial mucosa, uterus, and cervix, as well as in the small intestine. Some of these differences in results between different groups could be due to variations in the environmental antigenic load to which different animal colonies are submitted or to differences in technique, but there is little doubt that there are discrepant findings between different groups of workers, some of which are doubtless due to lack of appreciation of the limitations of technique and method. There are numerous circumstances in which large numbers of labelled cells may be found in such a large capillary bed as the lungs without there being any indication or interpretation of 'homing', merely that transit is slow or delayed.

One agreed site in which cell traffic experiments have confirmed that cells primed against gut antigens do lodge appears to be the mammary gland (Roux et al., 1977; Love and Ogilvie, 1977; Rose et al., 1978).

Chapter 6
Lymphocyte Traffic in Disease

6.1 LYMPHOCYTE TRAFFIC IN EXPERIMENTAL MODELS OF DISEASE

There are few studies of lymphocyte recirculation in experimental models of disease. These few studies, however, are of considerable importance because, by virtue of the experimental nature of the work, it is possible to analyse more than one component of the recirculating system simultaneously. For instance, in the most extensive of these studies (Bullock, 1976a,b) of lymphocyte circulation in chronic infection with *M. lepremurium* in rats (Section 6.1.4) it is clearly demonstrated that failure of the lymphocytes to circulate to the thoracic duct lymph is due to their progressive sequestration in the spleen, with progression of the infection. This is the study closer to clinical situations where lymphocyte sequestration might occur in a lymphoid organ with deceptive peripheral lymphocytopenias and immunodeficiency (see Section 6.2).

6.1.1 Thymic aplasia

Studies of the migration of ^{51}Cr-labelled lymph node, thymus and bone marrow cells from Balb/c-*nu* lymphoid donors in congenitally athymic nude recipients demonstrated that the donro cells distributed in reduced percentages to the spleen, lymph nodes, bone marrow, and small intestine of the nude mice when compared to the distribution in normal recipients (Gillette, 1975). These differences did not appear to be the result of lack of the thymus *per se*, since in control experiments designed to investigate the migration of the cell populations in mice that had been irradiated and thymectomized (B mice), no differences were observed between the distribution of the labelled cells in control and B mice. Further control experiments were done to control the possibility that histocompatibility differences between the injected Balb/c-*nu* cells and the *nunu* recipients might be responsible for the modified lymphoid cell migration in nude recipients (Gillette, 1975). The data indicated that H-2 antigens were not major factors in determining the behaviour of Balb/c-*nu* cells in nude recipients.

It was concluded from the results of these experiments that elements within the lymph nodes required for normal migration of recirculating lymphocytes are probably absent in lymph nodes and spleens of nude mice. The nature of these elements remains obscure, however. Regretfully, no data were available regarding the distribution of the labelled cells to the lung, where the cells might have been 'trapped'. Only a few of the cells were trapped in the lung, and the reasons why that might have occurred remain unclear.

These experiments illustrate well, however, the importance of multiple component analysis in studies of this kind; the results may be relevant to recent findings on the distribution of immunologically competent cells in cases of congenital immunodeficiency in man.

6.1.2 Autoimmunity

Studies of the patterns of migration of ^{51}Cr-labelled lymph node and spleen cells from NZB mice aged 1, 2, 3, 5 and 12 months have shown that in the 3 month-old spleen there is a decline in the proportion of recirculating cells, and that between 5 and 12 months there is a corresponding decrease in the percentage of recirculating cells in lymph nodes (Zatz *et al.*, 1971). The change in the relative numbers of recirculating and non-recirculating subpopulations in the 3 month-old spleen precedes the reported onset of the autoimmune haemolytic anaemia; in the lymph node, it parallels the development of the autoimmune process.

The reduction in the proportion of recirculating lymphocytes in the lymphoid organs of NZB mice at the same time that the autoimmune haemolytic anaemia develops may reflect the change known to occur in the balance of T and B cell populations in the lymphoid organs of mice from this strain (East *et al.*, 1965; Cantor *et al.*, 1978).

In addition, one of the pathological features of NZB mice is the accumulation of lymphoid cells in non-lymphoid organs such as the lung and the liver. It has been suggested that the progressive accumulation of recirculating cells in the 'wrong place' (ecotaxopathy) could lead to depletion of the immunologically competent cells from the lymphoid organs and to the anomalies of immunological function known to occur in this strain of mice (de Sousa, 1978a). Recent work from Cantor and co-workers (Cantor *et al.*, 1978) has shown that there are imbalances of T cell sets in the spleens of NZB mice (Fig. 6.1). It is not known whether the imbalances found in one lymphoid organ reflect the existence of a similar imbalance in the total lymphoid population or whether they result from the selective redistribution of some lymphoid cell sets in non-lymphoid sites. It seems necessary to reexamine many of the results of the early experiments using the new tools available for selection of lymphoid cell sets, to determine whether abnormalities of circulation of selected cells sets can be related to the development of autoimmunity and to other abnormalities of immunological function concurring with the autoimmune disease.

Recently, hepatic lesions of an autoimmune type, characterized by lymphocyte infiltration and destruction of endothelial and fat storage cells, have been induced experimentally in the mouse by repeated injections of neuraminidase-treated spleen lymphoid cells (Kolb-Bachofen and Kolb, 1979). As mentioned earlier,

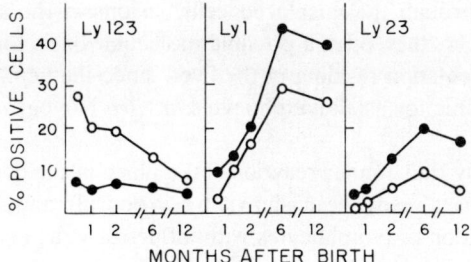

Figure 6.1 The ontogeny of Ly T cells sets in the spleen of NZB (●──●) and Balb/c (O──O) mice. Modified from Cantor et al. (1978)

asialolymphocytes fail to circulate normally and a small proportion persists in the liver, probably as the result of stereo-specific interactions between a D-galactose recognizing lectin-like receptor on liver cells and β-D-galactose residues uncovered by the neuraminidase treatment (Chapter 4.5). In a light microscopy and ultrastructural analysis of the changes taking place in the liver, following five weekly injections of asialolymphocytes, Kolb-Bachofen and Kolb (1979) demonstrated the persistence of infiltrating lymphocytes in the liver (Table 6.1) in close contact with hepatocytes after having destroyed capillary structures (Plate 19). Contact to hepatocytes occurred by extending lymphocytic microvilli into invaginations of liver cells (Plate 19, 3c), whereas hepatic microvilli that formerly extruded into the space of Disse were retracted (Plate 19).

These observations constitute a significant contribution to the field of the pathology of lymphocyte maldistribution; they illustrate for the first time in an experimental model how factors modifying normal lymphocyte migration can

Table 6.1 Autoimmune reactions against liver cells after injection of syngeneic asialolymphocytes. Data from Kolb-Bachofen and Kolb (1979)

Lymphocytes (no. of cells)	Neuraminidase treatment	No. of cell transfers*	No. of recipients	Autoimmune lesions in liver
Spleen (2×10^7)	−	5	4	− (c)
Spleen (2×10^7)	+	5	4	+++ (a)
Spleen (2×10^7)	−	1	4	− (c)
Spleen (2×10^7)	+	1	4	++ (b)

*Recipients received lymphocytes once weekly; animals were sacrificed 7 days later.
(a) Numerous lymphocytes were found infiltrating into the organ after having destroyed cápillary structures locally.
(b) Many lymphocytes were found in the capillary lumen adhering to sinusoidal lining cells. Some lymphocytes had destroyed endothelial cells and were in close contact with hepatocytes.
(c) No sign of lymphocytic infiltrations.

cause, indirectly, through the misplaced cells, lesions at the site of lymphocyte infiltration. Moreover, they offer a possible molecular basis for the expansion of the lymphocyte population residing in the liver, since the hepatic lectin has been shown to be mitogenic for asialolymphocytes *in vitro* Novogrodsky and Ashwell, 1977).

Finally, it is likely that similar reactions take place in the course of viral infections *in vivo*; it has already been shown by Woodruff and Woodruff (1976a, 1976b) that incubation of lymphocytes with influenza virus or Newcastle disease viruses (NDV) leads to desyalylation and to similar abnormalities of distribution of the virus-exposed cells (see below).

6.1.3 Newcastle disease virus infection

The size of the recirculating pool of lymphocytes decreases markedly in mice and rats challenged with Newcastle disease virus (Woodruff and Woodruff, 1972). In a study of the effect of virus inoculation on the distribution of [^{51}Cr]-labelled thoracic duct lymphocytes in the rat, Woodruff and Woodruff demonstrated that inoculation of a dose of 10_{50} NDV immediately after infusion of the labelled cells significantly reduced the 2 hr recovery of radioactivity from the lymph nodes of the recipients, without influencing recovering from the other compartments examined, namely lymph nodes, spleen, liver or lungs. When the virus was administered 4 hr before cell transfer, there was a significant decrease in lymph node recovery with a concomitant increase in spleen recovery. This effect was transient, and by 48 hr after cell transfer recovery of radioactivity in the lymph nodes of the virus-inoculated animals had increased and was not significantly different from recovery in the lymph nodes of control animals.

The exact mechanisms by which NDV challenge alters the circulation of lymphocytes is not known. Woodruff and Woodruff suggested that the virus may act directly on the lymphocytes since these cells have receptors for NDV (Woodruff and Woodruff, 1972). Moreover, in further studies of the fate of TDL inoculated *in vitro* with NDV (Woodruff and Woodruff, 1972), it was shown that the labelled cells behaved in a manner similar to that of labelled lymphocytes treated *in vitro* with neuraminidase (see Chapter 4.5 and section above).

It must be emphasized that the perturbation of lymphocytes caused by viral treatment was transient and by 48 hr the migratory pattern to the lymph nodes of virus-inoculated recipients was not significantly different from that in controls. This recovery probably depends on regeneration of lymphocyte surface components.

6.1.4 Murine leprosy

In a series of careful studies of the recirculation of lymphocytes in rats infected with *M. lepremurium*, Bullock (Bullock, 1976a,b) demonstrated that in the infected animals there is a significant decrease in cell output from the thoracic duct and an impairment of the recirculation of ^{51}Cr-labelled TDL from uninfected syngeneic donors (Fig. 6.2) infused intravenously. The failure of lymphocytes to recirculate normally did not seem to be due to factors in the serum of the infected rats. The recirculation of labelled cells from infected animals infused into uninfected recipients that received serum injections prior to the infusion period was similar to the recirculation of labelled cells from infected rats into recipients that had not received serum, and in both cases the results were not significantly different from the recirculation pattern of normal cells.

In additional experiments to determine whether the inoculation of large numbers of killed organisms caused an impairment of lymphocyte traffic, it was found that in rats infected with killed microorganisms the amount of radioactivity recovered in the thoracic duct lymph was 20–30% below control levels. This effect appears to be minimal in contrast to the considerable magnitude of the disturbance of lymphocyte traffic induced by the inoculation of living organisms. To determine the nature of the defect, Bullock examined the distribution of the radioactivity in the organs of the recipients (Bullock, 1976b). Significantly higher numbers of labelled cells were recovered from the spleens of the infected rats than from control rats (Table 6.2). Moreover, splenectomy increased the number of cells in the blood (Fig. 6.3) and the lymph nodes. In the absence of the spleen, there was a compensatory hepatic uptake of labelled TDL. The retention of labelled cells in the spleen was not due simply to hypersplenism, since labelled TDL recirculated normally in rats rendered splenomegalic by repeated injections of methyl cellulose intraperitoneally for 12 weeks prior to infusion.

The sequestration of recirculating lymphocytes in this form of chronic infection

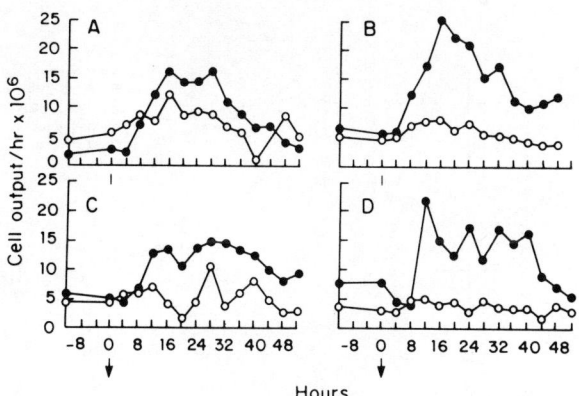

Figure 6.2 Abnormal lymphocyte recirculation in murine leprosy. Cell output in thoracic duct lymph after intravenous administration of syngeneic TDL to four matched pairs of control (●——●) and infected (O——O) rats. Preparatory reduction in cell output before cell infusion at time 0 (↓) achieved by TD fistulization in day 3. Cell output/hr x 10^6 estimated from 4 hr collection intervals. Slightly modified from Bullock (1976a)

Table 6.2 Radioactivity recovered from sham splenectomized rats*

| | Time after ^{51}CrTDL infusion | | | |
| | 12 hr | | 24 hr | |
Organ/fluid	Normal	Infected†	Normal	Infected†
Blood	1.1 ± 0.1	0.9 ± 0.2	1.5 ± 0.3	1.0 ± 0.2
Nodes				
Total	2.8 ± 0.26	1.6 ± 0.26	4.2 ± 0.3	3.0 ± 0.0
Cervical	0.3 ± 0.03	0.3 ± 0.02	0.6 ± 0.04	0.5 ± 0.04
Axillary	0.4 ± 0.06	0.2 ± 0.06	0.6 ± 0.06	0.4 ± 0.08
Abdominal	0.2 ± 0.03	0.1 ± 0.04	0.3 ± 0.07	0.2 ± 0.09
Spleen	21.3 ± 0.5	25.9 ± 1.0	14.9 ± 1.0	24.2 ± 0.77
Liver	14.2 ± 0.4	17.1 ± 0.6	9.1 ± 0.5	14.3 ± 6.0
Urine	3.7 ± 0.3	4.7 ± 1.0	7.7 ± 0.3	9.8 ± 4.0

*Mean of three experiments. Data from Bullock (1976b).
†Each animal was injected intravenously with 0.6 ml of an inoculum containing 1×10^9 *M. lepremurium* microorganisms. Rats killed at 18 weeks of infection.

differed from the non-specific 'lymphocyte trapping' seen after antigen administration (see Chapter 4.4) in several respects. In the antigen model the so-called lymphocyte trapping can be detected within hours after antigen administration but it is transient, disappearing within hours. By contrast, the lymphocyte sequestration observed in *M. lepremurium* infection is of much slower onset (2–6 weeks post infection), is far more marked, and appears to persist throughout the course of infection.

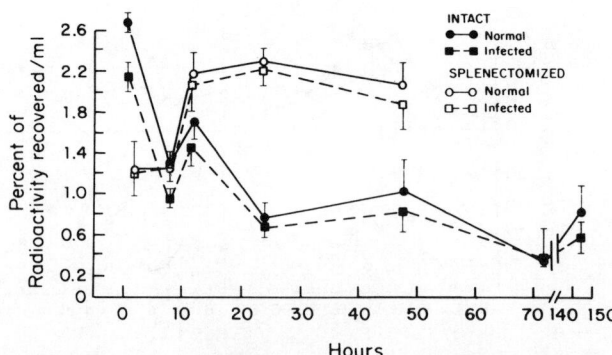

Figure 6.3 Effect of splenectomy on radioactivity recovered from peripheral blood after infusion of ^{51}Cr-labelled TDL. Samples were obtained from intact rats, normal or infected, at 1, 2, 8, 12, 24, 48, 72, and 145 hr; from splenectomized rats, normal or infected, at 2, 8, 12, 24, and 48 hr. Symbols represent mean data of three experiments. Splenectomy increased also the amount of radioactivity recovered from the lymph nodes of infected rats. Slightly modified from Bullock (1976b)

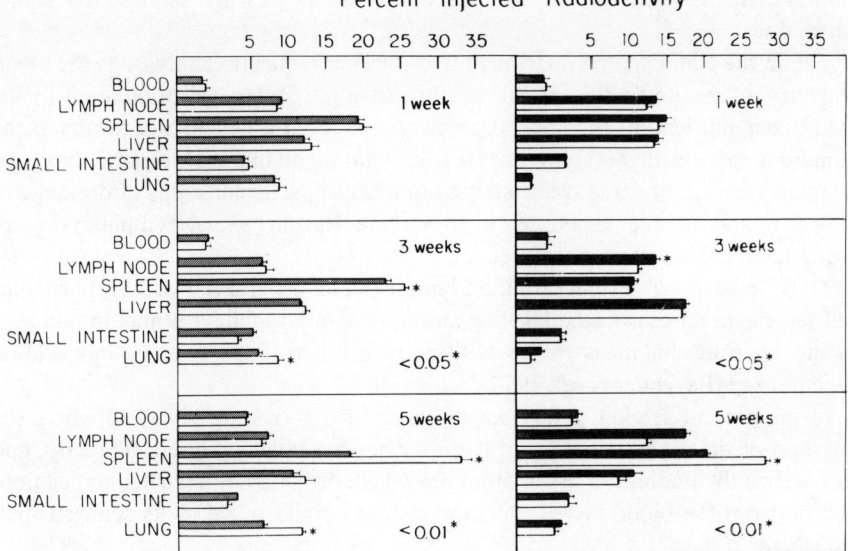

Figure 6.4 Changes in distribution of ^{51}Cr mouse lymph node cells in syngeneic recipients treated with subcutaneous injections of Fe-citrate (totalling 1.5 mg per week). The two separate sets of bars represent two separate experiments. Each bar represents the mean of 4–8 animals (+1 SD) for group of control (■) or Fe-citrate (□) treated mice. The most consistent, statistically significant (*) result was the finding of splenic sequestration of the transferred cells in mice that had received iron for 5 weeks

6.1.5 Iron overload

Following the suggestion that iron and iron-binding proteins participate in the mechanism of lymphoid cell maldistribution (de Sousa, Smithyman and Tan 1978), we examined patients with iron overload due to thalassemia intermedia and found imbalances of T cell subsets in the peripheral blood (Kapadia et al., 1980). In addition, we have also examined the effect of experimental iron overload in mice on the distribution of ^{51}Cr-labelled lymph node cells. At 5 weeks of treatment with daily injections of Fe-citrate, a significant spleen sequestration of the labelled cells was observed (Fig. 6.4).

6.2 LYMPHOCYTE MALDISTRIBUTION SYNDROMES (ECOTAXOPATHIES) IN MAN

The facts of direct relevance and possible application to the analysis of clinical problems were those described in the previous section relating to the circulation of lymphocytes in experimental models of disease. Although few experiments have been undertaken with clinical problems in mind, those that have been done illustrate well the fact that lack of lymphocytes in one compartment of the recirculatory pathway does not signify exclusively an absolute absence of lymphocytes but generally it signifies that lymphocytes are sequestered somewhere else.

Yet, in the clinic, the compartment that is more frequently analysed is the blood and very often the finding of the absence of a particular cell population in the blood does not lead to the question: where else could it be? As the results of the numerous experiments on lymphocyte traffic during an immune response indicate, lymphocytes can be mobilized in large numbers to particular areas of drainage of antigens, and as the experiments on murine leprosy show, lymphocytes are sequestered at sites of chronic infection.

Thus, in cases of peripheral blood lymphopenia, generalized or of a particular cell set, the practice of radiolabelling and tracing of lymphocytes may in fact lead to the accurate diagnosis of the position of a lesion. Such practice has seldom been utilized (Lavender *et al.*, 1977).

In the present section, a number of clinical situations are reviewed where the question of the maldistribution of lymphocytes has been analysed indirectly, and summarize the findings in other situations where depletion of a particular cell population from the blood is well documented and could relate to its sequestration elsewhere.

The term ecotaxopathy has been suggested to define syndromes of lymphocyte maldistribution (de Sousa, 1978a).

6.2.1 Hodgkin's disease

Hodgkin's disease is a progressive disorder of the lymphoid system often accompanied by lymphopenia and deficits of cell-mediated immunity (Hansen and

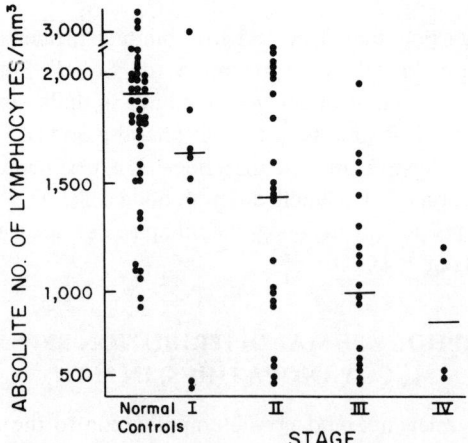

Figure 6.5 Relationship of absolute lymphocyte count to stage of disease in a group of adult patients with Hodgkin's disease. (Mean count for controls: 1,912/mm³.) Data from Case *et al.* (1976)

Good, 1974; Kaplan, 1976). Early findings of low numbers of peripheral blood T lymphocytes in patients with HD which were used to explain that deficiency (Jondal et al., 1972) were not confirmed; in adults, however, a progressive blood lymphopenia parallels progression of the disease (Young et al., 1972; Case et al., 1976) (Fig. 6.5).

Does a blood lymphopenia reflect an absolute decrease in numbers of circulating lymphocytes or simply their sequestration in some other tissue compartment?

With the advent of splenectomy as part of the staging procedure of the disease, it became possible to answer this question with some precision. From studies of peripheral blood and spleen both in children (de Sousa et al., 1977; de Sousa et al., 1978) and in adults (Kaur et al., 1974; Matchett et al., 1973; Payne et al., 1976), it became apparent that unusually high numbers of T cells are present in spleen of patients with HD, with simultaneous peripheral blood depletions. Differences in immunological function of peripheral blood and spleen cell populations were also detected. Thus, after stimulation with non-specific mitogens, peripheral blood lymphocytes from patients with Hodgkin's disease generally fail to respond to PHA, whilst spleen cells from the same patient respond normally to stimulation by the same mitogen (Fig. 6.6).

This dichotomy in mitogen responses of peripheral blood and spleen cell responses was interpreted as the result of a possible maldistribution of one particular T cell subset (Moretta et al., 1976). More recently, Gupta and Tan (1980), in a study of distribution of T lymphocyte subsets in the peripheral blood

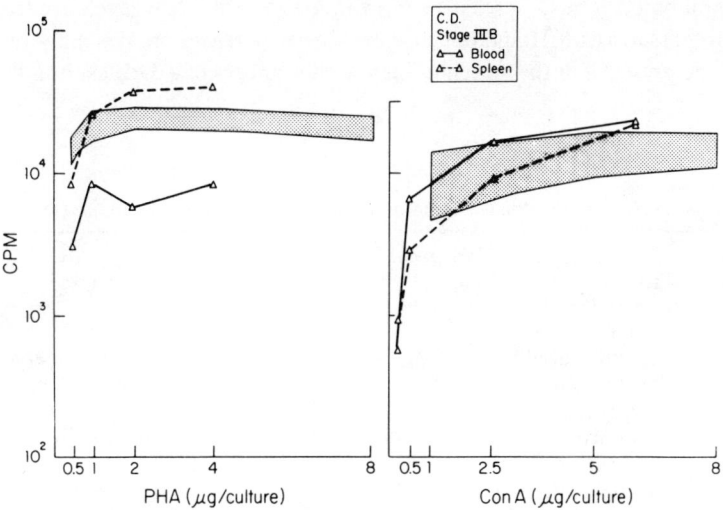

Figure 6.6 Representative example of the differences observed between peripheral blood and splenic lymphocyte responses to PHA and Con A in untreated Hodgkin's disease. Although in this case (Stage IIIB) the spleen was involved, similar differences are observed in uninvolved spleens. Data from Tan et al. (1978)

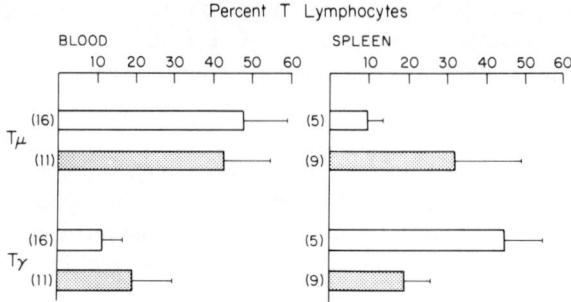

Figure 6.7 Comparative analysis of distribution of Tμ and Tγ cells in control (□) and Hodgkin's disease (▨) blood and spleen. Results expressed as per cent of T lymphocytes. Data from Gupta and Tan (1980)

and spleen of children with Hodgkin's disease, have found that the majority of E-rosette forming cells present in the spleen belong to the T 'IgM' cell subset, namely Tμ cells (Fig. 6.7). Concomitant depletions of the same T cell subsets occurred in the peripheral blood of the same patients. A similar imbalance of Tμ and Tγ cell populations in the peripheral blood of Hodgkin's disease patients was reported earlier by Romagnani et al. (1978). A summary of the results from the two groups is presented in Table 6.3.

The finding of an imbalance of T cell subsets in the spleen and blood may have functional implications other than the failure of some immunological responses in peripheral blood. Thus, increased serum IgG and serum IgA levels are frequently found in patients with Hodgkin's disease. These increases are probably the reflection of the presence in the spleen of increased numbers of a T cell subset known to

Table 6.3 Maldistribution of T cell subsets in Hodgkin's Disease

Cell set or subset	Group	Peripheral blood	Spleen	Reference
ERFC	HD		67.5 ± 10.5	Gupta & Tan* (1980)
Tμ	HD untreated	23.4 ± 3.4	ND	Romagnani et al. (1978)
	HD treated	17.8 ± 2	ND	
	Control	37.5 ± 1.4	ND	
	HD untreated	43.0 ± 12	32 ± 17	Gupta & Tan (1980)
	Control	48 ± 11	10 ± 4	
Tγ	HD untreated	16.9 ± 2	ND	Romagnani et al. (1978)
	HD treated	18 ± 1.7	ND	
	Controls	10.3 ± 0.7		
	HD untreated	20 ± 10	19 ± 7	Gupta & Tan (1980)
	Controls	12 ± 5	45 ± 10	Gupta & Tan (1980)

*Control 35 ± 8.

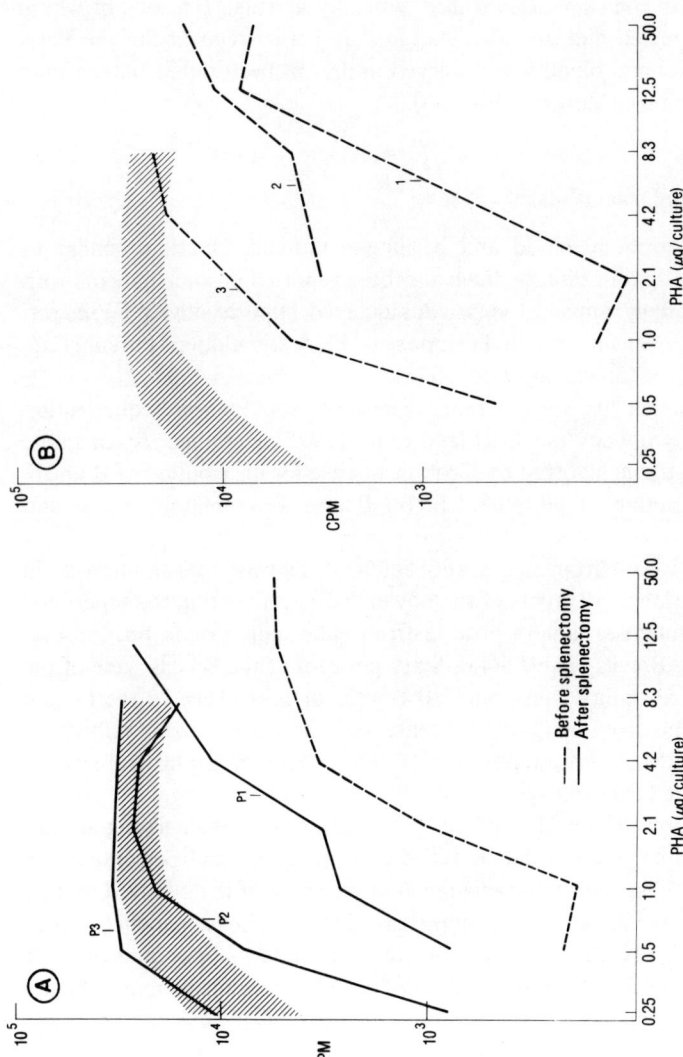

Figure 6.8 Effect of splenectomy on the PHA response. PHA dose response curves of peripheral blood lymphocytes from two Hodgkin's disease children of same sex (M), age (5 years), clinical stage (IA), and histopathology (lymphocyte predominant). Both patients received radiotherapy (4,000 rad) confined to a small area of the neck (irradiated field of 10 cm^2 over the area involved by the disease). Note that recovery of the response to values within the control range (shaded area: mean ± 1 SD) occurred more rapidly in the splenectomized patient (A). A-dose response curve prior to splenectomy and therapy and at 2 (P1), 14 (P2) and 18 (P3) months after diagnosis. B-dose response in non-splenectomized patient at 9 (1), 13(2) and 22(3) months after diagnosis. Data from de Sousa, Smithyman, and Tan, (1978)

participate in regulation of immunoglobulin synthesis by B cells (Moretta *et al.*, 1977).

Finally, if an organ is acting as a site of sequestration of immunologically competent lymphocytes, function should return to normal after removal of the sequestering organ. In a comparison of the PHA responses between two childhood patients of the same age, staged clinically as stage I-A, one of whom had been splenectomized and the other had not, an earlier recovery of the PHA response in the peripheral blood was observed in the splenectomized patient than in the non-splenectomized 'control' (Fig. 6.8).

6.2.2 Gastrointestinal tract disease

Abnormalities of peripheral blood and peripheral immune function, similar to those reported in Hodgkin's disease, have also been reported in some patients with Crohn's disease, namely impaired cutaneous delayed hyposensitivity (Williams, 1965; Jones *et al.*, 1969) and impaired response to PHA stimulation (Parent *et al.*, 1971; Guillou *et al.*, 1973; Sachar *et al.*, 1973).

To determine whether the bowel lesions themselves could act as sequestration sites of circulating lymphocytes, Strickland *et al.* (1975) examined frozen tissue sections of resected tissue involved by Crohn's disease for distribution of B and T cells and the distribution of peripheral blood B and T lymphocytes pre- and postoperatively.

In tissue sections both from ileum and colon, there was a clear increase in lymphocytic infiltration in all layers of the bowel wall except within the superficial epithelium. In the mucosal lamina propria from either colon or ileum, the predominant cells were B cells (Table 6.4a). Sixty per cent of the B cells were of the IgG class, 30% were of IgA class, and 10% were of IgM class. In the lamina propria of intestine involved by Crohn's disease, only 25–30% of the lymphocytes were T cells. In the deeper layers, however, T cells accounted for 60–70% of the lymphocytic infiltrate (Table 6.4a).

If indeed the sections of bowel involved by Crohn's disease were acting as sites of T cell ecotaxopathy, this should be reflected in numbers and percentages of peripheral blood T cells, and should change after resection of the involved section of the bowel. This was indeed the case in the two Crohn's disease patients studied by Strickland *et al.* (1975). Thus, at the time of surgery, both patients had decreased proportions and absolute numbers of T cells, while the proportions and numbers of B cells remained within the normal range (Table 6.4b). Two to six months after surgery, T cell proportions and numbers returned to normal; B cell values remained normal. These results indicate that there is indeed a clearcut T cell maldistribution in Crohn's disease.

In a separate study of the faecal recovery of autotransfused [^{51}Cr]-labelled peripheral blood lymphocytes in patients with Crohn's disease and seven patients with untreated coeliac disease, Douglas *et al.* (1976) found substantial higher faecal loss of radioactivity in the patients' groups than in nine normal subjects (Fig. 6.9).

Table 6.4a Lymphocyte populations in resected bowel from patients with Crohn's Disease. Data from Strickland et al. (1975)

Specimen	Mucosal lamina propria			Submucosa and muscularis		
	Degree of lymphocyte infiltration	B cells (%)	T cells (%)	Degree of lymphocyte infiltration	B cells (%)	T cells (%)
Crohn's colitis	Severe	70	30	Severe	40	60
Crohn's colitis	Severe	75	25	Severe	30	70
Control colon or ilieum	Moderate	50	50	Mild or absent	70	30

Table 6.4b Peripheral blood lymphocytes in two patients with Crohn's Disease before and after intestinal resection. Data from Strickland et al. (1975)

Cell set	Patient 1		Patient 2		Normal controls (means ± 1 SD)
	Preoperative	Postoperative	Preoperative	Postoperative	
T cells					
%	42	66	19	59	64 ± 11
No. (cells/mm^3)	570	1,815	481	1,273	1,629 ± 546
B cells					
%	12	14	17	7	13 ± 5
No. (cells/mm^3)	163	385	430	151	334 ± 202

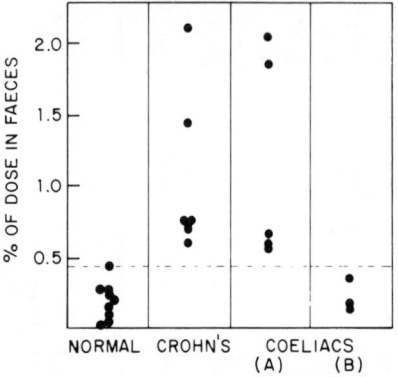

Figure 6.9 Five-day faecal excretion of ^{51}Cr in normal subjects or in subjects with Crohn's disease and untreated coeliac disease (A). The coeliac patients in remission (B) on a gluten-free diet did not differ from normal. – – – – upper limit of normal. Slightly modified from Douglas et al. (1976)

By contrast, faecal loss was comparable to the control subjects in three coeliac patients in remission on a gluten-free diet (Fig. 6.9). In addition, measurements of distribution of radioactivity were made using an external counter. In contrast to normals, where counts steadily decreased over the week following administration of the labelled cells, in all patients studied an increasing amount of radioactivity was recorded over the umbilicus.

6.2.3 Chronic liver disease

Studies of peripheral blood lymphocyte populations have demonstrated decreased T lymphocyte concentrations in alcohol-related liver disease (Bernstein et al., 1974; Thomas et al., 1976), in lupoid and hepatitis B virus induced chronic liver disease (De Horatius et al., 1974; Thomas et al., 1976), and in primary biliary cirrhosis (Thomas et al., 1976). Although these decreases occur concomitantly with per cent increases in 'null' cells, and the changes may be related to the presence of serum inhibitors influencing rosette formation (Chisari and Edgington, 1975), imbalances of peripheral blood and liver lymphocyte distribution have been demonstrated in cases in which lymphocytes were isolated from both sources in individual patients (Sanchez-Tapias et al., 1977).

Isolated cells separated from liver specimens obtained by aspiration needle biopsy were identified by E-, AE- or H-rosetting, by myeloperoxidase staining, and by morphological examination. The characteristic staining and rosetting features of each cell type are summarized in Table 6.5. The results of the comparison of lymphocyte populations found in liver and peripheral blood in a number of chronic liver diseases are summarized in Table 6.6.

Table 6.5 Method of identification of cells isolated from liver tissue (Sanchez-Tapias et al., 1977)

Cell type	Morphology	E-rosetting	EA-rosetting	H-*rosetting	Peroxidase
Hepatocytes	+	−	+	−	−
T lymphocytes	−	+	−	−	−
Activated T lymphocytes	−	+	−	+	−
B lymphocytes	−	−	+	−	−
K lymphocytes	−	−	+	−	−
Monocytes	+	−	+	−	+
Granulocytes	+	+ (occasional)	+	−	+

*Activated T cells were identified by their ability to form rosettes with fresh group-O rhesus-negative human erythrocytes (H cells, Sheldon and Holborow, 1975).

The percentage of lymphocytes identified as T cells (E-rosette forming) in liver biopsy specimens was significantly higher than in peripheral blood ($p < 0.0001$) in patients with alcoholic hepatitis and HB_sAg positive and negative chronic active hepatitis. No significant differences were noted between liver and peripheral blood in fatty liver, inactive cirrhosis, chronic persistent hepatitis, and primary biliary cirrhosis (Table 6.6).

The percentage of activated T cells was significantly higher in the liver than in the blood in patients with alcoholic hepatitis, HB_sAg positive and negative chronic hepatitis, and primary biliary cirrhosis. No differences in percentages of activated T cells were found in the other chronic disorders examined, namely patients with fatty liver, inactive alcoholic cirrhosis, and chronic persistent hepatitis.

The finding of activated T cells in the liver in active hepatocellular disease but not in inactive disease raises the possibility that a T cell mediated immune reaction is occurring in the liver of patients with active liver disease. The fact that the percentages of these cells found in the blood of the same patients are within the normal range (Table 6.6) indicates that the process of activation takes place in the liver as high proportions of T cells are presumably exposed to either a mitogenic or a native or denatured antigenic component of the liver or, in the case of hepatitis B virus induced disease, to a viral antigen.

In the case of HB_sAg positive and negative chronic active hepatitis, the percentage of EA-rosette forming cells (B and K lymphocytes) was significantly higher in the liver than in peripheral blood. This was not so in all other groups studied (Table 6.6). Since both B and K lymphocytes participate in antibody mediated cytotoxicity these findings are compatible with the possibility that this is the mechanism operating in the pathogenesis of the disease (Cochrane et al., 1976).

Recent in vitro studies of the mechanism of liver cell cytotoxicity in chronic active hepatitis have shown that preincubation of normal mononuclear cells with serum from CAH patients renders the normal cells cytotoxic. This effect is

Table 6.6 Comparison of lymphocyte populations in liver and peripheral blood (M + SEM). Data from Sanchez-Tapias et al. (1977)

Disease group	No.	%E−RFC			%EA−RFC			%H−RFC		
		Liver	Blood	p value	Liver	Blood	p value	Liver	Blood	p value
Alcohol-induced										
Fatty liver	4	69 ± 4	63 ± 1	NS	30 ± 2	33 ± 1	NS	8 ± 2	3 ± 1	NS
Inactive cirrhosis	4	65 ± 12	40 ± 2	NS	28 ± 8	24 ± 1	NS	7 ± 1	3 ± 1	NS
Hepatitis ± cirrhosis	7	62 ± 1	42 ± 1	<0.001	32 ± 4	28 ± 4	NS	20 ± 2	2 ± 2	<0.001
HB_s + ve hepatitis										
Chronic persistent	6	59 ± 3	70 ± 6	NS	36 ± 6	25 ± 6	NS	5 ± 2	2 ± 1	NS
Chronic active	5	72 ± 4	44 ± 4	<0.001	43 ± 3	30 ± 4	<0.05	26 ± 5	2 ± 1	<0.001
HB_s − ve hepatitis										
Chronic active	7	67 ± 5	48 ± 3	<0.01	40 ± 5	26 ± 2	<0.02	13 ± 5	2 ± 1	<0.05
Cholestasis										
Extrahepatic	5	72 ± 3	—	—	37 ± 8	—	—	11 ± 2	—	—
Drug-induced	3	63 ± 3	—	—	28 ± 1	—	—	6 ± 3	—	—
Primary biliary cirrhosis	4	62 ± 8	56 ± 2	NS	38 ± 10	30 ± 3	NS	29 ± 7	2 ± 1	<0.001
Controls	15	—	65 ± 2	—	—	31 ± 2	—	—	2 ± 1	—

specifically inhibited by addition to the serum of minute amounts of a membrane lipoprotein fraction of human liver, indicating that the majority of the antibody in the serum is directed against antigen determinants on the hepatocyte surface.

Whether cells are activated as they circulate through the liver, or whether antibody-coated cells are selectively sequestered in antigen-rich areas, this is a clear illustration of how lymphocyte maldistribution can occur and participate in the pathogenesis of a disease.

6.2.4 Skin diseases

Diseases characterized by lymphocyte or polymorphonuclear leukocyte infiltrations of the skin, namely mycosis fungoides, Sézary syndrome, lichen planus, and psoriasis, have been studied extensively with regard to characterization of the lymphoid cell type present in the skin and microenvironmental changes occurring in the skin which could account for the abnormal lymphoid or myeloid cell migration to the disease sites.

The techniques used in the above studies range from detection of selected cell populations *in situ* or in suspension to electronmicroscopy and chemotaxis, using skin extracts as chemoattractants.

6.2.4.1 Mycosis fungoides and Sezary syndrome

Most of the work on lymphocyte distribution in skin in man has dealt with mycosis fungoides and Sézary syndrome, diseases characterized by a predominantly lymphoid cell infiltrate of skin. Both from studies based on the mechanical extraction of cells from tissue homogenates (Tan *et al.*, 1975; Lutzner *et al.*, 1975) and from the *in situ* characterization of the cells constituting the cutaneous infiltrates using specific antisera (Schmitt *et al.*, 1979; Chu and MacDonald, 1979), it is clear that the cells infiltrating the skin in these diseases are T cells. Simultaneous analysis of peripheral blood and skin cell populations are rare, but there is one reported Sézary case in the literature (Lutzner *et al.*, 1975) in which exacerbations of the skin lesions occurred with decreases of the peripheral blood lymphocyte count (Fig. 6.10), indicating that there was a redistribution of circulating cells between blood and skin which could be associated with the state of the disease. Studies of the peripheral blood in patients with mycosis fungoides (MacKie *et al.*, 1976; Nordqvist and Kinney, 1976) have shown that MF patients have significantly reduced levels of circulating T cells and a high level of lymphocytes possessing neither marker (null cells). In the study of Nordqvist and Kinney, the finding of high null cell values was associated with stage of the disease; only one of seven patients with Stage II mycosis fungoides had low T cell and high null cell values as compared to five of six patients with such findings in Stages III and IV (Table 6.7).

Assuming that the finding of decreased numbers of circulating T cells reflects the abnormal migration of the same cells to the skin, one obvious question

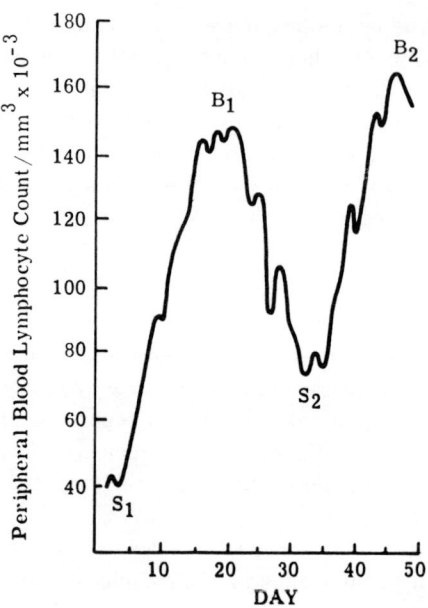

Figure 6.10 Spontaneous cyclic pattern of peripheral blood lymphocyte counts in a patient with mycosis fungoides. At points B_1 and B_2, skin involvement was improved, while cutaneous infiltration was most marked at the points of lower lymphocyte counts (S_1 and S_2). Reproduced from de Sousa (1978a) from original data of Lutzner et al. (1975)

follows: are there other changes in the skin that could be 'responsible' for the selective T cell maldistribution?

As discussed in Chapter 3, an association has been found between particular reticulum cell types and T or B lymphocytes within separate T or B cell areas of the spleen and lymph nodes. The ultrastructure features of the interdigitating reticulum cell found in association with T cells and of the dendritic reticulum found within B cell areas were summarized in Table 3.1. In an investigation of the ultrastructure of the skin of patients with mycosis fungoides, Goos and co-workers (Goos et al., 1976) have found IDC in the skin and speculated whether this finding constituted the morphological basis of T lymphocyte homing to the skin (Plate 20).

More recent studies of the malignant cells in cutaneous T cell lymphomas have focused on the functional characterization of the T cells. Both in patients with overt Sézary syndrome (Border et al., 1976; Siegal and Siegal, 1977) and in patients with aleukaemic cutaneous T cell lymphomas, i.e. mycosis fungoides and

Table 6.7 Rosette forming cells (T cells), lymphocytes with surface immunoglobulins (B cells), and cells without any marker (null cells) in patients with mycosis fungoides and Sézary's syndrome skin test. Reactions to recall antigens and to DNCB in patients with mycosis fungoides and Sézary's syndrome. Data from Nordqvist and Kinney (1976)

Case no.	Stage	Rosette-forming cells (T cells) (%)	Ig pos. cells (B cells) (%)	Null cells (100 − %T + %B) (%)	Skin tests to recall antigens	DNCB challenge
1	II	41	69	−1	Pos.	Pos.
2	II	29	40	31	Neg.	Pos.
3	II	71	30	−1	Pos.	Neg.
4	II	71	31	−2	Pos.	Pos.
5	II	64	25	11	Pos.	Pos.
6	II	68	26	6	Neg.	Neg.
7	II	56	39	5	Neg.	Pos.
8	III	43	29	28	Pos.	Neg.
9	III	44	19	37	Neg.	Neg.
10	III	31	32	36	Neg.	Neg.
11	III	30	14	57	Neg.	Neg.
12	IV	41	25	33	Neg.	Neg.
13	IV	63	30	7	Neg.	Neg.
14	Sézary's syndrome	13	12	75	Neg.	Neg.
15	Sézary's syndrome	33	8	59	Neg.	Neg.
Healthy controls (13)	Mean	61	29	13		
	Range	48–77	17–37	6–20		
Patients with various skin disorders (15)	Mean	64	27	13		
	Range	47–78	16–37	0–18		

Neg., absence of reaction. Pos., reaction to one or more recall antigens.

others not histologically classifiable as mycosis fungoides (Broder et al., 1976), malignant T cells obtained from the peripheral blood in the leukaemic cases, and from involved lymph nodes in the aleukaemic cases, have been shown to have 'helper' function, i.e. to facilitate normal B cell differentiation into immunoglobulin-secreting plasma cells. An illustration of the helper effect of T cells obtained from involved lymph nodes of patients with mycosis fungoides (from Broder et al., 1976) is shown in Fig. 6.11.

In this study, chromosome analysis of the lymph node T cells pointed to the monoclonality of the cells involved, insofar as no normal karyotypes could be detected and all proliferating cells had distinguishing chromosomal abnormalities. When T cell enriched fractions from the patients with cutaneous T cell lymphomas were added to normal B cells, an increase occurred in the numbers of

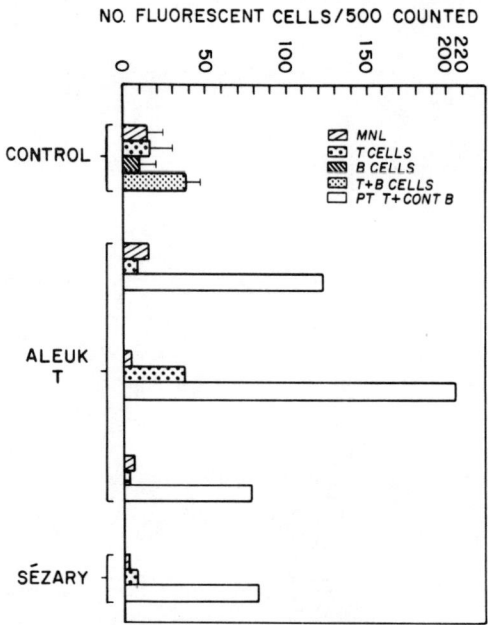

Figure 6.11 Demonstration of helper activity of T cells removed from three patients with aleukaemic cutaneous T cell lymphomas (Aleuk. T) and one patient with Sézary syndrome. The bars in the first group represent the mean numbers of fluorescein-labelled cells detected in the control mononuclear leukocyte (MNL) fractions: number of labelled cells seen after PWM stimulation of unseparated MNL, T and B cell enriched fractions (± 1 SD). White bars represent numbers of fluorescein-labelled cells obtained when neoplassic T cells were co-cultured with control B cells. Slightly modified from Broden et al. (1979)

normal B cells with identifiable intracytoplasmic immunoglobulin exceeding that observed in comparable co-cultures of normal T and B cells (Fig. 6.11).

There were no details of the actual serum immunoglobulin levels in the patients from whom the lymph node cells were removed, and therefore the exact significance of those observations to immunological dysfunction in the patients themselves is not clear from this study.

In our study of peripheral blood lymphocyte sets and serum immunoglobulin levels in patients with mycosis fungoides, we did find statistically significant higher serum levels of IgE in the patient group than in the control group, and higher (but not statistically significant) serum IgA levels in patients with mycosis fungoides (Mackie *et al.*, 1976). More recently (Joyner *et al.*, 1979), a case of T cell cutaneous lymphoma, clinically diagnosed as Sézary syndrome, has been reported in association with an immunoglobulin A type kappa M component monoclonal gammopathy.

6.2.4.2 Other skin diseases: lichen planus and psoriasis

Lichen planus. Studies of the cutaneous infiltrate in lichen planus, using specific anti-T cell antiserum or E-rosette formation on tissue sections (Alario *et al.*, 1978; Bjerke and Krogh, 1978), have also demonstrated that T cells constitute the predominant component of the skin infiltrate.

Psoriasis. Psoriasis is often characterized by an intense inflammatory cell infiltration of the skin, consisting of mononuclear cells and polymorphonuclear leukocytes. Subcorneal microabscesses and spongiform pustules develop, containing neutrophils that have migrated through the epidermis to the subcorneal space.

In vitro studies of the chemotactic activity of extracts of psoriasis scales (Langhof and Muller, 1966; Tagami and Ofugi, 1976; Lazarus *et al.*, 1977; Dahl *et al.*, 1978) have indicated that some component in the scale extract is indeed truly chemotactic for PMN and monocytes (Dahl *et al.*, 1978).

In addition, psoriasis scales were also found to be chemokinetic for PMN. The nature of the chemotactic and chemokinetic component in the extracts remains unknown. Tagami and Ofugi had suggested that the chemotactic activity might be due to a complement component, C3A (Tagami and Ofugi, 1976). Purified C3A, however, has no chemotactic activity for human leukocytes (Fernandez *et al.*, 1978). Many other components in the exfoliated scale could act as chemotactic agents, including factors derived from bacteria known to be present in the lesions (Marples *et al.*, 1973; Aly *et al.*, 1976) or polymorph-derived products resulting from cell death in the lesions.

6.2.5 Connective tissue diseases

One of the pathological and diagnostic features common to all connective tissue disorders is the accumulation of mononuclear cells and plasma cells in non-lymphoid organs. Thus, the histopathology of rheumatoid arthritis (RA) is characterized by a chronic inflammatory reaction of the synovial membrane containing small lymphocytes, polymorphs, plasma cells, and monocyte-like cells. In progressive systemic sclerosis (PSS, scleroderma) perivascular aggregates of lymphocytes are commonly found in skin, synovium, and internal organs; lymphocyte aggregates and plasma cells in the thyroid constitute part of the histopathology of Hashimoto's disease and are found in internal organs of patients with systemic lupus erythematosus (SLE).

Simultaneous studies of peripheral blood and tissue lymphocytes have been carried out in rheumatoid arthritis (Froland et al., 1973; Winchester et al., 1973; Vernon-Roberts et al., 1974; Sheldon et al., 1974; Brenner et al., 1975; van de Putte et al., 1976; Galili et al., 1979) and other forms of arthritis (van de Putte et al., 1976; Galili et al., 1979). A number of studies have focused on possible mechanisms of the peripheral blood lymphocyte depletion (lymphopenia) found in patients with SLE (Williams et al., 1973; Winchester et al., 1974; Winfield et al., 1975; Utsinger, 1976; Scheinberg and Cathcart, 1974; Hamilton and Winfield, 1979).

6.2.5.1 Rheumatoid Arthritis and other forms of arthritis

Studies of the proportions of T and B lymphocytes in peripheral blood and synovial fluid in patients with RA have shown some discrepancies regarding, in particular, the percentages of B cells recovered from the synovial fluid (Table 6.8).

Table 6.8 T and B cells in blood and synovial fluid (SF) of patients with arthritis

Form of arthritis	Percentage of cells				Reference
	T		B		
	Blood	SF	Blood	SF	
Rheumatoid	27.7	30.6			Froland et al. (1973)
	68.8	78.6	18.2	7.9	Sheldon et al. (1974)
		Not specified[a]			Winchester et al. (1973)
	38	49	44	43	Vernon-Roberts et al. (1974)
	69	76	18	16	Brenner et al. (1975)
	66.4	82.4	10.5	1.5	van de Putte et al. (1976)
Non-rheumatoid					
SLE	55	44	17	9	Brenner et al. (1975)
JRA	58	43	20	19	
Group II[b]	65.8	80	9.2	1.8	van de Putte et al. (1976)
Group III[c]	63.5	83.5	9.7	1.2	

[a] 4–23 fold reductions in % B lymphocytes, when compared to blood; up to five fold enrichment of T lymphocytes over levels in blood.
[b] Two cases of psoriatic arthritis, two seronegative JRA, one adult seronegative HLA–B 27 positive polyarthritis, one HLA–B 27 negative sacroilitis and arthritis, one case with polyarthritis, vasculitis, and hypocomplementia.
[c] Three cases of crystal synovitis, two ostearthrosis, two traumatic arthritis, one pigmented villonodular synovitis.

Table 6.9 Mononuclear phagocytes contaminating isolated lymphocyte preparations.* Data from van de Putte et al. (1976)

	PB	SF	p value
Group I (n = 12)	5.2	8.2	NS
Group II (n = 7)	2.0	9.2	<0.05
Group III (n = 8)	6.9	19.9	<0.05
Controls (n = 10)	4.0	–	–

*Percentages of isolated lymphocyte preparations. Mean values calculated by analysis of variance after angular transformation of individual data. PB, peripheral blood; SF, synovial fluid.
Group I: includes rheumatoid arthritis patients.
Group II: arthritis of unknown origin.
Group III: arthritis not immunologically mediated, i.e. crystal synovitis, traumatic arthritis, osteoarthrosis, and pigmented villonodular synovitis.

In all studies the majority of cells present in synovial fluids from rheumatoid or other forms of arthritis were T cells (Table 6.8). In some studies the percentage of T cells in synovial fluid were similar to those in blood (Utsinger, 1975), but in the majority of cases they were higher than in the peripheral blood of the same patients (Froland et al., 1973; Winchester et al., 1973; Sheldon et al., 1974; Vernon-Roberts et al., 1974; Brenner et al., 1975; van de Putte et al., 1976).

The variation in the percentages of B cells found in synovial fluid (Table 6.8) is probably attributable to differences in the surface marker probe used to identify these cells, and also to failure to correct for numbers of monocytes also present in the synovial fluid suspensions. An example of the mononuclear phagocyte contamination of lymphocyte preparations obtained from synovial fluids is shown in Table 6.9 from the work of van de Putte et al. (1976).

In a more recent study of the state of activation of the T cells in synovial fluids and paired peripheral blood, Galili and co-workers (1979) have shown that a large

Table 6.10 Comparison between synovial and blood lymphocytes*

Characteristics	No. of cases tested	Synovial fluid lymphocytes Mean ± SE	Range	Blood lymphocytes Mean ± SE	Range
[^{3}H-] thymidine incorporation (cpm)	10	2,000 ± 488	750–5,200	173 ± 47	60–550
Percentage of stable E-rosettes	27	15 ± 2.4	6–55	0	
Attachment to synovial fluid monocytes†	8	27 ± 4.7	18–42	0	
Attachment to blood monocytes*	8	16 ± 2.3	9–31	0	

*Data from Galili et al. (1979).
†Number of T cells attached to 100 monocytes.

proportion of the T cells in the synovial fluid are activated, as indicated by their capacity to form stable E-rosettes, to attach to synovial fluid and blood monocytes and by a high {^{3}H}-thymidine incorporation (Table 6.10).

As pointed out by van de Putte, 'The meaning of the relative increase of T cells and the relative decrease of B cells in synovial fluid remains speculative, one possibility is that the predominance of T cells in extravascular fluid (Manconi et al., 1978, see also Chapter 5) is an expression of their recirculation pattern' (van de Putte et al., 1976). This possibility will be discussed in greater detail later (Chapter 8).

6.2.5.2 Systemic lupus erythematosus

The question of lymphocyte maldistribution in SLE is largely speculative, since in only one study the simultaneous analysis of T and B cells in peripheral blood and in one other compartment (the joint) was carried out in five SLE patients with joint effusions (Brenner et al., 1975). In this study, the mean percentages of T and B cells in peripheral blood ($55 \pm 11\%$ and $17 \pm 5\%$, respectively) were higher than the corresponding ones found in the synovial fluids ($44 \pm 7\%$ and $9 \pm 4\%$, respectively). The mean percentages of null cells were high both in the synovial fluid (47%) and in the peripheral blood (38%).

Systemic lupus erythematosus is included here, however, because the lymphopenia generally associated with the disease (Scheinberg and Cathcart, 1974) and accentuated during episodes of active disease (Utsinger, 1976) has been the subject of carefully designed prospective studies (Winchester et al., 1974; Winfield et al., 1975; Utsinger, 1976). The results of these studies have demonstrated the existence of a strong correlation between the level of cold reactive antilymphocyte antibodies present in the serum of these patients and the peripheral blood lymphocyte counts in the same patients (Winfield et al., 1975; illustrated in Fig. 6.12). In addition, it has been shown that the total lymphopenia observed in SLE patients is attributable to decreases in peripheral blood T and B lymphocytes (Table 6.11), but the clearcut drops observed during disease activity are due largely to decreases in T cell numbers (Utsinger, 1976; see Table 6.11). This observation prompted the analysis of the specificity of the cytotoxicity of the antibodies for selected T or B subpopulations (Table 6.12, from Utsinger, 1976). Marked cytotoxicity was found for both cell populations. In a study of the nature of the cold reactive antibodies present in SLE it was established that the antibodies are primarily IgM in class (Winfield et al., 1975). More recently, it has become apparent that the anti-T lymphocyte antibodies present in SLE serum are directed against, and capable of detecting, selected T cell subpopulations (Koike et al., 1979; Strelkauskas et al., 1979). It seems likely that in in vivo, the autoantibodies are not acting by direct lymphocytolysis, but perhaps by promoting maldistribution of selected T cell sets, presumably to the liver or spleen. The functional implications of maldistribution of T cell sets to the spleen could become an important part of the further development of autoantibody synthesis and, consequently, of the disease itself.

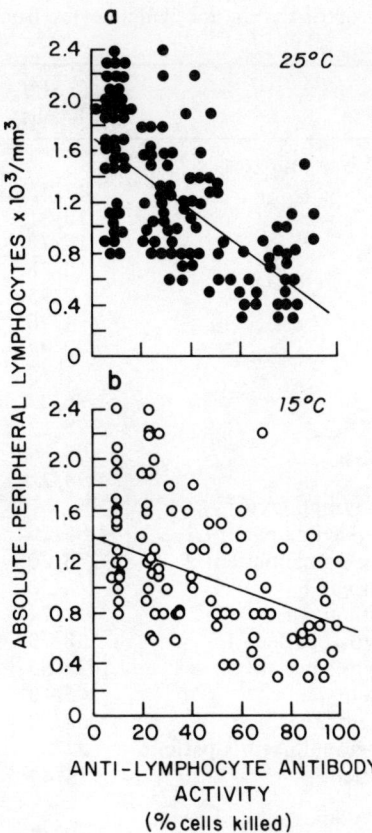

Figure 6.12 Inverse linear correlation between serum cytotoxicity and peripheral lymphocyte counts in SLE. a, Data obtained with undiluted serum assayed at 25°C against PBL ($r = 0.6667$). b, Data obtained with serum diluted 1:4 in 15°C assays ($r = 0.4664$). Slightly modified from Winfield et al. (1975)

Table 6.11 Peripheral blood lymphocytes/cmm in SLE patients during points of disease stability and activity. Data from Utsinger (1976)

Group	N*	Total	T	SIg
(a) Disease stable	142	1,721 ± 73	843 ± 78	386 ± 49
(b) Disease active	70	1,109 ± 129	418 ± 62	321 ± 39
(a) vs. (b)		$p < 0.005$	$p < 0.0005$	NS
Normals	184	2,320 ± 176	1,685 ± 61	663 ± 84

*Number of determinations.

Table 6.12 Cytotoxicity of SLE sera for lymphocytes from different sources. Data from Utsinger (1976)

Target cells	% SIg/% T cells*	% cytotoxicity ± SD
Normal peripheral blood lymphocytes		
PU	11/85	64 ± 8
WY	13/81	62 ± 9
JF	12/79	74 ± 11
RF	13/78	55 ± 8
PU purified T	2/95	59 ± 11
WY purified T	1/96	63 ± 7
JF purified T	2/97	74 ± 8
RF purified T	1/95	73 ± 7
PU purified B	96/2	78 ± 6
WY purified B	98/1	65 ± 7
JF purified B	95/1	66 ± 4
RF purified B	94/2	68 ± 12
Patient peripheral blood lymphocytes		
Chronic lymphatic leukaemia patient 1	85/10	74 ± 9
Chronic lymphatic leukaemia patient 2	73/20	68 ± 7
Multiple myeloma patient 1	8/70	62 ± 6
Multiple myeloma patient 2	7/74	65 ± 9
Infectious mononucleosis patient 1	28/70	68 ± 11
Infectious mononucleosis patient 2	25/65	72 ± 13
Viral pharyngitis patient 1	55/40	74 ± 11
Viral pharyngitis patient 2	68/29	72 ± 12
Waldenstrom's macroglobulinaemia patient	21/65·	69 ± 9
Mycosis fungoides patient	14/84	64 ± 12
Organ lymphocytes		
Foetal thymus	6/94	66 ± 11
Adult spleen	24/70	65 ± 13
Adult lymph node	33/55	71 ± 10
Cell lines		
IM — 1	B cell line	58 ± 9
IM — 9	B cell line	62 ± 14
T5 — 1	B cell line	65 ± 11
DG	B cell line	57 ± 10
BU — 1	B cell line	52 ± 11
UM — 56	B cell line	74 ± 8
UM — 61	B cell line	71 ± 15

*Per cent of the mononuclear cell population.

6.2.5.3 Progressive systemic sclerosis (PSS, scleroderma)

Progressive systemic sclerosis is a generalized connective tissue disorder characterized by inflammatory, fibrotic and degenerative tissue changes. Vascular lesions are found in the skin, synovium, and internal organs (Rodnan, 1972). Antitissue antibodies are detected in patients with PSS (Rothfield and Rodnan, 1968; Jordan et al., 1971), although their significance to the pathogenesis of the disease remains unclear, and lymphocyte accumulation in tissues is a pathological feature of the disease (Barnett, 1974; Fleischmajer *et al.*, 1972; Rodnan and Medsger, 1966).

Neither the aetiology of the disease nor the mechanism of accumulation of lymphocytes in tissues is understood. In an *in vitro* study of the production of MF by peripheral blood lymphocytes of PSS patients and of patients with other connective tissue disorders and with the CREST syndrome, Kondo *et al.* (1976) found that lymphocytes of patients with diffuse scleroderma did respond to extracts of normal and PSS skin. Two of 16 PSS patients had migration indices below 2 SD of the normal range in contrast with one of 10 CREST patients or one of 13 patients with other connective tissue disorders. Moreover, in an immunofluorescence study of PSS skin biopsies, the same authors characterized the majority of the lymphocytes in cutaneous infiltrates as T lymphocytes. The mechanism of the T cell accumulation in non-lymphoid tissue in this, as in other diseases, remains unclear, but the fact that T lymphocytes accumulate in sites of disease activity may contribute to the pathogenesis of the disease since it is known that substances derived from activated lymphocytes can stimulate collagen synthesis by fibroblasts (Johnson and Ziff, 1976).

6.2.6 Central nervous system diseases

The pioneering studies of Kabat and co-workers (1950) of the protein, gammaglobulin and albumin content of cerebrospinal fluid in neurological disease, including 100 patients with multiple sclerosis, demonstrated the existence of high levels of IgG in this disease. Later it was shown that the IgG in CSF is oligoclonal (Link, 1967, 1972) and that lymphocytes isolated from CSF have the capacity to synthesize it *in vitro* (Sandberg-Wollheim, 1974). It is thought that lymphocytes present in CSF in MS patients derive from lymphocyte infiltrates in the meninges and perhaps also from the lymphoid aggregates found within active demyelinating plaques (Adams, 1977).

Separate experimental studies of viral encephalitis demonstrated the importance of T cells in development of the specific immune inflammatory response to the viruses (Hapel and Gardner, 1974) and in the development of the disease itself (Doherty and Zinkernagel, 1974).

The possibility of simultaneous analysis of the cellular content of peripheral blood and CSF in man has led to several studies of T and B cell distribution in neurological diseases, as part of the process of clarifying their pathogenesis (Sandberg-Wollheim and Turesson, 1975; Fryden, 1977; Kam-Hansen *et al.*, 1978; Kam-Hansen, 1979). Multiple sclerosis, aseptic meningitis, and optic neuritis were investigated.

6.2.6.1 *Multiple sclerosis (MS)*

Patients with MS had significantly higher percentages of T cells in CSF than in blood (Sandberg-Wollheim and Turesson, 1975; Kam-Hansen *et al.*, 1978). B cell

Table 6.13 Frequency and distribution of lymphocytes containing the three Ig classes in peripheral blood and cerebrospinal fluid (CSF) of six patients with multiple sclerosis. Data from Sandberg-Wollheim and Turesson (1975)

Source of cells	Frequency of Ig-positive cells		Ig class distribution of Ig-positive cells			χ/λ ratio
	% Ig	% IgG	% IgA	% IgM	% IgG	
CSF	0.40	0.40	1	0	99	Not done
	0.50	0.50	1	0	99	Not done
	0.61	0.47	17	6	77	0.5
	0.45	0.39	12	2	86	2.7
	0.74	0.60	19	0	81	2.3
	0.42	0.33	12	11	77	1.9
Mean	0.52	0.45	10.3	3.2	86.5	1.9
Blood	0.35	0.05	87	1	13	1.0
	0.25	0.06	55	23	22	1.0
	0.21	0.05	53	20	27	1.2
	0.07	0.02	55	19	26	1.6
	0.02	0.01	50	23	27	1.6
	0.19	0.06	50	20	30	1.3
Mean	0.18	0.04	58.3	17.5	24.2	1.3

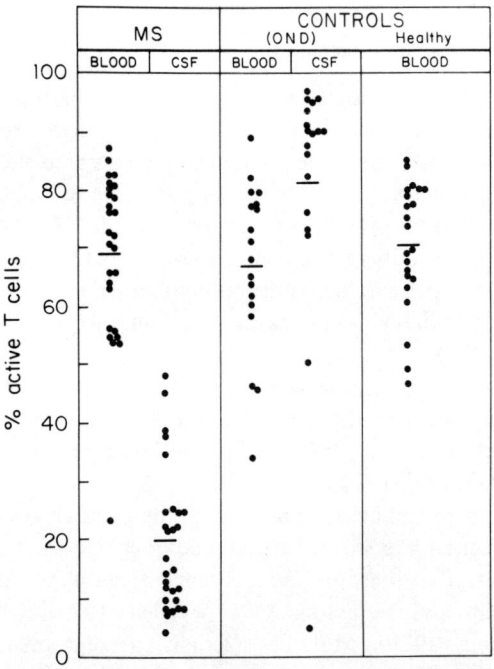

Figure 6.13 Percentages of active T cells in the CSF and blood in multiple sclerosis (MS), in controls with other neurologic disease (OND), and in healthy persons. MS patients studied: 28; OND: 18; controls: 23. Slightly modified from Kam-Hansen (1979)

values determined as cells with surface Ig, on the other hand, were lower in CSF than in blood in one study and not different in another. Ig-containing cells, however, were found in larger numbers in CSF than in blood (Sandberg-Wollheim and Turesson, 1975). The immunoglobulin class distribution of the Ig-containing cells in CSF was as follows: IgG > IgA > IgM (see Table 6.13). These findings corroborate earlier findings of increased amounts of IgG in the CSF of patients with multiple sclerosis (Kabat *et al.*, 1950; Link, 1972).

The finding of large percentages of E-rosette forming cells in CSF has been looked at further, with a view to defining the subpopulation of T cells present in CSF. Using the active rosette test described by Wybran and Fudenberg (1973), believed to be a better indicator of cell-mediated immunocompetence than total E-rosette formation, Kam-Hansen has shown that the percentages of active E-rosette forming T cells in CSF in multiple sclerosis patients are in fact lower than those found in the peripheral blood of the same patients and lower than those found in patients with other neurological diseases (Fig. 6.13) (Kam-Hansen, 1979).

6.2.6.2 Aseptic meningitis

T cell values were also significantly higher in CSF in patients with aseptic meningitis than in peripheral blood (Kam-Hansen *et al.*, 1978; Fryden, 1977). Lower B cell values were observed in CSF than in blood. No differences were observed

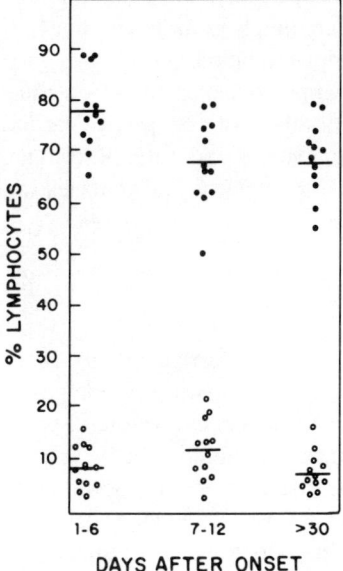

Figure 6.14 Percentages of T (●) and B (○) cells in blood from 12 patients with acute aseptic meningitis during the course of disease. Data from Fryden (1977)

between T cell or B cell percentages between patients with mumps meningitis or other forms of aseptic meningitis (Fryden, 1977). In a prospective study of 12 patients with aseptic meningitis (Fig. 6.14) in whom the percentages of T and B lymphocytes in the peripheral blood were estimated in consecutive samples drawn at 1–6 days, 7–12 days, or more than a month after onset of infection, a slight, not statistically significant rise in B cells was seen in the blood at the same time that a significant decrease ($p < 0.001$) of the mean value of T cells was found from the first to the second week of infection (Fryden, 1977). From the second to the third observation, a significant decrease ($p < 0.05$) of B cells was observed while no further changes occurred in T cell values. The difference between declining slopes of the mean values of T and B cells (Fig. 6.14) may represent another illustration of their different tempos of circulation.

6.2.7 Pulmonary diseases with pleurisy

Simultaneous determinations of the percentage and total T and B cell count in peripheral blood and pleural fluid were carried out by Petterson and colleagues (Petterson et al., 1978) in patients with pleurisy of various aetiologies, namely pulmonary tuberculosis, pulmonary malignancy, connective tissue diseases, non-specific pleurisy, and congestive heart failure (Table 6.14). In all patients except those with pulmonary tuberculosis, the percentages of T lymphocytes in pleural fluid were similar to those in peripheral blood. In pulmonary tuberculosis, both the percentage and the absolute numbers of T lymphocytes were significantly higher in pleural fluid than in peripheral blood.

The percentage of B lymphocytes, on the other hand, was lower in peripheral blood in all patients except those with congestive cardiac failure. Statistically significant reductions in percentage and total B cell numbers were observed in patients with tuberculosis, pulmonary malignancies, and non-specific (probably 'viral') effusions (Table 6.14).

6.2.8 Solid tumours

Two types of studies have been carried out to characterize the origin of the lymphoid cells infiltrating solid tumours. Percentages of T and B cells have been determined in suspensions of lymphocytes isolated from biopsy material using E-rosette formation and surface immunoglobulin as surface markers of T and B lymphocytes (Jondal and Klein, 1975). Proportions of T and B cells have also been estimated in tumour tissue sections using specific anti-T and anti-immunoglobulin antisera and counting the numbers of fluorescent cells detected by staining (Husby et al., 1976). With both techniques T lymphocytes were found to predominate in the tumour tissue.

Although a significant reduction in peripheral blood T cell numbers is known to occur in a proportion of the patients with solid primary and metastatic cancer (Potvin et al., 1975; Husby et al., 1976), this decrease has not been clearly related

Table 6.14 Total number of lymphocytes (mean ± SD) and percentages of T and B lymphocytes (mean ± SD) in peripheral blood and pleural fluid. Data from Petterson et al. (1978)

Diagnosis	Total lymphocytes × 10⁹ L	T lymphocytes Total number × 10⁹ cells L (%)		B lymphocytes Total number × 10⁹ cells L (%)	
Pulmonary tuberculosis (11)					
Blood	2.2 ± 0.9	59.5 ± 8.5‡	1.3 ± 0.6*	27.0 ± 5.5‡	0.6 ± 0.2‡
Pleural fluid	4.1 ± 3.3	78.5 ± 9.0	3.2 ± 2.4	5.0 ± 3.5	0.2 ± 0.1
Pulmonary malignancy (6)					
Blood	1.9 ± 0.7	60.0 ± 5.0	1.1 ± 0.4	29.0 ± 7.9‡	0.5 ± 0.2†
Pleural fluid	2.3 ± 1.3	69.0 ± 17.5	1.5 ± 0.8	7.5 ± 5.0	0.2 ± 0.1
Connective tissue disease (3)					
Blood	3.2 ± 3.0	51.0 ± 6.5	1.5 ± 1.3	37.5 ± 2.0‡	1.2 ± 1.1
Pleural fluid	2.7 ± 0.9	60.5 ± 10.5	1.6 ± 0.5	6.5 ± 5.5	0.2 ± 0.2
Non-specific pleurisy (6)					
Blood	2.8 ± 1.2	59.0 ± 15.5	1.6 ± 0.5	32.5 ± 9.0‡	0.9 ± 0.5*
Pleural fluid	1.6 ± 0.6	64.5 ± 19.0	1.0 ± 0.4	11.5 ± 6.0	0.2 ± 0.2
Congestive cardiac failure (4)					
Blood	1.9 ± 0.7	58.5 ± 17.5	1.1 ± 0.5	21.5 ± 17.5	0.4 ± 0.2
Pleural fluid	1.3 ± 0.2	69.0 ± 14.5	0.9 ± 0.3	14.5 ± 13.0	0.2 ± 0.2
Controls (24)					
Blood	2.0 ± 0.9	66.0 ± 8.0	1.3 ± 0.5	19.0 ± 5.0	0.4 ± 0.2

*$p < 0.025$.
†$p < 0.005$.
‡$p < 0.001$ by Student's t-test.

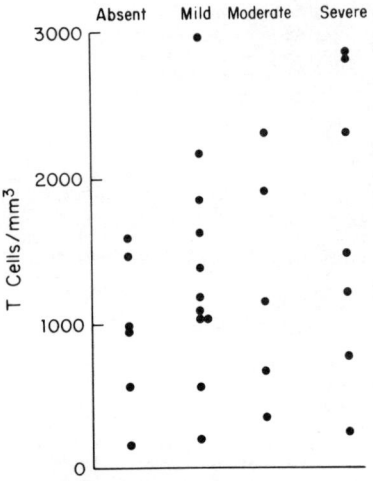

Figure 6.15 Relationship between peripheral blood T cell numbers (cells/mm^3) and degree of lymphocyte reaction at tumour margins in 30 patients with malignant tumours. Decreases in peripheral blood T cell counts in this case could not be related to lymphocyte infiltration of tumour estimated in tumour tissue sections using specific anti-T antiserum and immunofluorescence. Data from Husby et al. (1976)

either to the extent of local tumour T cell infiltration (Fig. 6.15) or to the presence of disseminated disease (Husby et al., 1976). These results differ from studies of distribution of labelled lymphocytes (Zatz et al., 1973) and of tumour-associated inflammatory cells (Russell et al., 1976a,b) during progression and (or) regression of Moloney sarcoma virus induced tumours in mice, in which a direct association was found between numbers of infiltrating T lymphocytes and tumour regression (Russell et al., 1976b; Fig. 6.16). Zatz et al. (1973) found that between 10 and 36 days after MSV inoculation, significantly higher numbers of labelled cells were found in the draining than in the contralateral nodes of virus-inoculated mice. The interval of greater regional lymph node localization (between days 17 and 28) corresponded to the time of tumour regression.

The question of lymphocyte migration patterns in tumour-bearing hosts is of paramount importance to the analysis of the effectiveness of immune mechanisms in tumour surveillance. Specifically sensitized cells with demonstrable cytotoxic properties *in vitro* may be of little use *in vivo* if sequestered somewhere along the recirculatory circuit.

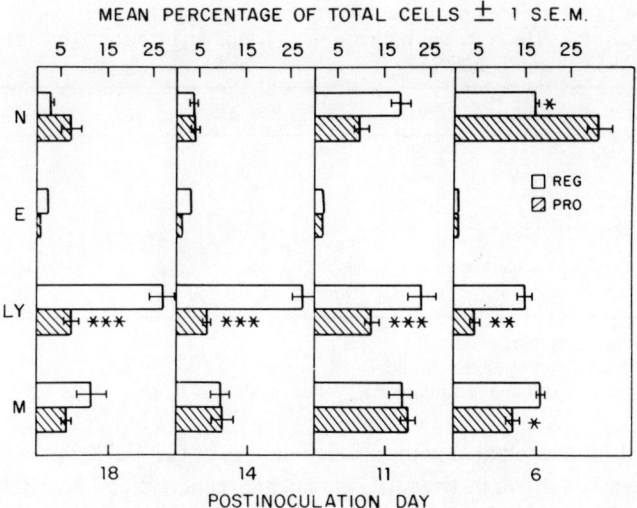

Figure 6.16 Principal inflammatory cell types found in regression (REG) and progressing (PRO) Moloney sarcomas shown as percentages of the total cells recovered following disaggregation of tumours with enzymes (using either a mixture of trypsin, collagenase, and DNAse or collagenase and DNAse, results pooled). Each bar represents the mean ($\pm$ SEM) of values obtained from the analysis of five or more individual tumours. N, neutrophils; E, eosinophils; LY, T lymphocytes; M, macrophages. Significant differences between percentages of infiltrating cells are indicated by the asterisks. *$p < 0.005$; **$p < 0.01$; ***$p < 0.001$. Slightly modified from Russell *et al.* (1976b)

6.2.9 Leukaemia

Direct tracer studies of the fate of labelled lymphocytes have been carried out in patients with chronic lymphocytic leukaemia (CLL) and in one patient with lymphosarcoma (Bremer, Wack and Schick, 1973; Bremer, Fliedner and Schick, 1973; Flad *et al.*, 1973). The results demonstrate an impairment of the circulation of B leukaemia cells from blood to central (thoracic duct) lymph. Following autotransfusion of *in vitro* [^{3}H]-cytidine-labelled peripheral blood lymphocytes, the first labelled cells appeared in the samples of lymph collected from the thoracic duct within the first 7 hr of transfusion (Table 6.15). A higher amount of radioactivity persisted in the blood of leukaemia patients than in healthy control subjects (Hersey, 1971; Brenner, Wack and Schick, 1973) or in the control lymphosarcoma patient (Figs. 6.17 and 6.18). Five minutes after completion of the autotransfusion in the lymphosarcoma patient, only 1.2% of the blood lymphocytes were found labelled, compared with 3–5% present in the leukaemic patients. These initial percentages decreased rapidly in most patients and within

Table 6.15 Labelled lymphocytes in thoracic duct lymph sampled 1–7 hr after autotransfusion in six patients with lymphocytic neoplasms. Data from Bremer, Wack and Schick (1973)

Patient	1 hr	2 hr	3 hr	4 hr	5 hr	6 hr	7 hr
A.U.	/	/	/	+	+	/	+
M.R.	/	/	/	+	/	/	+
M.S.	/	+	+	/	/	/	/
U.S.	+	+	+	+	+	+	+
C.M.	−	+	+	+	/	+	+
A.O.	/	/	/	/	+	/	+

/ no lymph samples collected.
− no labelled lymphocytes found.
+ presence of labelled lymphocytes.

1 hr levelled off at a plateau with labelling indices of 0.2–0.5% in the LSA patient and between 2 and 6% in the CLL patients (Brenner, Wack and Schick, 1973). However, in a separate study including patients with similar initials and lymphocyte counts (Flad et al., 1973), much higher percentages of labelled cells were found in the blood of the leukaemic and LSA patients 2 days after transfusion (Table 6.16; Flad et al., 1973). These values are closer to those obtained in earlier studies of the presence in the blood of [^{3}H]-cytidine (Stryckmans et al., 1968) or [^{51}Cr]-labelled lymphocytes in normal and leukaemia subjects (Hersey, 1971). The estimated half-times for residence of cells in the circulation obtained in the latter study (Hersey, 1971) of normal and CLL patients are 1.7 and 5 days respectively (Fig. 6.17).

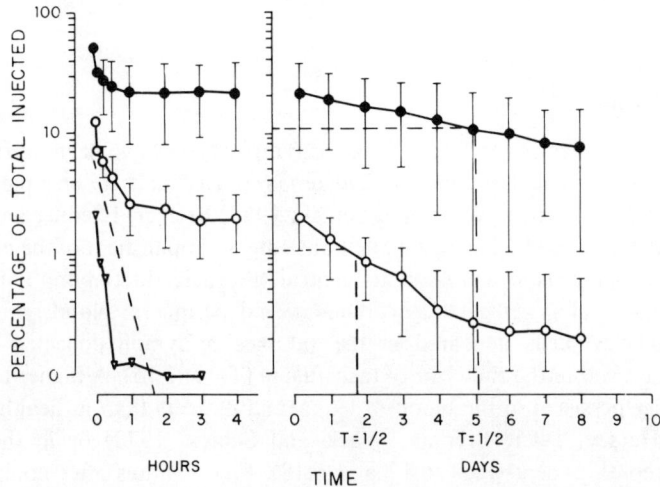

Figure 6.17 Survival of autotransfused ^{51}Cr-labelled lymphocytes in normal subjects (O) and chronic lymphocytic leukaemia (●) patients. Δ——Δ indicates the rapid clearance from blood of heat-killed cells. Slightly modified from Hersey (1971)

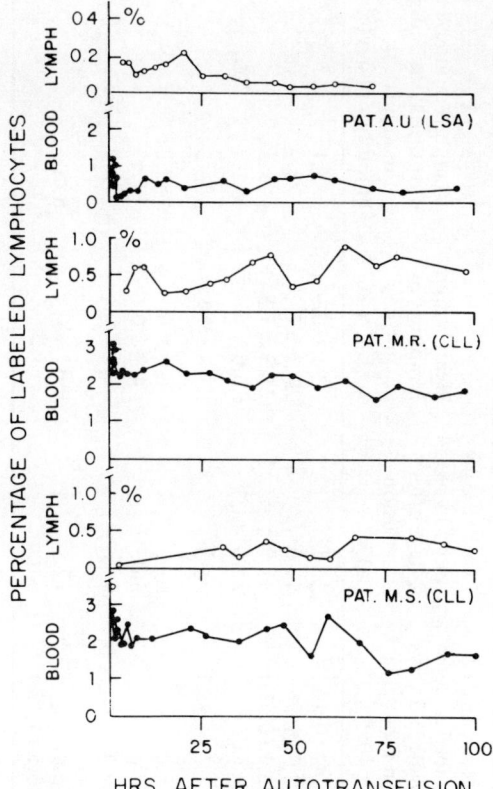

Figure 6.18 Changes in the percentage of labelled lymphocytes in peripheral blood and thoracic duct lymph after autotransfusion of |³H|-cytidine-labelled blood lymphocytes in two patients with CLL (M.R., M.S.) and one with lymphosarcoma (A.U.). See also Table 6.16. Slightly modified from Bremer, Wack, and Schick (1973)

Recovery of labelled cells in thoracic duct lymphs was higher (4.8%) in the LSA patients within the first 2 days after autotransfusion (Table 6.16) than in the leukaemia patients (ranging from 0.2% to 0.6%). The amount of radioactivity recovered in the lymphosarcoma patient (4.8%) is very close to the value obtained in an earlier study of lymphocyte recirculation in two patients with chronic renal insufficiency (4.6%) (Revillard et al., 1968).

Estimated numbers of thoracic duct lymph lymphocytes collected per day in three of the four leukaemic patients included in Flad et al.'s study (Flad et al., 1973) were markedly lower than the estimated numbers collected in the LSA patient and in three other non-leukaemic patients (Table 6.16).

In addition, studies of the lymphocyte count in the peripheral lymph of patients

Table 6.16 Recovery of autotransfused [^{3}H]Cyt-labelled lymphocytes in the thoracic duct lymph. Data from Flad et al. (1973)

Patient	Diagnosis	Labelled lymphocytes transfused $\times 10^{-9}$	Recovery of labelled cells within 2 days in lymph $\times 10^{-8}$	Labelled cells found in blood 2 days after transfusion (%)	Mean lymph lymphocyte output/day $\pm$ SEM $\times 10^{-9}$	Lymph lymphocyte output/day as % of total circulating blood lymphocytes
M.R.	CLL	4.0	0.7 (0.4%)	22.1	2.1 ± 0.9	5.1
U.S.	CLL	26.7	2.7 (1%)	49.0	72.7 ± 7.2	23.2
C.M.	CLL	68.2	3.3 (0.5%)	31.9	21.3 ± 1.8	3.5
C.S.	CLL	176.0	n.d.	23.0	36.6	1.9
A.U.	LSA	2.5	1.2 (4.8%)	5.3	65.8 ± 19.2	306.0
W.H.	Sclerodermia	n.d.	n.d.	n.d.	6.7 ± 0.9	152.2
K.H.	M. sclerosis	n.d.	n.d.	n.d.	4.9 ± 0.6	37.7
H.G.	Myatrophic lat. sclerosis	n.d.	n.d.	n.d.	7.5 ± 0.5	75.0
4 haematol. normals		0.5–1.7	n.d.	12.1	n.d.	n.d.
1	Renal failure*	7.6	3.5 (4.6%)	n.d.	—	—

*Data from Revillard et al. (1968).
n.d., not done.

Table 6.17a Number of blood lymphocytes, percentage of B lymphocytes and composition of peripheral lymph in patients with CLL. Data from Engeset et al. (1974)

	Blood			Lymph				Ratio
Cannulation no.	Lymphocyte count/µl	B lymphocytes (%)	Days of cannulation. In brackets, pretreatment morning samples	Flow (ml/hr)	Lymphocyte count/µl	Lymphocyte output/hr $\times 10^3$	B lymphocytes (%)	Lymphocyte counts (blood/lymph)
39	93,000	90	8(3)	1.20	92	111	4	1,011
38	77,000	96	7(2)	1.28	40	51	2–3	1,940
35	28,900	95	4(1)	0.20	824	165	<1	35
37	21,000	90	8(1)	0.91	302	274	5	70
29	17,000	95	6(3)	1.10	120	132	50	141
93	16,000		4(3)	2.00	30	60		537
21	9,600		2(1)	0.82	15	12		658
76	3,200	3	9(5)	1.02	85	87		38
23	3,000		2(1)	2.42	22	54		136
10	2,800		2(1)	1.58	86	136		32
88	2,100		4(3)	1.40	18	28	<1	115
Mean	24,873			1.27	149	101		428

Table 6.17b Number of blood lymphocytes, percentage of B lymphocytes and composition of peripheral lymph before treatment in patients with solid tumours. Data from Engeset et al. (1974)

Cannula-tion no.	Blood			Lymph				Ratio
	Lymphocyte count/μl	B lympho-cytes (%)	Days of cannu-lation. In brackets, pretreatment morning samples	Flow (ml/hr)	Lymphocyte count/μl		Lymphocyte output/hr $\times 10^3$	Lymphocyte counts (blood/lymph)
87	3,213		3(1)	0.54	191		104	17
61	2,842		5(2)	0.84	137		115	21
15	2,696		2(1)	1.80	29		52	95
85	2,520		3(2)	1.85	128		237	20
33	2,470	18	11(5)	1.18	207		243	12
90	2,400		6(5)	0.36	114		42	21
89	2,124		4(3)	0.68	47		32	45
77	1,242	4	2(1)	2.14	133		285	9
Mean	2,438			1.17	123		139	30

with B cell leukaemia with abnormally high peripheral blood lymphocyte counts (Table 6.17a) and of patients with solid tumours (Table 6.17b) have shown that in most leukaemia patients the lymphocyte output in peripheral lymph is either within the range of or lower than that of patients with solid tumours (Engeset *et al.*, 1974).

All of the above results point to an impairment of lymphocyte recirculation in CLL. Whether this reflects the B cell nature of the leukaemic cells studied or whether malignant B cells recirculate even more poorly than normal B cells is yet to be ascertained in man.

In an experimental study of the tempo of recirculation and tissue distribution of murine leukaemia B cells, Warnke *et al.* (1979) have shown that leukaemic B cells recirculated much more poorly than control spleen B cells. Tracing FITC-labelled leukaemic and control spleen cells, they have found that the concentration of leukaemic cells in the thoracic duct lymph, 24 hr after intravenous injection, was roughly 1,000 times less than that observed after injection of normal splenic B cells. Greater numbers of leukaemic cells were present in the spleen and liver than lymph nodes. Within the spleen, they were distributed predominantly in the marginal zone and in B cell areas (Warnke *et al.*, 1979).

6.2.10 Thoracic duct drainage as a therapeutic tool

One other clinical development deriving from the principles and techniques of lymphocyte circulation is their application to the therapy of diseases requiring immunosuppression. Thoracic duct drainage in man is an effective surgical measure of depletion of circulating lymphocytes (Tilney and Murray, 1968; Revillard *et al.*, 1968; Girardet and Benninghoff, 1977). It has been used successfully as a supportive measure of immunosuppression in kidney transplantation (Tilney *et al.*, 1970; Sarles *et al.*, 1970; Franksson *et al.*, 1976). It has also been used with some measure of success in diseases resistant to other forms of immunosuppressive therapy, i.e. glomerulonephritis (Bonomin *et al.*, 1970; Ravnskov *et al.*, 1977) and SLE manifested as severe cutaneous vasculitis (Nyman *et al.*, 1977). Finally, thoracic duct drainage has been attempted in diseases in which lymphocytes themselves have been implicated in the pathogenesis of the lesions, particularly in rheumatoid arthritis (Wegelius *et al.*, 1970; Paulus *et al.*, 1973), again in the SLE case mentioned above (Nyman *et al.*, 1977), and in myasthenia gravis.

6.2.11 Glomerulonephritis (GLN)

In Ravnskov *et al.* series (Ravnskov *et al.*, 1977), nine patients with various types of severe glomerulonephritis were treated with drainage of the thoracic duct drainage ($n = 8$) and/or plasmapheresis ($n = 6$) without any other form of concomitant immunosuppressive therapy. Generally, there was prompt clinical improvement reflected in a temporary regression of the albuminuria and decreases of serum creatinine levels to 84% of the value measured immediately before drainage was started. After the treatment was stopped, however, the creatinine increased gradually during the next 3 months or immediately after treatment in eight of the patients followed, and only in one patient with membranoproliferative GLN the effect of serum creatinine lasted 8 months after thoracic duct drainage and plasmapheresis.

In another series (Bonomini et al., 1970), cases resistant to azathioprine and prednisone therapy were first drained and then treated further with the two drugs. The chief effect of the thoracic duct fistula consisted in the disappearance of the resistance to the immunosuppressive therapy, the mechanism of the phenomenon remaining unclear.

6.2.12 Rheumatoid arthritis

Marked clinical improvement has been reported in patients with rheumatoid arthritis who had thoracic duct fistulas. In one case (Paulus et al., 1973), improvement was observed during the first 2 weeks of drainage and persisted until about 6 weeks after the fistula was discontinued.

In another series of six patients with severe classical RA and one with JRA (Wegelius et al., 1970), the immediate response was good in three of the first five, fairly good in two, and no effect was found in the clinical course of the JRA patient. In four of the patients the remission lasted for several months. When exacerbation of the disease occurred cytostatic therapy was administered with good responses.

6.2.13 SLE

Immunosuppressive therapy by thoracic duct lymph drainage has been reported in at least one case of SLE with cutaneous vasculitis unresponsive to oral prednisone and azathoprine. After 1 week of drainage, obvious clinical improvement of the skin component of the disease was noticed. This continued during the 10 week period of thoracic duct drainage and then steroid treatment was reduced from 120 mg/day to 60 mg/day. There was, however, no evidence of change in the patient's lupus nephritis as judged by serial 24 hour urinary protein, creatinine clearance, and pre and post drainage kidney biopsies.

Twenty-two weeks after drainage, at the time of publication of the case report, the patient had had no recurrence of the cutaneous vasculitis or need to increase the daily intake of prednisone (Nyman et al., 1977).

Chapter 7

Clues, Concepts, and Possible Answers from other Systems

A. S. G. CURTIS

7.1 INTRODUCTION

The purpose of this chapter is to construct a vantage point for the reader from which he or she may be able to look around to see the larger biological landscape within which lymphocyte movement lies. We hope that this vantage point may be used by the reader chiefly as a means to espy the road ahead. We do not know the road ahead but are fairly sure that it lies somewhere in the landscape we shall present. Part of this chapter is devoted to looking at a particular area that the author feels personally to be of some importance, and similarly the main author Maria de Sousa devotes the rest of the book to her own particular part of the landscape. I hope that one matter will emerge strongly from our texts: namely that we shall draw attention to those regions that may have been hidden as it were in the folds of the hills, to the questions that have not been asked because the answers have been assumed, and to those questions that may be important though no one has thought that so far.

7.2. CELL–CELL RECOGNITION SYSTEMS

Lymphocyte circulation lies clearly in the area of biology termed cell–cell recognition. Thus the first enlargement of our mental landscape is to look at the whole field of cell–cell recognition and to search for similarities and for the results of investigations on related systems.

In all recognition systems we can distinguish four stages of the process:

1. Production, release, and transport of the recognition signal
2. Reception of the signal
3. Activation of an effector system in the receiving cell
4. Production of the result.

For instance, a chemotactic substance might – at the moment we have to write rather hypothetically – be secreted by a given cell, diffuse through the medium, and be received by a plasmalemmal protein on the target cell. Binding of the chemotactic signal to the molecule might then start a process which would reorient the microfilaments within the cell so that the final overt result would be that the cells would start to move towards the source of the signal molecules.

In some cases the signal and receptor molecules appear to be either very similar or even identical so that it seems inapposite to write of one cell signalling and the other receiving. Such cases are found in systems in which insoluble cell surface components are probably able to react directly with each other. Consequently it seems appropriate to term such molecules mutual receptors.

In studying lymphocyte positioning, as in studying other morphogenetic processes, we are still largely at the level of seeing results and trying to discover which effector systems operate to produce the results. For instance, at the moment it is unresolved whether cell adhesion, specific or otherwise, chemotaxis, or more complex types of cell behaviour effect the sorting out of T and B cells into their respective dependent areas in spleen and nodes. This does not mean that it is idle and illogical to investigate the more molecular aspects of the system, namely to discover the identity of the signal and of the receptor or the effector systems. Problems are often best attacked from both ends. It does mean that at the moment we can at best only make a series of sketches of more or less probability of the whole recognition process in any given biological situation.

We can obtain, however, a firm conceptual framework to guide this discussion by considering how many main types of recognition system might be possible physicochemically.

Recognition systems can be divided into two main classes. First, those systems in which the signal molecule is transmitted in soluble form and is bound by the receiving cell. All the classical hormone systems are of this type. The receptor molecule may be either at the cell surface or internally positioned.

The second class comprises those systems in which both the recognition signal and its receptor are insoluble. This simple physical constraint has very important biological effects, because it has the consequence that signal and receptor must be borne at the surface of the cells involved, and that cell contact must be established for recognition to operate. It should be noted that at the moment few systems have been shown unequivocally to be of this type, though many proposals and models have been put forward in which such a scheme is used. 'Mutual' receptor systems, if they exist, will be of this type, with a molecule on one cell surface having some form of complementarity for one of the same type on another surface. A variant of this model is the receptor–ligand system (see Fig. 7.1) in which each plasmalemma of recognizing cells carries a receptor site which will not bind the site on the other surface because it is identical. A ligand molecule which is at least bivalent can bind to each receptor. The ligand molecule might be soluble but in the presence of appropriate cells will be bound tightly to the plasmalemma, so that it will in effect be insoluble. Few systems of this type have been identified unequivocally, but the mating-type systems in yeasts and in Chlamydomonads

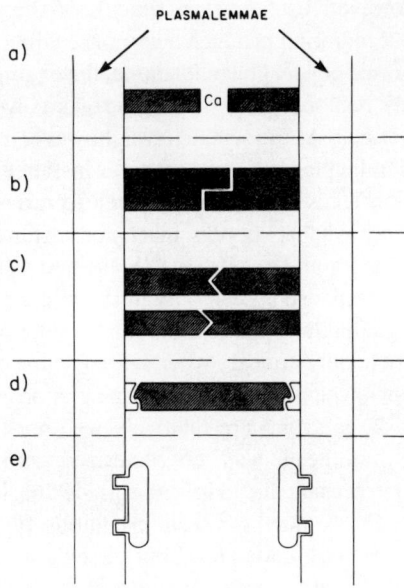

Figure 7.1 Hypothetical models of the various ways in which receptor–signal interactions at the cell surface might modify cell adhesion. (a) Macromolecules (black) attached to or part of the plasmalemmae bind to each other through the action of calcium ions. This type of interaction might be either specific or non-specific. Calcium might play a role in any of the reactions shown in (b) to (e). (b) Each surface of the interacting cells bears mutual receptors which interact to effect specific adhesion. If all cells bear the same type of receptor or if the interaction is not sterically specified the adhesions will be non-specific. (c) Each surface bears two types of recognition molecule; one might be termed a receptor and the other a signal. (d) Receptor sites on each plasmalemma bind more or less specifically a ligand molecule. (e) Each surface binds more or less specifically a signal molecule which acts to change the adhesiveness of that surface without directly bridging from one surface to another

have been clearly shown to belong to this second class (Crandall, 1978; Wiese and Wiese, 1978), with differing insoluble receptor and signal substances on male and female gametes.

Other physical constraints on recognition systems can be conceived though they lead to systems that are inherently improbable (see discussion by Curtis, 1978a,b).

This classification of recognition systems can, I feel, be usefully continued by considering the other end of the process, namely the sort of effects that result from recognition. The range of cell processes and type of behaviour that might be or have been shown to be affected by recognition is obviously very large (see list in Curtis, 1979a) but in the context of the present chapter can, of course, be limited to those types of behaviour that position cells, which are effects at least largely on adhesion and movement, the two interrelated processes that will determine how cells position. It is, however, useful to consider how the effects are displayed. Many simple forms of recognition produce a response which is limited to the level of each single cell that responds. A given hormone, for example, stimulates protein synthesis in a cell; this response does not directly involve further interactions between it and any other cell. At the second level, however, pairwise interaction of cells is found. This may take place at a distance, for instance when one cell emits a chemotactic signal which leads the responding cell to move towards the first. It may also take place only when two cells meet, for instance in the mating-type systems of some algae and some yeasts (see Wiese and Wiese, 1978). The third level is one in which the response is seen only in the interaction of relatively large groups of cells. It is arguable that positioning cannot take place between pairs of cells, and that the response only appears when large groups of cells are involved.

The classical hormones which produce the same response in the cell whether it is isolated or part of a large group are relatively well understood insofar as the nature of the signal has been well characterized and the receptor often characterized (see Cuatrecasas and Hollenberg (1976) for review). Pairwise interactions of cells such as may be seen in mating-type systems or in the chemotaxis of cells are less well understood but in several cases the nature of the signal molecule and of the receptor are known, e.g. Wiese and Wiese (1978).

When, however, we consider positioning systems in animals, we are still at the stage where we do not know whether recognition processes of the type outlined above are involved at all. The reason for this is that the cells may be using much simpler systems which do not necessarily involve any interaction of specific signal molecules with receptors. Obviously we should look at these systems before returning to attempts to explain positioning in terms of highly specific molecular mechanisms.

7.3 PATTERNING SYSTEMS – IS THERE SPECIFIC CONTROL OF THE MOVEMENT OF CELLS?

It is appropriate that we should ask whether mixtures of two or more cell types have any intrinsic ability to establish pattern starting from a random arrangement. Much of the evidence that they have this ability comes from studies on sorting out in aggregates of vertebrate embryonic tissue (see Steinberg, 1963; Townes and Holtfreter, 1955), while studies of the natural disaggregation and subsequent reaggregation that the embryos of the annual fish (Wourms, 1972) undergo and of the aggregation of slime moulds and subsequent sorting into stalk and spore cells (Garrod *et al.*, 1978) also support the idea that mixtures of cells have this ability. Studies on the reaggregation and sorting out of cells of two species of sponge are less convincing evidence because the process probably does not occur in nature and because no clear positioning of one cell type with respect to the other takes place.

However, despite this fairly convincing set of demonstrations that cell populations can display the ability to set up patterns *de novo*, it is still possible to explain such behaviour without recourse to mechanisms that require highly specific molecular interactions. Steinberg (1963, 1970, 1978a,b) has championed the view that the morphogenetic movements seen in embryos and in sorting out in aggregates simply represent the attainment of a minimum surface free energy charge situation by cell adhesions. He showed (Steinberg, 1963) that there is a sorting-out hierarchy whereby different pairs of cell types taken from a set of 14 or so cell types always sort out in a constant manner such that one type 'low' down on the list always sorts out internally to any one above it. The existence of this hierarchy suggests that sorting out is controlled by some graded quantitative property shared by all the cells in the system. This observation is, I think, one of great importance. Steinberg suggested that the graded property is cell adhesiveness. The evidence that this is indeed so has been very hard to obtain and has led to arguments as to the methods that should be used to measure cell adhesion. Steinberg argued that the graded differences in adhesion would lead to sorting out and positioning in the same manner as differences in surface free energy control the relative positions of adherent immiscible oil droplets. However, it is unclear whether such a mechanism would, in fact, operate in a multi-component system such as an aggregate. This hypothesis has been further criticized by Harris (1976).

Another explanation which does not require specific recognition is that of contact guidance. In the adult or even in the late embryonic stages of an animal, there is already a great deal of cell positioning and orientation of extracellular material such as collagen. This positioning and orientation might be used to provide clues for very simple mechanisms to operate upon to position newly arriving cells. For instance, the organization of reticular cells in the lymph node might provide the orientation necessary to lead B and T cells into separate areas. Weiss suggested a considerable while ago (Weiss, 1941) that the extension of axons to definite normal anatomical connections with sensory cells, other nerve cells or muscle cells might simply be controlled by the cells being 'contact guided' along some preexisting structure to their normal goals. Horder and Martin (1978) have revived this idea to a considerable extent and suggested that such a mechanism determines regeneration of the optic nerve axons to the tectum in experiments upon amphibia and fish. This hypothesis has, of course, the unsatisfactory feature that it simply pushes the process which establishes topographic placing of cells in the organism back to an earlier stage.

There are four systems which display features typical of cell recognition systems but which do not involve selective or directed cell movement as a mechanism in producing positioning. However, it is appropriate to give them consideration because they may, in fact, operate to produce positioning.

First, there may be random movement of cells say from one site to all parts of the body followed by selective survival in only one site. Willis (1952) suggested that this might account for the selective distribution of secondary tumours. If the migration and settlement is random, an apparent selectivity can be imposed on this by the death of the majority of the cells and their survival in a few sites only.

Willis viewed survival as being due to the special nutrition available at special sites for certain cell types. It might well have been viewed as the presence of generalized cytotoxic mechanisms, perhaps lymphocyte controlled, at all but a few special sites. In either case, there is little or no evidence that such specialized systems exist. It is, however, particularly pertinent that Meyer (1964) demonstrated that just such a mechanism must operate in the apparent specific migration of primordial germ cells to the gonads from their extra-embryonic site or origin. Meyer showed that many primordial germ cells locate in other tissues but then die. Presumably the occasional survival of such cells may account for the existence of teratoma. It should be borne in mind that such specific systems controlling the position of cell death or cell survival are quite properly classed under cell recognition systems. Other instances of positioned areas of cell death are known (see Saunders, 1966), which play important roles in normal development; in these other instances there is little or no involvement of cell migration in association with the phenomena.

Second, it is easy to confuse those mechanisms which lead to cells acquiring new and patterned positions with those that merely ensure that certain types of differentiation only take place in certain positions. Wolpert (1969), for example, has suggested that most of the various tissues which are placed in different parts of the body differentiated *in situ* rather than migrated into position. Clearly the very early differentiation into ectodermal plus mesodermal elements rather than endodermal elements arises before cell displacements take place. Once gastrulation takes place, however, cell migration both by the mass movement of cells and by their individual movement becomes common. Examples are given in Table 7.1. Thus though the topographical control of differentiation without cell movement may be of great importance, involving perhaps as Wolpert suggests systems that

Table 7.1   Positioning phenomena in embryogenesis

Movement by individual migration of cells
    Neural crest emigration giving rise to:
        Pigment cells in epidermis, etc.
        Chromaffin cells in adrenals
        Sympathetic and parasympathetic nervous systems
        Hyoid and related cartilages
    Population of bone marrow by stem cell populations
    Population of thymus by lymphocyte T cell precursors
    Migration of primordial germ cells to gonads

Selection of precise position by cell processes
    Selection of connections by nerve cells with each other and with muscle cells

Movement by cells moving in coordinated populations
    Gastrulation in nearly all Metazoa
    Movement of blocks of precardiac mesoderm over endoderm to form heart in chickens (Rosenquist, 1970)
    Movements of sheets of cells as in sternum formation (Fell, 1939)

provide positional information, other systems that move and position cells are also clearly of great moment in morphogenesis. It seems appropriate at this point to indicate that I am using the term 'positioning' to cover those phenomena that move or result in the movement of cells to definite selected positions, while 'positional information' refers to the instructions about differentiation that a cell acquires as a result of the position that it holds in the animal body. Clearly, the acquisition of 'positional information' is also to be considered as a cell recognition process.

The third mechanism which might be regarded as effecting positioning is that which controls the folding of cell sheets. Surprisingly little attention has been given to the control of the direction of folding, even though in recent years a good deal of research has been directed towards discovering the mechanism by which folding takes place. The embryologists of the period from 1930 to 1955 described many situations in which folding was either abnormal (e.g. exogastrulation), incomplete (as in spina bifida), or occurred at an inappropriate site (e.g. archencephalic inductions by mesoderm in spinal cord regions). They were not in command of techniques which would have allowed them to analyse the situations further. It is, however, of considerable interest to note that specific folding patterns are induced in neural plate tissue by specific areas of mesoderm (see Balinsky, 1965). The ensuing folding changes the topographical relationships of presumptive nerve cells and ectoderm and places the nervous system in its correct place as a hollow tube. Clearly, the process or processes that ensure that folding of a particular target tissue takes place in a given site at a particular time under the instruction of a second tissue are to be classed as cell recognition processes.

The fourth mechanism that can control positioning is that which produces topographical oriented cell division, ensuring that the cleavage planes of dividing cells are constant or nearly so. The most beautiful examples are, of course, seen in the division of certain invertebrate eggs, but we should bear in mind that a similar mechanism operates in the normal cell division in the epidermis, ensuring that daughter cells lie external and internal to one another. Little is known about the control of the plane of division in animals, though it might be quite reasonable to relate it to the positions of microfilament bundles and microtubule arrays.

Thus we should remember that positional death, 'positional information', and positional control of folding and of division planes are all mechanisms involving cell recognition systems which can produce results that might exactly resemble the effects of positioning of moving cells and cell masses. It is only when the actual processes that produce certain cell types in certain positions have been observed that we can decide between these alternatives. Table 7.1 lists some of the embryonic processes in which cell movement is used to effect positioning, while Table 7.2 lists similar events in adults and in a variety of pathological situations. Examination of Table 7.1 shows that the positioning of moving cells must play a major role in normal embryogenesis. I propose to confine further discussion to this area of positional phenomena, mainly because it is clear that it is the one that

Table 7.2 Positioning phenomena in the adult body (including pathological effects)

Movement by individual migration of cells
    Lymphocyte recirculation and segregation into T and B dependent areas in lymphoid organs
    Leukocyte localizations in sites of inflammation, etc.
    Fibroblast movement into wounded areas
    Metastasis

Movement by cells moving in coordinated populations
    Epithelial and endothelial movement during wound repair

---

is relevant to lymphocyte positioning. Lymphocytes apparently do not show positional death or folding nor are their division planes seemingly of any significance. It is true that the actual type of lymphocyte differentiation may be controlled by the local environment, but this is only a background to their circulation. Thus we can conclude that positioning by cells does indeed occur *de novo*. However, it is less clear that specific recognition processes act for both the Steinberg hypothesis and contact guidance might explain the positioning of cells.

7.4 EFFECTOR SYSTEMS FOR CELL POSITIONING AND CELL BEHAVIOUR

Two main routes exist for the transport of cells from one part of the body to another:

(i) through blood or lymph vessels, and
(ii) by penetration between groups of cells or between cells and intracellular structures.

The first route will normally be used for all migrations, whether of single cells or of groups of cells, in the first stages of the movement for blood vessels or lymph vessels can only be entered from the surrounding tissue by infiltration between the endothelial cells.

Surprisingly little is known about the problems that may exist for cells moving between other cells or between other cells and the surrounding extracellular materials such as collagen. The cells presumably move using their own locomotory apparatus. Intercellular space in the average adult mammalian organism is fairly extensive (Curtis, 1967), but we have little accurate idea of the average space between cells save that a great deal of it appears in electronmicrographs as a gap of between 7 and 50 nm in width. If a cell moves between two other cells, is it able to exert sufficient mechanical strength both to move the surrounding cells far enough apart to push through and break any molecules or more complex junctional structures that may join them?

Alternatively, cell surface associated enzymes, in particular proteases (Reich *et al.*, 1975), may be used to lyse such molecules. Observational evidence shows that cells, including lymphocytes, leucocytes, macrophages, and many neural crest derived cells amongst others, are able to penetrate between cells whose appearance in electronmicrographs suggests reasonably strong adhesion, for instance endothelia. It is probable that infiltrating cells cannot open the close junctional structures termed zonulae occludentes since white blood cell types are not found in the lumen of the kidney tubule: a site surrounded by such structures. When oriented movement takes place, it is conceivable that the cells follow the line of least resistance. I am not aware of any example for which this has been shown to be the case, but it is worth considering that it might act to lead cells from one site to a very definite secondary site.

Any selectivity that may be imposed on the transport system can act either on the direction of migration or in deciding at which point migration is stopped. Few systems, however, could act to determine the direction of migration in the bloodstream or lymph because of the rapid flow and good mixing in that flow. Chemotactic or chemokinetic mechanisms would be unlikely to act in the fast flow. It is, however, possible that electrophoretic effects might act radially to separate cells with different surface charge, because streaming potentials (see Kruyt, 1952) should be set up in blood vessels both by the movement of the medium against the charged walls and by any lagging of cells in the flow. These potentials might act to impose a radial motion on the cells. Otherwise, the two systems that might act to produce a selectivity are:

(i) adhesion to specialized endothelium, as is believed to occur at the high endothelium in lymph nodes (see Chapter 8.1), and
(ii) mechanical obstruction to blood or lymph flow such that cells larger than ordinary blood cells could not penetrate beyond the obstruction.

The first of these two mechanisms is discussed at length both in this and in other chapters. The second mechanism has been put forward in attempts to explain the apparent selectivity of siting of certain secondary tumours, in particular by Wood (1964) and Zeidman (1961). If a particular organ has small capillaries, it may trap tumour cells which are too large or too rigid to infiltrate between the walls of the capillaries.

Once we turn to consider cell movements within and between tissues, we find a larger potential range of mechanisms that might act to effect positioning. The relatively narrow fluid-filled spaces between cells might provide an ideal situation for chemotaxis or chemokinesis to act. A cell moving between two or more cells will almost certainly overlap at least two cell lengths in the direction of its progress from time to time. In consequence, a cell may be able to detect differences in its adhesion between the two cells and thus move in the direction of the more adhesive contact. This provides a second general type of mechanism for orienting and directing cell movements. Thirdly, positioning may result, either if a particular region is non-adhesive to a particular entering cell type, in which case the cell type is unable to invade that region, or if, as is more commonly thought to be the case, a particular site provides so strong an adhesion for an entering cell that it is

Table 7.3 Contact inhibition of movement

(a) Overlap ratio measurements

Cell type A	with	Cell type B	Overlap ratio	Reference
Normal cells				
Embryonic chick ventricle fibroblasts		Themselves	0.12	Abercrombie (1975)
Embryonic chick ventricle fibroblasts		Mouse MC1M sarcoma	0.55	Abercrombie & Heaysman (1976)
Embryonic chick ventricle fibroblasts		Mouse BAS/56 sarcoma	0.40	
Embryonic chick ventricle fibroblasts		Mouse 311 sarcoma	0.37	
Embryonic chick ventricle fibroblasts		Mouse SZ_3B16 melanoma	0.26	Abercrombie (1975)
Embryonic chick ventricle fibroblasts		Human MM96 melanoma	0.11	Stephenson & Stephenson (1978)
Embryonic chick pigmented retinal epithelia (PRE)		Themselves	0.02	Middleton (1973)
Human thyroid		Themselves	0.1–0.19	Projan & Tanneberger (1973)
Human skin fibroblasts		Themselves	0.09	Stephenson & Stephenson (1976)
Human skin ?		Themselves	0.04–0.11	Projan & Tanneberger (1973)
Mouse neonatal muscle fibroblasts		Themselves	0.18	Abercrombie *et al.* (1968)
BHK cells		Themselves	0.18–0.29*	Turbitt & Curtis (1974)
Tumours				
Follicular adenocarcinoma		Themselves	0.91	Projan & Tanneberger (1973)
Ovarian cystoma			0.56	
Pulmonary carcinoma			0.47	
Thymoma			0.63	
Granulosa cell tumour		Themselves	0.02	
Fibrosarcoma		Themselves	0.09	Abercrombie & Heaysman (1976)
Mouse MC1M		Themselves	0.25	
BAS/56		Themselves	0.25	
311		Themselves	0.34	
SZ_3		Themselves	0.10	
Hamster Py BHK		Themselves	0.25–0.45*	Turbitt & Curtis (1974)

trapped at that place. These reactions should be visible at the level of the individual cell in terms of cell behaviour. The main form of cell behaviour is contact inhibition of movement. It is arguable that contact guidance (Weiss, 1941) and contact retraction (Weiss, 1961) are but special cases of contact inhibition (see Dunn, 1971). In essence, all forms of cell behaviour so far described for the interaction of two or more cells lead to the distribution of the cells in a particular

Table 7.3 (*continued*)

(b) Film analysis, movement analysis, and orientation measurements

Cell type A	with	Cell type B	Contact inhibition	Reference
Nerve cell extensions		Themselves	√	Dunn (1971)
Nerve cell extensions		Themselves	√	Ebendal (1976)
Pigmented retina (embryo chick)		Themselves	√	Parkinson & Edwards (1978)
		Choroid	√	
BHK and Py BHK cells			√	Erikson (1978)
Rat fibroblasts and sarcoma		Themselves	√	
		Each other	Non reciprocal c.i. low for tumour cells	Vesely & Weiss (1973)

*Expressed as cells per counting area (1.8×10^{-8} m^2)

relationship to each other. Contact inhibition of movement (Abercrombie and Heaysman, 1954) is basically a phenomenon in which two cells, on making contact by their movement, paralyse further movement towards each other. This paralysis does not take place until a fairly extensive contact as seen by phase contrast microscopy has been made. The locomotory machinery for a fibroblast or an epithelial cell moving in a particular direction is controlled from the front end of the cell, so that contact paralyses movement that might lead to one cell overlapping or underlapping the other. This contact does not paralyse movement that might be set up in some other part of the periphery of either cell. As a result, if space is available for each cell to move into, on either side, they will then move apart. As a consequence of contact inhibition of movement, cells tend to monolayer and to move into free space in a tissue culture. It is probable, however, that the same phenomenon serves to prevent the cells moving too far apart. Abercrombie and Gitlin (1965) showed that if fibroblasts by chance move ahead clear of the outgrowth of fibroblasts in a culture, then their locomotion stops.

It seems likely that the presence of a second fibroblast close behind keeps the one in front moving steadily away, owing perhaps to the operation of contact inhibition of movement. Thus contact inhibition serves to orientate monolayer cells and to form them into confluent sheets. A list of cells that show and do not show contact inhibition of movement is given in Table 7.3. Contact guidance and contact retraction appear to be special instances of contact inhibition of movement. The test for contact inhibition is that overlapping or underlapping is less frequent than would be expected for random packing of the cells. The opposite type of behaviour has been named 'contact promotion' of movement. It means that cells prefer to move on each other rather than on other surfaces. This term was introduced by Curtis (1960). Only a few instances of this form of behaviour have come to light, the most notable being of lymphocytes on reticulum cells in culture

(Haston, 1979). However, it is likely that cells in an aggregate can show this type of behaviour.

Unfortunately it is hard to see the relevance of these studies to positioning in the embryo or to cell infiltration. The main reason for this is that little is known about the differential behaviour that a cell may show towards two different cell types from *in vitro* studies. In these studies cell behaviour is usually examined when the cells have the choice between a plastic or glass substrate (albeit serum-coated) and another cell of their own type. Abercrombie and his co-workers have made fairly extensive studies of interactions between fibroblasts and various tumour cells (see Abercrombie, 1975; Abercrombie and Heaysman, 1976) but these are unfortunately of little relevance to studies of positioning of normal cells. It would be of great interest to have more studies of the behaviour of groups of cells on culture substrates. Furthermore, invading tumour cells and possibly lymphocytes can alternate rapidly between contact inhibition and contact promotion. Studies of cell behaviour in culture have failed to provide evidence for the action of specific adhesion or selectivity operating in the disposition of cells. The reason for this probably lies in a failure to carry out appropriate experiments rather than its non-existence.

7.5 EXPERIMENTAL DEMONSTRATION OF SELECTIVITY IN CELL ADHESIONS

Selectivity of a cell for its adhesion between two other cells, one of its type and one of another type, could provide an important basis for positioning. A variety of mechanisms (see later) could act to produce this selectivity, and it is important to note that some of these mechanisms could lead to precise patterned positioning while others might simply do no more than incline a cell to association with one of its own type rather than with an unlike cell. Positioning which arises in a group of randomly arranged cells of two or more types requires the operation of a patterning system. Positioning in which cells simply accrete to a previously positioned cell by some form of selectivity in their adhesion requires no patterning system. So we should ask whether experimental systems demonstrate an ability for *de novo* positioning or whether they merely test whether cells will accrete to a preexisting pattern. In the latter case, possible mechanisms that the cells may have for *de novo* positioning may be concealed.

The basic problem is whether the selectivity simply acts to bias the preference for adhesion towards a particular combination of two cells rather than another or whether it also selects position. Chemotaxis, for instance, might select position and thus automatically select the particular partner a cell might have. The specific adhesion of like cells to each other in a mixture would as far as I can see (Curtis, 1978a,b, 1979; see also Curtis, 1967; Steinberg, 1962) select partners but would not select position. Thus when we use a particular experimental system we should enquire whether the system demonstrates positioning or merely selectivity of partner cells. If it only does the latter, it does not disprove the existence of a positioning mechanism, it merely fails to reveal it. Conversely, as we shall see, some experimental systems reveal positioning but do not clearly reveal the mechanism behind it.

Cell biologists have usually assumed that when two vertebrate cell types are aggregated together they unite into the initial aggregate in a random pattern and later sort out into discrete tissues. If this is true, it is a beautiful example of positioning arising *de novo*. Unfortunately there are very few investigations which show whether this assumption is true or false. Elton and Tickle (1971) found that very early aggregates of chick embryonic tissue formed from two cell types contained these two types but that they were already sorted out to some extent. Curtis (1974, 1978a) found that aggregates could be random in composition proportions for two cell types at times as early as 1 hr after the start of aggregation but that non-random compositions could be obtained if the cells were allowed to condition the medium. I also found that aggregates at 8 hr tended to be random in arrangement of cell types as far as could be judged selectively and this corroborates Steinberg's (1970) observations. Studies of the aggregation of two cell types thus appear to indicate that positioning takes place but do not reveal whether adhesion is involved in positioning because the cells have already become adhesive in order to form aggregates. Obviously in cases in which two cell types will not adhere to each other but form separate aggregates from the start of aggregation, selective or specific cell adhesion must play an important if not paramount role in the process. It is, however, arguable that such results are not relevant to positioning studies because no positioning occurs. Such instances are, however, rare and in many cases, for example with several sponges, aggregation initially occurs between cells indiscriminately. Only later do the cell masses separate into different aggregates. In some experimental situations, e.g. Moscona (1962), aggregation can be manipulated so that it is specific from the start, but such studies may still be irrelevant to positioning studies.

Clearer methods of establishing whether selectivity occurs in cell adhesion have been devised. In three of these methods cells are presented with a preformed substrate of sheets or balls of one cell type and the degree of adhesion between like cell suspensions and cell substrates is compared with that between unlike cell suspensions and substrates. These are:

1. The collecting aggregate system (Roth and Weston, 1967)
2. The collecting cell lawn, in which cell suspensions are allowed to settle on to monolayers of cells
3. The 'natural cell lawn', in which the sheet-like nature of certain tissues is used as a substrate (Barbera, 1975). Tissue 'slices' (Stamper and Woodruff, 1977) have also been used.

In two methods the nature of the initial adhesions formed is studied:

4. The initial aggregate cell type composition (IAC method; Curtis, 1974) in which the cell types in very early 2, 3, 4 and 5 cell aggregates and so on are studied using some appropriate cell type marker. If the proportion of the various

Table 7.4 Selectivity in the formation of adhesions

Cell types	Technique	Selectivity	Reference
Sponge			
Various species	CA	Species-specific	McClay (1971)
Strain types in *Ephydatia*	KAS	Specific control of adhesion	Curtis & Van de Vyver (1971)
Other species	KAS	Non-specific	Curtis (1970a)
Echinoderms			
Lytechinus and Tripneustes embryos	CA	Specific control of adhesion	McClay & Hausman (1975)
Embryonic chick tissues			
Neural retina and liver	CA tissue spec.	Tissue specificity	Roth & Weston (1967)
Neural retina and liver	KAS, IAC	Tissue specificity under defined conditions only, often not	Curtis (1974); Elton & Tickle (1971)
Neural retina and liver	CL	Tissue specificity	Walther et al. (1973)
Neural retina and liver plus mesencephalon	CA	Tissue specificity	McGuire & Burdick (1976)
Neural retina to optic tectum	CT	Ventral retina to dorsal tectum, dorsal retina to ventral tectum, but low specificity	
Neural retina to optic tectum	KAS	No specificity	Jones (1977)
Various embryonic tissues	CA	Tissue specificity	Roth et al. (1971)
BHK and 3T3	CL	No specificity	Walther et al. (1973)
Mouse kidney and teratoma	CL	Tissue specificity	Walther et al. (1973)
Polymorphs, human and calf, to endothelia and various cell lines	CL	Preference for endothelia	Hoover (1978)
Mouse fibroblasts, different H-2 type	CL	Preference for their own H-2 type	Bartlett & Edidin (1978)
Embryonic chick pigmented retina, neural retina, and choroid	CL	Choroid collects PRE preferentially	Buultjens & Edwards (1977)
Lymphocytes, murine	KAS	Specificity under defined conditions, specific endothelial cells	Curtis & de Sousa (1973)
B and T cells	IAC		Curtis & de Sousa (1973)
Circulating lymphocytes tonnode cells	CTS		Stamper & Woodruff (1977)

CA, Collecting aggregate
CL, Collecting lawn
CTS, Collecting tissue slice
CT, Collecting tissue surface
IAC, Specificity in initial aggregates
KAS, Kinetic assay of specificity

types in the aggregates is biased from that in the original suspension, selectivity may be taking place.

5. The kinetic assay of specificity (Curtis, 1970a,b; Curtis and de Sousa, 1975; Jones, 1978), though only given this name recently (Curtis, 1979a, 1979b), achieves the same result as method 4 by studying the rate of aggregation. If cells adhere specifically then collisions with other types will be ineffective and the rate of adhesion will decline.

All these methods have at times given indications that cell adhesion can be specific, or at least selective (Table 7.4). Methods 1–3 produce cell layers, etc., that may be able to condition the medium, while cell products can be added to the medium to test if they have any effect in methods 4 and 5. It is particularly interesting that methods 4 and 5 only produce evidence for selectivity when cell products have been added to the medium.

The selectivity that has been demonstrated in these experiments has usually been simply interpreted as being due to the action of specific adhesion. Is it possible to explain the sorting out seen in aggregates in terms of specific adhesion? The behaviour of sponge cells – cells which sort out into specific aggregates – might be accounted for by specific adhesion though it is not necessary to use this explanation. Again, specific adhesion could account for the accretion of cells on to a preexisting pattern of cells such that the appropriate cells to which adhesion is to be made are already in the right place. For instance, the sorting out of lymphocytes into T and B dependent areas in the lymph nodes and spleen could be due to the entrant cells forming specific adhesions with existing features of the nodes. This specific adhesion might be with reticulum cells or with lymphocytes already in place. However, it is, I feel, very difficult to explain the formation of pattern *de novo* that is seen in aggregates on the basis of some form of specific adhesion. The reason for this difficulty is that the existence of specific mechanisms of adhesion does not specify the pattern that will be taken up by one cell type with respect to another. Specific adhesion might produce systems in which cells sort out into separate groups each composed of one type but it does not provide a system which specifies that cell type A will always enclose cell type B. It is just remotely possible that cells might exist with various specific groupings arranged in a pattern over their surfaces such that they ensure that the whole structure can be assembled in one patterned way – this seems extremely unlikely. This defect in concepts of specific adhesion has been appreciated by Steinberg (1962) (see also Curtis, 1962). Specific adhesion would, of course, explain the adhesion and accretion of moving cells to prepositioned structures. Conversely, self-patterning mechanisms of cell positioning could also act in the presence of prepositioned structures.

7.6 PATTERNING POSSIBILITIES IN RECOGNITION SYSTEMS: THEORIES EXPLAINING POSITIONING AND PATTERNING

Four theories have been proposed to explain the positioning and patterning seen by the control of cell movement in multicellular animals. They are:

1. Specific adhesion
2. Chemotaxis
3. The interaction modulation theory (Curtis, 1974, 1978a,b), in which the specific control of adhesion by diffusible agents is suggested.
4. The differential adhesion theory due to Steinberg (1963, 1970).

If we correlate these theories with the different physical models for recognition put forward on p. 165 we obtain the following correspondence:

Specific adhesion = insoluble signal and receptor (mutual receptor theory)
Chemotaxis = soluble signal: insoluble receptor
Interaction modulation theory = ditto
Differential adhesion theory (no specific recognition process).

I have already suggested that there are great difficulties in explaining *de novo* positioning when the specific adhesion theory is used. This can be stated in physical terms as the simple consequence that there is no vectorial change from place to place in a mass of cells in any property that might affect cell movement if a system of cell surface-bound mutual receptors is proposed. Soluble signal : insoluble receptor systems have, however, considerable potentialities for setting up a system of information in the environment that will trap cells in particular positions.

When we turn to consider chemotaxis, we are immediately provided with a system that could provide positioning *de novo*, for instance in an aggregate. Specific adhesion would, of course, explain the adhesion and accretion of moving cells to prepositioned structures. Conversely, self-patterning mechanisms of cell positioning could also act in the presence of prepositioned structures. On the simplest hypothesis about chemotaxis, it would be expected that the only patterns that could be set up would be ones in which the various different cell types would be arranged radially (Edelstein, 1971). Steinberg (1964) has criticized the application of chemotaxis in theories of sorting out by claiming that radial patterns are the only ones that would result, while in fact the patterns are that one cell type encloses another. Obviously the only basis for the generation of gradients in an otherwise unordered aggregate of cells will be the diffusion out of cellular products and the diffusion inwards of various metabolites. Ideally, we would expect that the gradients would be symmetrically and radially arranged in a spherical aggregate. However, local random accumulations of one cell type at one place in the initial random aggregate are inevitable and this, together with defects of diffusion, could well modify the gradients so that they cease to be wholly radial. Chemotaxis or chemokinesis thus provides a system that would tend to segregate one cell type internally and the other externally.

Clearly, recognition systems which depend upon the diffusion of a soluble signal and which produce cellular responses such as chemotaxis would provide a means of positioning cells both *de novo* and to a preexisting structure. The system is unlikely to operate in fast-flowing media, but could easily operate in tissue systems that are already prepositioned, as well as in aggregates. The relatively thin interstices between cells would tend to hold chemotactic gradients in a stable form.

The interaction modulation theory was first proposed by the author of this chapter in a simple form (Curtis, 1974) and later discussed more fully (Curtis, 1976, 1978a,b). It is closely related to chemotactic theories. The basic proposal is that cells secrete soluble diffusible recognition molecules that specifically interact to reduce the adhesion of a range of unlike cells. It is worth noting that an inverse theory to this might be proposed, namely that the diffusible molecules specifically increase the adhesion of certain target cells. However, the experimental evidence favours the former version. The theory contains elements of the theory of specific adhesion in that it would be expected that cell adhesion would appear to be specific until the experimenter could dissociate the specific control system from the response of the cells. It also contains elements of the chemotactic theory in that the signal molecule is thought to be diffusible. The response of the range of unlike cells that can respond to the signal is thought to be a reduction in adhesion to any surface. Thus, the adhesion mechanism is not in itself specific but the control is.

The reader should note that the chemotactic theory and the interaction modulation theory may be very closely related indeed. Dierich *et al.* (1977) have suggested that changes in adhesion may result from chemotactic agents, and this is reinforced by the work of Smith *et al.* (1979), who found that chemotactic agents reduced the adhesiveness of target cells. Approaching from the other side, Wilkinson and Curtis (in press) have shown that a pure interaction modulation factor which decreases the adhesiveness of B lymphocytes to surfaces stimulates chemokinesis of these cells. The chemotactic theory also proposes specific control of a cell property, the direction of movement, by soluble diffusible molecules, while the IMF theory proposes that a similar mechanism controls the final position of cells by determining whether they will prefer to make adhesions at one site or another.

I have referred already to the differential adhesion hypothesis which Steinberg proposed (1963) and now return to this. In essence, this suggests that the driving force by which one cell type leaves the surface of an aggregate is due to the difference in interfacial free energies of the two (or more) cell types involved. Steinberg (1962, 1970, 1975) suggested that this driving force would lead to the system (all the cells in the aggregate) tending towards the minimum free energy configuration. If the interfacial free energy between A type cells be written σ_{aa}, that between B type cells σ_{bb}, that between A and B cells σ_{ab}, and σ_{ao}, σ_{bo} are interfacial tensions of A and B with the external medium, the cells should, if they behave like droplets of immiscible oil in forming and breaking adhesions, adopt an equilibrium defined by $\sigma_{ao} + \sigma_{ab} > \sigma_{ab} > \sigma_{ao} - \sigma_{bo}$. Simple, somewhat inexact rules (see Phillips, 1969) suggest that if $\sigma_{ab} < \sigma_{aa} + (\sigma_{bb}/2)$, then cell type A will accumulate internally while it will be surrounded by B. This hypothesis requires, I believe, that large numbers of discrete units (cells) behave like small numbers of oil droplets and that the cell contacts bring extensive areas of surface into molecular apposition. The answer to the first of these points is not known while the second requirement, if such it be, is not borne out by examination of electronmicrographs of the contacts. However, two features of the theory have the strong support of experiment. The first of these is that the theory explicitly predicts constant patterns, whereas, as we have seen, the theory of specific adhesion fails to obtain this prediction. The second is that it suggests that pattern formation arises *de novo* simply as the consequence of the graded value of a single property, interfacial free energy, that the various cell types in an aggregate possess in different measure. Steinberg (1964) showed that there is a hierarchy in the sorting out of various types in an aggregate. The hierarchy is constant and strongly suggests that a quantitative property varies from one tissue type to another. Phillips *et al.* (1977) also showed experimentally that when centrifugal deformation of aggregates was carried out, cells were drawn into the surface layer to expand it and that they returned reversibly inside the aggregate when the centrifuge was stopped. This is an interesting observation which suggests that interfacial or internal rheological properties of cells may be of much more importance in determining tissue shape than we have suspected heretofore. However, the observation, though agreeing with one of the contentions made by Steinberg about cell movement in aggregates, is as Harris (1976) pointed out not diagnostic between Steinberg's theory or any other.

It seems appropriate to return to the interaction modulation and chemotactic theories to examine how they might explain the hierarchy of sorting out. It seems to me that the simple answer to this question is that the graded property would on these theories become the diffusibility of the signal. It should be borne in mind that at first sight it would be difficult to imagine large differences in diffusibility of two different signals unless they were of very different molecular weight. This point has been made by Crick (1970), who has considered how the putative signals involved in setting up differentiation gradients might act. However, it should be remembered that two mechanisms probably exist to sharpen and differentiate between two gradients. First, the signal will be bound to target cells; consequently in regions containing other cell types the signal will diffuse through largely unaffected to steepen its gradient in regions containing cells that carry receptors. The second mechanism is the likelihood that the cells that bind the signal will both synthesize new receptors and may also destroy the signal. Consequently the problem must be seen not merely as one of physical diffusion but also of the density of binding sites per unit volume and the rate of turnover and freeing of these sites.

The differential adhesion hypothesis predicts that the most adhesive cells will locate internally in the aggregate. The interaction modulation hypothesis and the chemotactic theories would see the process rather differently, and though the theory of sorting out on the IMF hypotheis has been described (Curtis, 1978a,b), it is appropriate to restate it here.

Imagine an aggregate in which two cell types have coaggregated in roughly equal proportions and in which they are arranged randomly. The concentrations of the IMFs that they produce will rise inside the aggregate soon after its formation; near the surface there will be a particularly sharp gradient in both IMFs because they will be lost to the outside. If one IMF is more diffusible than the other, its concentration in the outer cell layer will be very low. Consequently, the adhesiveness of the cells it reacts with will not be reduced. Remember that IMFs as known at present diminish the adhesiveness of an unlike cell type. The other IMF will be at a relatively higher concentration and its target cell will have its adhesiveness reduced. As a consequence, that cell type whose adhesiveness is reduced will either fall out of the aggregate (a phenomenon that is seen regularly) or will become motile so that it can move into the aggregate. Thus unlike the differential adhesion hypothesis, the first stable layer of adhesive cells will form at the outside of the aggregate. It will be most interesting to check whether this is true: the histological appearance of aggregates suggests that it might be. Once a non-randomness in cell disposition is established, the process becomes autocatalytic. The peripheral layer of cells will be bordered on its inward side by a high concentration of the IMF that it makes and a low concentration of the other IMF: thus cells of its own type will become adhesive and be trapped as they approach this layer. Similarly, the other cell type will become purified and more adhesive. Finally (see Fig. 7.2), the aggregate will be sorted out and the two cell

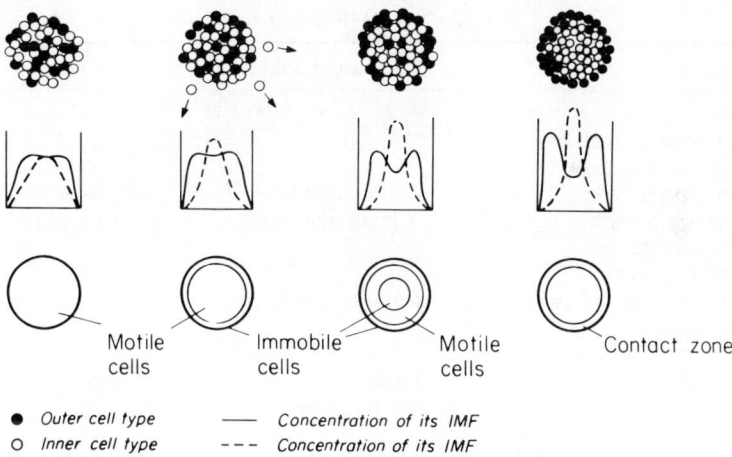

Figure 7.2 Diagram to explain the sorting out of aggregates in terms of the interaction modulation theory. The top row shows a summary of the experimental observations during sorting out. The middle row shows how the two cell types establish gradients of their IMFs whose initially different slopes are determined by the different diffusibilities of the IMFs. These gradients then show positive feedback to the final forms as a result of the movement of cells to their sorted-out positions. The bottom row shows main areas of cell movement during sorting out on this hypothesis. In any region where there is a considerable difference in concentrations of the two IMFs, cells of the type opposite to that producing the greatest concentration of IMF will become less adhesive and will leave that region

types will be joined by a junction of low adhesiveness, whereas the differential adhesion hypothesis predicts that this junction will be of intermediate adhesiveness. If aggregates are made with very varying proportions of the two cell types, sorting-out patterns may be reversed because the relative concentrations and diffusion difference of the two IMFs may be changed; this behaviour has been observed (Wiseman *et al.*, 1972) and used as support for the differential adhesion theory.

7.7 INTERACTION MODULATION AND THE CONTROL OF CELL POSITIONING

7.7.1 Evidence for the interaction modulation theory

There are three main stages in the demonstration that an interaction modulation system operates to control cell positioning.

First, the effect of secreted cell products on the adhesion of an unlike but related cell type (for instance B lymphocyte products on T lymphocyte adhesion) should be tested. The simplest test to use is medium conditioned by actively metabolizing cells. If a reduction in adhesion of a range of target cells is found, this is evidence that an IMF system may operate. Further work should lead to the

Table 7.5 IMF-like factors

Producing cell type	Decreasing adhesion of	Reference
Sponges		
Ephydatia fluviatilis (freshwater sponge)		
Alpha strain type	Delta strain type	Curtis & Van de
Delta strain type	Alpha strain type	Vyver (1971)
Hymeniacidon sp. (marine sponge)		
27 non-coalescent paired individuals	Non-coalescent partner	Curtis (1979b)
Embryonic chick tissues		
Neural retina	Liver	Curtis (1974)
Liver	Neural retina	
Mouse, human, rat lymphocytes		
B lymphocytes	T lymphocytes	Curtis & de Sousa
T lymphocytes	B lymphocytes	(1973, 1975)
T lymphocytes	Leukocyte	
T lymphocytes	Macrophage	
T lymphocytes	Allogeneic T cells	Curtis (1979c)
Macrophages	Allogeneic macrophages	
Lymphocyte	Leukocyte	Lomnitzer *et al.* (1976)
Liver	Lymphoid cells	Fichtelius (1964)
? in serum	Lymphocytes or macrophages	Martineau & Johnson (1978)

Table 7.6 Do IMF systems affect display of selectivity in cell adhesion?

System	Type of assay*	Result	Both IMF tests	Reference
Two strain types of *Ephydatia fluviatilis*	KAS	+	ND	Curtis & Van de Vyver (1971)
Chick embryonic neural retina and liver	IAC	+	+	Curtis (1974); Hoover quoted in Curtis (1974)
Mouse B and T lymphocytes	KAS IAC	+	ND	Curtis & de Sousa (1975)
Chick embryonic retina	KAS (no IMF)	−	ND	Jones (1977)

+ selectivity found with IMF present.
− selectivity not found with IMF present.
ND not done.
Both IMF tests refer to use of IMFs from both cell types simultaneously.
*See Table 7.4, for details of assay description.

purification and concentration of the activity. Table 7.5 shows a range of systems on which this test has yielded definite decreases in adhesion.

Second, addition of the IMF to a system containing the cell type that produces it and another target cell type which tests selectivity of cell adhesion should show this, because the IMF will depress the adhesion of the target cell type. The crucial distinction of this result from those in which a factor has specifically stimulated the adhesion of its own type is to test whether addition of both IMFs to a system containing both producer cell types enhances or destroys specificity. This test has been very rarely done, but with IMFs specificity will diminish because the adhesiveness of both cell types will be lessened. Results are shown in Table 7.6.

The third test is, I believe, the crucial one for any hypothesis about positioning. This is to show direct association of IMF molecules with a positioning system that produces them by demonstrating that abnormally low or high concentrations of the factor *in vivo* alter positioning. The results of the test are summarized in Table 7.7.

Table 7.7 Alteration of positioning: association with IMF-like factors

Sponge	
Hymeniacidon sp.	
Association of IMF production and effects on adhesion with graft rejection and non-coalescence	Curtis (1979)
Embryonic chick tissue	
Reversal of sorting-out positions in aggregates	Curtis (1978a)
Reversal of sorting out on filters using gradients of IMF	
Lymphocytes	
Alteration of recirculation of injected labelled lymphocytes by T IMF	
Release of B lymphocytes from spleen on injection of T IMF	Davies & Curtis (in preparation)

This short section summarizes the main evidence in favour of the IMF theory available at present. The data for lymphocytes, which are the most extensive with the best characterized factors, are discussed more fully in the final section of this chapter.

7.7.2 Examples of positioning systems

7.7.2.1 Propigment cells in urodele amphibians

The first example is one in which it is believed that chemotaxis provides the main positioning system. I make no apology for the fact that this work was completed by Victor Twitty (1944), more than 30 years ago (see also Lehman and Youngs, 1959). It has been overlooked, and though the experiments could be repeated nowadays with some technical improvements, the work is of classic quality and should inspire biologists, particularly in North America, to return to it and extend it.

The propigment cells, promelanophores and proxanthophores, are of neural crest origin and migrate from that tissue as single cells as neurulation finishes. Some of the neural crest cells go to other sites to form other tissues (see Noden, 1978), but here I shall consider the propigment cells which reach the dermis, probably by a migration through solid somite tissue (see Weston, 1963).

In *Triturus rivularis*, the melanophores are initially diffused over the flank with a gentle dorso-ventral gradient over which they decrease in number per unit area as one moves ventrally. In other words, the flank shades from dark brown to pale brown from top to bottom. In *Triturus torosus*, the melanophores are arranged initially in the same manner. Later they concentrate into a dense lateral band which runs longitudinally high on the flank of the animal. In *Ambystoma mexicanum* (Lehman and Youngs, 1959) the flank is initially covered evenly and fairly densely with melanophores. Later these segregate into a number of rather irregularly placed vertical bars with the yellow xanthophores in between.

Twitty (1944) carried out simple experiments in which cultures of the larval pigment cells in peritoneal fluid were observed. He noted that *rivularis* pigment cells tended to form cultures of very sparsely arranged cells which gave the appearance of repelling each other. With *torosus* cells in culture, a tendency to aggregate appeared after the cells showed a tendency to overdisperse. He pointed out that this *in vitro* behaviour would exactly explain the *torosus* pattern. He also carried out various xenogeneic grafts which suggest complex interactions between tissues of different species. Twitty and Niu (1948, 1954) showed that the confinement of the cells in situations in which they might condition the medium and set up diffusion gradients led to the overdispersal of the cells, which suggests that a chemotactic (negative) or chemokinetic (positive) system might be in action. Thus Twitty (1949) was able to account for the initial dispersal of the propigment cells over the flanks of these urodeles by their mutual spacing out due to the secretion of chemotactic or kinetic substances that led to the cells moving down gradient. In

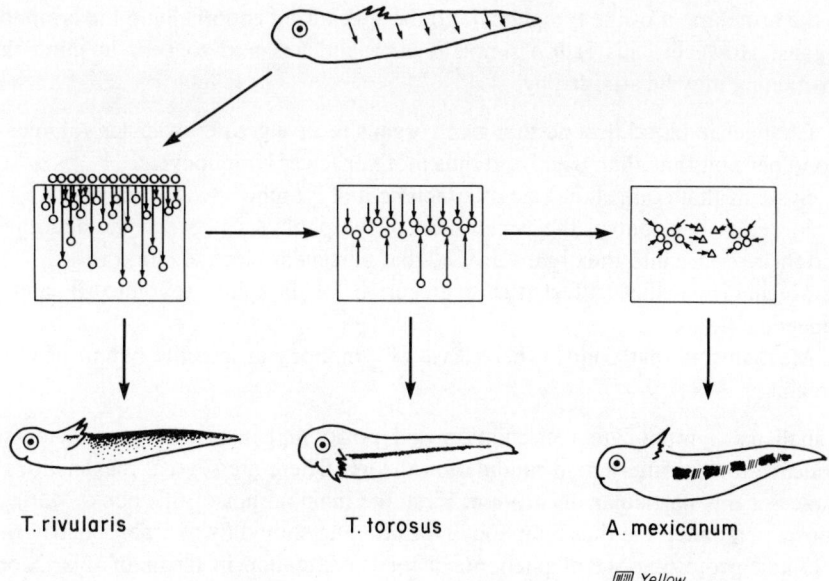

Figure 7.3 Cell interactions in the pigmentation of the flank of urodeles. The propigment cells migrate down the flank from the neural crest, see top of diagram. Twitty and Lehman and Youngs showed that in *Triturus rivularis* migration is due to negative chemotaxis between the propigment cells and this tends to spread them over the surface of the flank in a graded, even distribution, see left-hand box which illustrates movement of cells on the flank. This gives rise to the *T. rivularis* type of pigmentation. Other species pass through this stage, but in *T. torosus* the initial negative chemotaxis is followed by a positive chemotaxis and aggregation related to the top of the underlying muscle blocks. The middle box shows this cell movement. This produces a lateral bar of pigmentation. *Ambystoma mexicanum* passes through this positive chemotactic stage but then the xanthophores and melanophores which have collected in a bar repel each other, probably by negative chemotaxis, and sort out into alternative black and yellow bars

torosus and in *A. mexicanum* there then followed a phase of positive chemotaxis such that the cells aggregated, with evidence in the latter species that the areas of high melanophore concentration became repellent to xanthophores so that they migrated into the areas in between the melanophore bands (see Fig. 7.3).

7.7.2.2 *Lymphocyte positioning: an example for the application of the interaction modulation theory*

All the other chapters of this book are eloquent testimony to the enormous capabilities of positioning that lymphocytes show. Instead of a single movement during the embryonic lifetime of a tissue and a steadfast maintenance of that position thereafter, lymphocytes, individual lymphocytes, may go through positioning processes time after time. It has often been supposed by tacit acquiescence that the main, perhaps the only, point at which lymphocyte positioning is controlled is at the attachment of the lymphocyte to the specialized endothelia in the lymphoid organs. However, this is too simple a view and we need to bear in mind that positioning may be attained by:

1. Changes in blood flow so that given organs receive greater or lesser volumes of blood per unit time than usual and thus more or fewer lymphocytes.
2. Systems that control the rate of attachment of lymphocytes to endothelia.
3. Systems that control the penetration of lymphocytes between the endothelia and their release into the organs around that particular piece of blood vessel.
4. Mechanisms that affect the segregation of lymphocytes into B and T dependent areas.
5. Mechanisms that control the release of lymphocytes into the lymph or blood stream.

I shall use lymphocyte recirculation and positioning to illustrate in detail the evidence for the interaction modulation theory. There are several reasons for the choice of this particular illustration. First, the main author of this book, Maria de Sousa, persuaded me that lymphocyte positioning should form a particularly suitable and promising set of phenomena for investigation in terms of this theory. Second, her hopes have been satisfied in quite a large measure so that, third, more is known about the role of interaction modulation factors in this system than in any other.

At first sight, it might seem that since positioning can take place in five different sites, the lymphocyte positioning system must be one of great complexity. However, it will appear that with the possible exception of those factors that affect blood flow, IMF systems might act in the remaining four levels. This possibility will be discussed later.

7.7.3 Initial evidence for the existence of lymphocyte IMFs

The initial evidence that B and T cells might interact by an IMF system came from experiments in which the kinetic assay of specificity was used (KAS system). This technique requires the measurement of the rate of adhesion of the cells from single cell suspensions into aggregates. If there is no specificity in cell adhesion and no interaction between the two cell types which might affect adhesion, we would expect that the adhesiveness for a mixture would be a mean of the adhesivenesses for the two cell types separately weighted for their proportions in the mixture. If adhesion was completely specific, all collisions between unlike cell types would be ineffective and as a consequence the average adhesiveness for the mixture would be much reduced. Precise equations for making these calculations are given in Curtis, (1970a). If the cells interact to reduce each other's adhesion, the reduction in adhesion might be either smaller or larger than that predicted for complete specificity of adhesion. In the former case, it would be impossible to make distinction between this hypothesis and a partial specificity of adhesion but a larger reduction in adhesion would be strong evidence for an IMF system. Results for such an experiment are shown in Fig. 7.4 in which those T and B

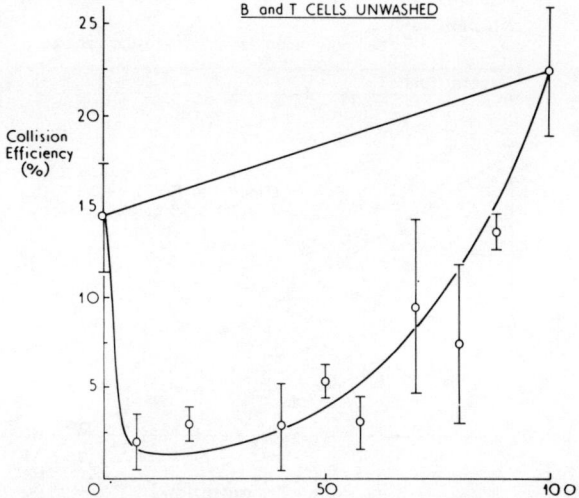

Figure 7.4 Adhesiveness (collision efficiency) for various mixtures of unwashed B and T cells. Vertical lines, SD. This demonstrates that factors in conditioned media depress the adhesion of the opposite cell type

lymphocytes, in media which they had conditioned, were mixed. The experimental results for cell mixtures show an adhesion even lower than that expected if adhesion were specific. When the experiment is repeated with cell suspensions that have been well washed immediately prior to the experiment, adhesion becomes raised to the mean value expected for mixtures without any specificity of adhesion.

This type of experiment gave Maria de Sousa and me (Curtis and de Sousa, 1973, 1975) reason to suspect that IMF systems might be involved in B and T cell interactions. The next stage of our work was to show that media conditioned by B and T cells respectively reduce the adhesion of T and B cells. In due course, this led to the purification of both factors and the development of an assay system and definition of units of activity (see Fig. 7.5, Curtis and de Sousa, 1975).

It appears that mouse thymocytes and peripheral T cells produce an IMF which is a small glycoprotein of molecular weight 10,000, potent in reducing the adhesion of syngeneic B lymphocytes and macrophage and neutrophil leucocytes. B lymphocytes produce a less well characterized IMF of approximate molecular weight 6,000 which at present is known to reduce the adhesion of thymocytes and peripheral T cells. The effect of those IMFs on the adhesion of other cell types has not been tested yet. Both factors have more marked effects on allogeneic cells; this is discussed later in the chapter.

It is possible to prepare antibodies against these factors. Use of the antibodies has shown that the T IMF glycoprotein is bound to the surface of target and producer cells. These cell types show a positive reaction with the antibody both in immune fluorescent staining and in complement-mediated lysis tests. Though this

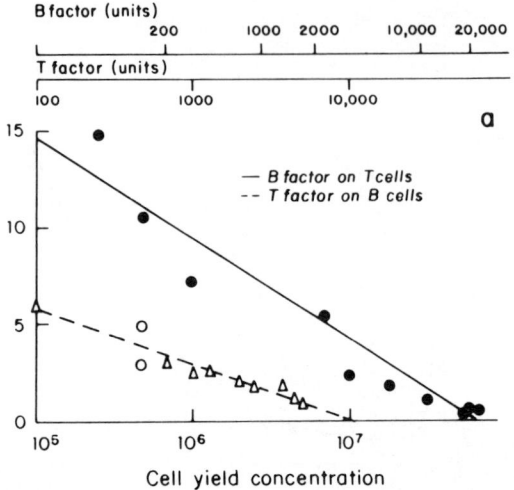

Figure 7.5 Dose-response curves for the effects of mouse T (thymic) and B factors on the adhesion of mouse B and thymus cells. Preparation of factors described in text. Ordinates, adhesiveness expressed as collision efficiency (%). Abscissae, concentration of factor applied. (a) Effects on heterologous cells. Cell yield concentration (abscissa) refers to concentration of factor in terms of the amount produced by that number of cells under conditions specified in text. Units of activity in upper abscissa. Values of adhesiveness in absence of factor: 22.6% for T cells and 11.7% for B cells. Vertical bars = 2SD

would appear to suggest a cell surface location for the material even in the producer cells, it is not impossible that binding is slight and transitory. Examination of other cell types and tissues for presence of the T IMF antigen in mice showed that the cells listed in Table 7.8 displayed surface binding of the T IMF. It might be argued that these observations are compatible with the theory that these other cell types are also producers of the glycoprotein. However, when animals were immunosuppressed with anti-lymphocyte serum for a period of nine days, during which the theta-positive population of cells virtually disappeared, this positive reaction for T IMF disappeared from all cell types. This suggests that the factor is produced by T cells and thymocytes and is bound to a small range of target cell types.

T and B IMFs can confer apparent specificity on cell adhesion. For instance, small aggregates prepared from well washed mixtures of B and T cells show no specificity in their compositon. Aggregates which are composed of both B and T

Table 7.8 Presence of T IMF antigen in CBA/ca mice

Thymocytes	Weakly positive on their surface: strong internally
Peripheral T cells	Weakly positive on their surface: strong internally
Peripheral B cells	Weakly positive: negative internally
Lymph nodes, spleen	All lymphocytes at least weakly positive T-dependent areas strongly positive (in sectioned material) Stromal cells negative
Macrophages	All positive
Leukocytes	All positive
Erythrocytes	All negative
Cerebral hemispheres	Many non-glial cells positive, all glia negative
Cerebellum	Glial cells negative, peduncular areas strongly positive
Eye	Rods and cones positive, all other layers including sclera and choroid negative
Liver	Very occasional positive cells (? lymphocytes, macrophages)
Kidney	Occasional positive cells in glomeruli
Heart	All components negative
Lungs	Alveolar surface positive, remainder negative
Intestine	Villi weakly positive
Skin	Epidermis negative, occasional positive cells in dermis

cells are more common than those consisting solely of one or other type (see Fig. 7.6). However, addition of B factor biases the aggregates so that they become impoverished in T cells, presumably because T cells are now of reduced adhesion. Addition of T factor biases the aggregates to compositions impoverished in B cells, presumably for the same reason. In the presence of both factors, aggregates hardly form but those that do are random in composition (see Fig. 7.6). This type of experiment shows that IMFs can specifically control adhesion. The results also show that such effects cannot be explained as a specific stimulation of adhesion, for if this were so aggregates in the final experiment should be present in large numbers and should be biased to being T or B rich.

I have the impression, subjective alone at present, that the effect of these IMFs is to reduce the adhesion of the cells to any surface to which they would normally adhere. It is important that this point should be confirmed because it has a marked bearing on the interpretation of the effects of these systems.

Lymphocytes which have been exposed to IMFs of the opposite type recover their adhesion once this factor is removed. This, together with the data on binding, the fact that the IMFs do not affect viability of cells, suggests that IMFs are either being removed from the cell surface or that new sites involved in adhesion are being generated continuously. Thus it is likely that the particular value of adhesiveness shown by a cell at any one time represents a balance between IMF binding and IMF removal by the cell.

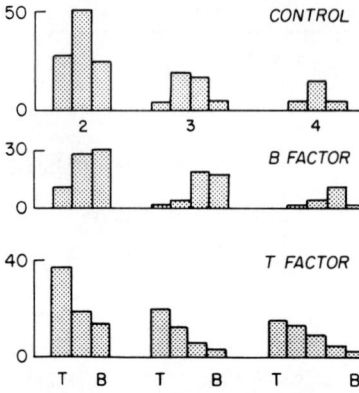

Figure 7.6 Composition of aggregates of B and T cells formed in absence (upper line) of any added factor and in presence of 200 units/ml of added B factor or 300 units/ml added T factor. The histograms for 2, 3, and 4 cell aggregates show the number of aggregates observed in each composition class. For 2 cell aggregates there are three composition classes, pure T (on left of each block), 50% B, and pure B. The letters T and B indicate the class solely composed of that type. For 4 cell aggregates, for instance, there are the following classes: 100% T, 75% T, 50% T, 25% T, 0% T

7.7.4 *In vivo* effects of IMFs

Although IMFs can be detected in body fluids such as serum, or in the supernatants from mechanically dissociated tissue or in peritoneal washings (Curtis, in preparation), the crucial test of their action in life is to show that injection of abnormal amounts or of cells treated with IMF leads to altered positionings of these cells.

The first experiments of this type have been recently completed, mainly by my colleague, Dr. M. Davies, and results have been reported (Curtis *et al.*, 1978). In essence these experiments are of three types:

1. Injection of T IMF intravenously followed by examination of white blood cell levels and changes in the B and T populations of various organs.
2. Injection of T IMF together with labelled lymphocytes to discover whether the circulation of these cells is altered.

3. Injection of labelled lymphocytes that have been previously treated with T IMF immediately prior to injection.

The effects of injection of 7,000 units of CBA/ca thymocyte IMF into a CBA/ca mouse (a quantity of about 20 ng) are fairly remarkable in that the population of B lymphocytes in the blood doubles while there is also a marked leucocytosis. The greater proportion of these two cell types comes from the spleen, whose B-dependent areas are probably almost emptied of cells. The effect of B lymphocytes persists for at least 24 hr after injection, while the neutrophil leucocytosis is less long lasting.

Injection of the factor with labelled lymph node lymphocytes produces some significant changes in their location after 4 hr, in particular increased accumulation in the nodes (see Table 7.9). A similar effect is found when the lymphocytes for injection are pretreated with the T IMF just before injection. If B lymphocytes are used instead of T rich lymphocyte populations, the node accumulation is depressed below that which is found in controls.

These results, though representing a very preliminary investigation of the roles of IMFs in lymphocyte circulation, show that these IMFs can indeed alter circulation in a marked manner – one of the essential demonstrations that has to be made for any theory of cell positioning.

It is worthwhile affording a small amount of speculation as to the manner in which these agents may be acting in the experiments. The thymocyte IMF injections lead to an increase in T cell entrance into nodes and perhaps to other organs. Since the factor does not make these lymphocytes more adhesive, the effect must have a more subtle explanation than the simple-minded idea that attachment to the high endothelium is the only step that controls traffic. Perhaps factor is transferred to the endogenous B lymphocytes to depress their adhesion so that there are now fewer competitors with the T cells for entry to the nodes. This conclusion is easily though not exclusively arrived at for those experiments in which T IMF was injected. It is harder to use this explanation for the experiment in which the cells were pretreated with the factor which was then removed. However, it should be remembered that these experiments were carried out with node suspensions which, though T rich, contain about 30% B cells. Obviously it is important to repeat such experiments with purer T and B populations. It should also be borne in mind that in the experiments with injected T factor, there was presumably a marked release of B cells into the blood. As a consequence, B cells would tend to lower the adhesiveness of T cells in the blood. At the moment, I feel that the conclusions that can be drawn are threefold:

1. T IMF glycoprotein can produce large changes in lymphocyte location.
2. The results cannot be interpreted in simple terms of the increase or reduction of adhesion in the treated type for the high endothelium. They suggest that a series of interactions, possibly of a feedback nature, take place in lymphocyte positioning.
3. The system lends itself to a wide range of further experiment.

Table 7.9 Effect of intravenously injected thymocyte IMF on the localization of ^{51}Cr-labelled lymph node cells

Time (hr)	Treatment	% labelled cells					Total recovery (%)
		Spleen	Liver	Peripheral lymph nodes	Mesenteric	Small intestine	
1	Control	28.5	13.05	3.1	1.64	2.07	68.0
1	Thymocyte IMF 122 7,000 units	32.0	16.0	1.97*	1.68	2.1	73.3
4	Control	31.05	11.78	5.18	2.84	2.72	61.7
4	Thymocyte IMF 122 7,000 units	36.08**	14.27**	4.29**	3.19	2.33	67.7
24	Control	17.98	10.36	8.62	9.18	6.4	57.2
24	Thymocyte IMF 122 7,000 units	19.28	10.30	8.51	9.02	6.08	57.5

p values of significance of difference: * < 0.05
** < 0.01

SD < 2.6%.

7.7.5 Effects of IMFs on T:B interactions *in vivo*

If IMFs act on lymphocyte distribution *in vivo*, it might be expected that they would also act on some lymphocyte interaction systems *in vitro*. For this reason, the effect of these IMFs on MLR, CML, and antibody synthesis *in vitro* has been investigated. Though T IMF has a suppressive effect on the MLR reaction, it has been hard to disentangle this from non-specific effects. However, the effects on CML and on antibody synthesis in the Mishell-Dutton system are clearer. Both B cell and T cell IMFs act as non-specific suppressors of antibody response to SRBC antigen in Mishell-Dutton type cultures. Suppression occurs both when the cells and the IMF are syngeneic or when they are allogeneic. If they are allogeneic the suppression is more extreme for a given dose of IMF. This result is entirely in agreement with the two features of IMF effects on target cells, namely that a syngeneic suppression of the adhesion of unlike lymphocyte types takes place as well as an allogeneic suppression of the adhesion of like lymphocyte types. Thus T cell IMF should suppress both T cells and B cells in an allogeneic situation while suppressing B cells alone in a syngeneic situation. The B cell factors appear to be good suppressors of CML systems.

7.7.6 Allogeneic effects of IMF's histocompatibility restriction and cell interactions

The effects on cell interactions in CML and T:B cooperation immediately suggest that there might be some type of genetic requirement for matching of source and reactant cell in IMF action. However, even before these findings, we already knew (Curtis and de Sousa, 1975) that IMFs would act on the adhesion of cell types allogeneic or even xenogeneic to the source of the factor. Examination of the data shows that the effects on allogeneic cells are more marked than would be expected simply because a T cell IMF was acting on a B lymphocyte population. I began to suspect that the extent of effect of any given lymphocyte type was a function both of the cell type difference (B as opposed to T and *vice versa*) and of the allogeneic difference. In a set of experiments (Curtis, 1980), I found that the effects of T IMF can also be seen in reducing thymocyte adhesion provided that the cells are mismatched at the H-2 D locus. These observations (see Table 7.10) were parallelled by examining the cytolytic activity of anti-T IMF antibodies in complement lysis of thymocytes. The antibodies only lyse those cells whose T IMF has the same genotype of H-2 D as the T IMF against which the antibody was raised. These results show that there is a clear H-2 restriction in thymocyte IMF action.

This result has considerable interest. First, it provides a clear support for the intimacy explanation (Zinkernagel and Doherty, 1974) of the H-2 restriction phenomenon. The intimacy explanation can now be reinterpreted as a requirement for cell adhesion which cannot be achieved when cells are mismatched at H-2 loci because of IMF interactions. Zinkernagel and Doherty found that the H-2 K locus was also involved in the restriction phenomenon in the cell-mediated lysis of fibroblasts, whereas I have found no involvement of the K locus in effects on

Table 7.10 H-2 relationship of IMFs. Allogeneic effects of IMFs on adhesion of thymus cells

Target cell strain type	IMF origin	Adhesion	H-2 mismatch	Congenic
A/WySn	A/WySn	9.4	None	–
	B10.AKM	0.03	IC, S, G, & D	No
	B10A.(5R)	9.0	K, 1A, & 1B	No
B10S.(7R)	B10S(7R)	8.4	None	–
	B10T.(6R)	8.3	All except D	Yes
B10G.	B10G.	10.7	None	–
	B10G.AKM	11.0	All except D	Yes
B10A.A	B10A.A	13.8	None	–
	B10A.(2R)	0.0	D only	Yes
	B10A.(4R)	2.1	All except K & 1A	Yes
	A/WySn	4.8	None	No
B10A.(2R)	B10A.(2R)	27.4	None	–
	B10A.A	0.0	D only	Yes
	B10A.(4R)	13.9	1B, 1J, 1E, 1C, S, & G	Yes
B10A.(4R)	B10A.(4R)	11.8	None	–
	B10A.(2R)	14.9	1B, 1J, 1E, 1C, S, & G	Yes
	B10A.A	0.0	All except K & 1A	Yes

IMFs were applied at 7×10^3 units/ml, or as the yield of 1×10^7 cells/ml for those IMFs not precisely assayed.

thymocyte adhesion or T IMF action. This second apparent discrepancy can be easily resolved in an interesting manner if we follow Bodmer's suggestion (1972) that the function of the histocompatibility genes may lie in cell recognition, in particular in cell positioning. If this hypothesis is correct, different tissue types must have their adhesion and movements controlled by different sets of gene products drawn from the histocompatibility gene set. The different cell types should interact using systems controlled by different sets of genes. If we now equate the phenomena seen or alternatively absent in allogeneic combinations with those seen in tissue interactions within one organism, we are claiming that investigation of allogeneic situations may give us a clue as to which genes are involved in tissue interaction within an organism. Thus we would expect that allogeneic requirements for genotype matching to obtain some particular cell interaction would vary according to the exact pair of cell types investigated. We have, in my laboratory, preliminary evidence that the K locus may be involved in B cell interactions and the Ir genes in macrophage–macrophage adhesion.

Three papers published in 1978 have investigated whether histocompatibility genes control fibroblast adhesion (Zeleny et al., 1978; Bartlett and Edidin, 1978) and liver and heart cell adhesion (McClay and Gooding, 1978). The first two papers report positive results though they are not of a very clear nature; the third paper reports negative results. Collecting lawn assays were used by the first two groups and collecting aggregate assays by the third group. It is of interest that

Bartlett and Edidin's results are indicative of a lowering of adhesion in allogeneic combinations – an expectation of the IMF theory. The rather indistinct results may be due to the type of assays used, in which cells would be relatively well washed free of any of the products that might confer cell selectivity. In addition, it is unfortunate that few allogeneic combinations were used by two of the groups while all three groups used strain combinations which would not allow any effect to be tied down to any particular locus or loci.

Thus we seem to be at the stage when evidence is emerging that cell recognition involved in cell positioning is brought about by IMF systems which either are part of or are involved in the system of histocompatibility antigens.

7.8 REINTERPRETATION OF FINDINGS ON SUPPRESSION

Bell and Shand (1975) found that injection of large numbers of TDL into the circulation of rats reconstituted with B cells produced a suppression in the response to antigen (see pp. 93 and 94). This result is one that forms a direct parallel with the experiments carried out by Davies in my laboratory using similar doses either of thymocytes or of T IMF. Their results can be directly predicted by our findings – namely that B:T cooperation would be suppressed by the T IMF normally secreted by the T cells or thymocytes. I should like to suggest that some forms of non-specific suppression can be explained in this simple manner.

Since antigenic stimulation of either B or T lymphocytes increases secretion of B or T factors, it is reasonable to suppose that antigeneic stimulation will in some situations stimulate apparently specific suppression systems, which are however specific only in the manner of their genesis.

7.9 ENVOI

The contents of this chapter show that the study of cell positioning is in a lively if controversial state. I find the theory of specific adhesion somewhat unsatisfactory because it does not predict *de novo* positioning systems, which despite this fiat clearly exist. However, there is a large body of evidence supporting the claim that there are cell surface receptors involved in cell positioning. It would be a tidy and happy solution to our problems should it turn out that these receptors are in fact receptors for IMF molecules which are used in positioning. It is also my belief that it is important at the present time to consider actual positioning mechanisms that operate *in vivo* because these alone can provide the acid tests of our theories. It is also important to link studies of positioning mechanisms to their genetical background, to cell behaviour studies, and to all findings of substances that occur *in vivo* and which might affect adhesion.

For instance, Maria de Sousa has suggested (see Chapter 8) that transferrin and lactoferrin may play important roles in lymphocyte behaviour. Recently, at her suggestion, I and my colleagues Lorna Breckenridge and Linda Fergusson have investigated the effects of these compounds on cell adhesion. The important finding is that the apo-forms of both proteins decrease cell adhesion very markedly. The probable interpretation of the effects of these proteins is that a very small amount of iron is bound in the Stern layer with marked effects on cell electrostatic forces of repulsion. These proteins or appropriate chelating agents in their apo-form such as DEPTA, CHDTA will remove this iron and make the cells less adhesive. Thus though it is probably unlikely that there are gradients on the apo-form of either protein in the body, the general adhesiveness of the circulating lymphocytes will be controlled in part by these two proteins and the iron status of the body concerned. Thus lymphocyte circulation might be modified by these agents: in a similar manner, the level of serum and tissue fluid proteases might well affect cell adhesion, and in turn circulation. For instance, it might be rewarding to investigate possible relationships between serum antitrypsin levels and lymphocyte circulation.

Finally, I feel that we should turn to looking at the factors controlling lymphocyte movements inside the nodes and their release from the lymphoid organs. Events in these two sites may be just as important as those that determine the binding to the high endothelium.

Chapter 8

A Circulation of Lymphocytes: Reflections on the Questions of How and Why

It is clear from the data presented in the previous chapters that the continuous circulation of lymphocytes between blood and lymph represents a major physiological event, demonstrable in fish and birds, which has acquired a considerable degree of complexity with evolution. This complexity is manifested particularly in three phenomena: (1) the physiological exclusion of lymphoid cells from non-lymphoid organs; (2) the exclusion of non-lymphoid cells from the lymph circuit, observed in mammals but not in fish or birds; (3) the selective sorting out within the lymphoid organs of distinct lymphoid cell sets observed in the chicken spleen and further perfected in the mammalian peripheral lymphoid organs (Chapter 4.3). The question of how these phenomena occur has been a subject of considerable interest in recent years. The question of why a continuous cell recirculation of this magnitude has evolved has not, in my view, received adequate attention. The argument for the existence of a continuous blood to lymph recirculation of lymphocytes being beneficial for the dissemination of immunological memory (Ford and Gowans, 1969; Ford, 1975; Sprent, 1977) is weakened by the fact that the blood circuit covers all parts of the body quite adequately and that species with a paucity of lymphocytes in the lymph (i.e. pig) mount vigorous secondary immune responses (Binns and Hall, 1966).

I have argued that of the three major cell types found to travel in the blood circuit, red blood cells, granulocytes, and lymphocytes, the reasons for circulation of the latter are still the least clear (de Sousa, 1976).

Lymphocytes have well-defined and distinct patterns of migration in the whole animal which lead them in large numbers to the liver in foetal life (see Table 8.5), to the spleen and peripheral lymph nodes in the neonatal period (Joel *et al.*, 1972). In the foetus, the recirculatory cells are already long-lived (Cahill and Trnka, 1980); they cannot be memory cells, nor can their pathway or recirculation be directed by any immunological stimulus (Pearson *et al.*, 1976). The ability to recirculate between blood and lymph is thus a physiological property of immunologically virgin lymphocytes; a major physiological system, it is in many respects reminiscent of the circulation of red blood cells. But whereas in the case of the red blood cell circulation the biochemical and molecular basis of its function are rigorously known, in the case of lymphocyte circulation much more is known of its immunology and immunochemistry than of its more general molecular biology or biochemistry.

This chapter is divided into two sections. In the first section, recent work on the question of how lymphocytes enter the lymph circuit and sort themselves out within the lymphoid tissues is reviewed and discussed. In the second section, the possibility that the circulation of lymphocytes represents a form of 'surveillance' not exclusively related to the development of specific immune responses is raised and discussed.

8.1 A CIRCULATION OF LYMPHOCYTES: HOW?

Recirculating lymphocytes emigrate from the blood into the lymph circuit, in lymph nodes, by crossing sections of postcapillary venules characterized in normal rodents by the presence of high, cuboidal, endothelial cells. The ultrastructural and enzymatic features of the high endothelium venules (HEV) of lymph nodes were described earlier (Chapter 1.4). In the present chapter the results of a series of *in vitro* experiments designed to characterize the specificity of the interaction of small lymphocytes with HEV are reviewed (Stamper and Woodruff, 1976, 1977; Woodruff *et al.*, 1977; Kuttner and Woodruff, 1979; Woodruff and Rasmussen, 1979).

These experiments were made possible by the development of an *in vitro* technique in which lymphoid cells are layered over glutaraldehyde-fixed sections of lymph nodes at 7°C. Under these conditions thoracic duct lymphocytes, lymph node, and spleen cells, but not bone marrow or thymus cells, adhere selectively to HEV.

The reaction is highly sensitive to temperature; it is maximal at 7°C, significantly reduced at 1 or 24°C, and not demonstrable at 37°C. It is more reliable when glutaraldehyde-fixed sections are used rather than fresh frozen sections (Woodruff and Rasmussen, 1979). It requires metabolically intact lymphocytes, it is calcium but not magnesium dependent, and it is inhibited by cytochalasin B but not by colchicine (Woodruff *et al.*, 1977). These findings indicate that circulating small lymphocytes do have surface determinants mediating HEV recognition and that the binding depends on contractible forces generated by cytoplasmic microfilaments (Woodruff *et al.*, 1977; Table 8.1).

The *in vitro* findings correlate well with observations made *in vivo* and presented earlier (Chapter 4.5, p. 82). Thus, trypsin-treated lymphocytes always fail to enter the lymph nodes *in vivo* (Woodruff and Gesner, 1968; Freitas and de Sousa, 1975), even when presented directly to a single perfused lymph node (Ford *et al.*, 1976). As discussed earlier (Chapter 4.5, p. 91), cytochalasin B-treated lymph node cells also enter lymph nodes in reduced numbers (Freitas and Bognaki, 1979). *In vivo* experiments using colchicine treatment have given conflicting results, but in one case it was found to have no effect on lymphocyte migration into lymph nodes (see Chapter 4.5, p. 92).

Table 8.1 Comparison between the effect of cytochalasin B and colchicine on adherence of TDL to rat HEV in lymph node sections. Data from Woodruff et al. (1977)

TDL treatment*			TDL–HEV adherence	
Drug	Medium	Conc. (μg/ml)	% of positive HEV	% of positive HEV with heavy TDL binding†
Colchicine	RPMI	0	79 ± 6‡	62 ± 10
		5	79 ± 4	55 ± 5
		40	77 ± 6	65 ± 6
Cytochalasin B	RPMI	0§	89 ± 6	84 ± 10
		10	0	0
	PBS	0	84 ± 8	57 ± 8
		10	10 ± 9	4 ± 4

*Incubations were performed at 37°C for 3 hr in experiments with colchicine, for 30 min in experiments with cytochalasin B in RPMI and for 5 min in experiments with PBS. The suspensions were then chilled to 7°C and the cells assayed immediately for HEV binding.
†With two or more adherent TDL.
‡Mean ± SE.
§1% DMSO present.

There is one recent aspect of the question of the specific lymphocyte interaction with HEV presently under investigation (Ford, Smith, and Andrews, 1978; Andrews et al., 1980) which constitutes the first indication that one component synthesized and secreted by the endothelium itself acts as a chemoattractant for circulating lymphocytes in vivo. Following selective labelling of HEV in lymph nodes removed from rats $2\frac{1}{2}$ hr after footpad injection of $^{35}SO_4$, a material has been purified from a lymph node homogenate which contains 30–40% of the radioactivity initially present in the lymph node pellet. The sulphated material, whose precise nature is not yet defined, when injected into the flank skin of rats at 2 hr before the intravenous injection of ^{51}Cr-labelled syngeneic thoracic duct lymphocytes, appears to induce a 3–7 fold increase in radioactivity compared to uninjected skin.

This sulphated compound is synthesized and secreted by HEV and thought to act as a signal to lymphocytes first to adhere and then to retract their microvilli (Andrews et al., 1980). These observations are in agreement with the suggestion first put forward by Wenk et al. (1974) that the Golgi apparatus of HE cells might produce material which was incorporated in the HE cell coat and could thus influence lymphocytes in the bloodstream. Both suggestions presuppose that only lymphocytes in the bloodstream are capable of recognizing such a molecule. Moreover, they do not take into account the fact that lymphocytes cross postcapillary venules in species with lymph nodes in which the endothelium does not have the striking high cuboidal appearance (Fahy et al., 1980) and in T cell depleted animals, in which the venules have an endothelium perfectly undistinguishable from other venules (see Fig. 1.9). If this represents an exclusive lymphocyte recognition process, it is neither a species nor a site specific event, since xenogeneic lymphocytes have been found to adhere to rat HEV *in vitro* (Butcher *et al.*, 1979) and rat TDL to adhere to myelinated areas of rat brain (Kuttner and Woodruff, 1979).

Finally, since T and B lymphocytes adhere equally well to HEV *in vitro* (Table 8.2) and are found equally associated with postcapillary venules *in vivo* (see Chapter 4.3), it seems rather surprising that T lymphocytes are present in excess of B lymphocytes in lymph nodes, in lymph, in extravascular fluids other than lymph (Manconi *et al.*, 1978), and in non-lymphoid tissue sites during responses characterized by the appearance of abundant perivascular mononuclear cell infiltrates. In addition, changes in the morphological appearance of endothelium from flat to cuboidal often follow rather than precede the crossing of endothelia by small lymphocytes in lymph nodes of T depleted animals and in non-lymphoid sites (see Chapter 1). Therefore, the alternative that the signal for lymphocyte crossing of venules comes not from the endothelium itself but from some tissue, lymph or extravascular component cannot and should not be ruled out at the present time. This, of course, raises the question of what component or components of lymph, tissue, or extravascular fluid could act as a signal that, under physiological conditions, influences T lymphocyte immigration into thymus-dependent areas of lymph nodes and spleen, and under pathological conditions influences T lymphocyte immigration into synovial fluid, cerebrospinal fluid, peritoneal exudates, pleural fluid, etc. (for review of T lymphocyte distribution in non-lymphoid sites in disease see Chapter 6.2).

One candidate, and the one for which evidence is most compelling, is the interdigitating reticulum cell found in thymus-dependent areas of normal and T cell lymphoma lymph nodes, and present in abnormally high numbers in T cell lymphomas of skin (Goos *et al.*, 1976).

The presence of IDC has not been sought in other conditions in which abnormal accumulation of T cells occurs, i.e. rheumatoid arthritis, pleural effusions in

Table 8.2 Effect of nylon wool non-adherent and adherent TDL concentration on binding of the cells to HEV *in vitro*. Woodruff (personal communication)

Overlaid TDL concentration ($\times 10^6$/ml)	TDL population*	% positive HEV/section†	% HEV with heavy TDL binding/section‡
15	Non-adherent	67 ± 3§	21 ± 6
	Adherent	65 ± 5	16 ± 3
5	Non-adherent	38 ± 7	12 ± 3
	Adherent	35 ± 8	11 ± 2

*Non-adherent TDL, 2% sIg$^+$; adherent TDL, 92% sIg$^+$.
†HEV with two or more adherent TDL.
‡HEV with six or more adherent TDL.
§Mean ± SE of three–four sections.

tuberculosis, PSS, etc. It is not clear whether the coappearance of T lymphocytes and IDC represents T cells following IDC or *vice versa*. Experiments reducing IDC numbers in lymph nodes should be followed by the tracing of labelled cells into lymph nodes. If the former reduces entry of the latter, then IDC could indeed represent a signalling mechanism for lymphocyte entry into the lymph circuit.

The possible biochemical basis for such hypothetical signalling is unknown.

8.2 A CIRCULATION OF LYMPHOCYTES: WHY?

In the closing section of this chapter, I wish to discuss the possibility that lymphocytes are equipped biochemically to participate in some form of physiological surveillance comparable in magnitude to the exchange of oxygen and CO_2 from haemoglobin; that under physiological conditions, this surveillance function keeps lymphocytes circulating within the boundaries of the lymphocyte system; and that under pathological conditions, developing in response to infection, malignant transformation, and tumour growth, or to some other assault such as exposure to metals and other environmental pollutants, lymphocytes leave their physiological path and accumulate at the disease site.

The basic assumption for this discussion derives from the conviction that the significance of the circulation of lymphocytes lies beyond a role in immune surveillance, even when at times it encompasses it. This conviction stemmed in part from the realization that if a system has evolved just to cope with recognition and elimination of 'forbidden' non-self elements within self, or environmental components toxic to self, it need not have acquired such large dimensions as those of the recirculatory pool of lymphocytes, nor did a long lifespan seem an indispensable prerequisite for its effectiveness as a defence mechanism. On the other hand, the existence of a lymph circuit which excludes other leukocytes but favours the traffic, growth, and lodging of malignant neoplastic cells did not seem a specially effective evolutionary step for host protection.

Thus, it seemed necessary to consider the alternative that recirculating lymphocytes, particularly T lymphocytes, are long-lived and have the capacity to cross endothelium readily (into lymph nodes and spleen, other non-lymphoid tissues, and lymph and other extravascular fluids) as a result of unique metabolic properties acquired in the physiological process of differentiation, independent of antigen.

As biochemists begin to recognize that the lymphoid organs do not consist of homogeneous cell populations as does a liver or a heart, and the need to analyse selected lymphoid cell populations becomes apparent, fine basic metabolic distinctions between cell types have started to be delineated. Some of these distinctions, like the association of the enzyme terminal transferase with T cells at a particular stage of differentiation, are already well established and are being used routinely as additional markers of T cell differentiation and in the diagnosis of T cell leukaemias and lymphomas (Silverstone *et al.*, 1978). Others are only now beginning to be examined. Of the latter, I attribute particular significance to the recent finding by a group of Japanese workers (Kobayashi *et al.*, 1979) of a higher

Table 8.3 Superoxide dismutase activity of T and non-T lymphocytes and granulocytes, with ratio of activity in parentheses. Data from Kobayashi et al. (1979)

Cell	Units/mg protein	Units/10^7 cells	Cyanide-sensitive fraction (%)
T lymphocytes	52.3 ± 3.3* (3.3)	27.6 ± 3.0 (4.2)	81.4 ± 4.4
Non-T lymphocytes	29.7 ± 4.6 (1.9)	15.6 ± 5.4 (2.4)	66.8 ± 10.7
Granulocytes	15.9 ± 3.7 (1.0)	6.5 ± 2.0 (1.0)	76.0 ± 5.4

*Mean ± 1 SD.

superoxide dismutase activity in T lymphocytes than in non-T lymphocytes or granulocytes (Table 8.3). Superoxide dismutase (SOD, EC 1.15.1.1) catalyses the dismutation of superoxide anion O_2- to less toxic hydrogen peroxide and molecular oxygen; it is an ubiquitous enzyme in oxygen-metabolizing cells and contributes to the protection of cells from the potentially harmful effect of the free reactive radical (McCord and Fridovich, 1969). Thus, its presence in higher amounts in T lymphocytes than in non-T lymphocytes or in granulocytes could contribute to the different lifespans of the different cell populations (Kobayashi et al., 1979).

My colleagues and I were interested in clues to a possible biochemistry of lymphocyte migration which could be common to the control of normal and pathological lymphocyte distribution. At first, on the basis of the finding of abnormally high numbers of T lymphocytes in the spleen of patients with Hodgkin's disease, in which abnormal numbers of lactoferrin-containing cells are present (de Sousa et al., 1978) and high amounts of ferritin are synthesized and secreted in the serum (Bieber and Bieber, 1973; Eshhar et al., 1974), we postulated that iron and iron-binding proteins might play a role in the control of lymphocyte maldistribution in disease (de Sousa et al., 1978) and in the control of normal lymphocyte circulation (de Sousa, 1978b).

It is implicit in this postulate that the lymphomyeloid system and its circulating components participate in the recognition and binding of metals as a protective device against metal toxicity and the preferential use of indispensable metals such as Fe or Zn by bacteria or transformed cells (de Sousa, 1978b).

8.2.1 Detectable Fe, other cations, and iron-binding proteins in sites of physiological and pathological lymphocyte migration

8.2.1.1 Small intestine

In Chapter 5, Parrott, discussing the question of the control of the numbers of effector cells in mucosal sites (Section 5.3, p. 117), noted how the differences in blood flow to proximal and distal segments of the small intestine (Parrott and Ottaway, 1980) coincided with similar differences in distribution of IgA-containing cells in the lamina propria, numbers of intraepithelial T lymphocytes, and blast cell migration. Thus, higher numbers of IgA-containing cells have been found in proximal than in distal sections of the small intestine in man (Crabbé and Heremans, 1966), in mice (Crabbé et al., 1970), calves (Porter et al., 1972), and in rats (Husband and Gowans, 1978). According to Parrott, there is also some indication that intraepithelial T lymphocytes are found in higher numbers in the proximal sections of the small intestine.

Studies of lymphocyte migration and antibody production within distinct segments of the small intestine and in antigen-free systems have led to the general conclusion that cell migration to the lamina propria occurs independently of an antigen stimulus, although antigen exposure plays an important role in the expansion of the lodging population (Halstead and Hall, 1972; Parrott and Ferguson, 1974; Husband and Gowans, 1978).

Following the postulate that lymphocytes migrate to sites of iron deposition, we looked at published data on the pattern of distribution of iron absorption in proximal and distal segments of the small intestine and compared them to the data on blood flow, blast cell migration, and distribution of IgA-containing cells. These data are summarized in Table 8.4. Studies of Fe absorption in the rat (Duthie, 1964) and in man (Wheby, 1970, data not shown) have demonstrated that Fe absorption parallels lymphocyte migration and distribution of IgA-containing cells insofar as it is highest in duodenum and jejunum and lowest in ileum (Table 8.4). In iron deficiency, however, the distinction between absorption at different small intestine segments is no longer apparent; iron absorption is extended to the caecum (Wack and Wyatt, 1959).

From studies of rejection of *Nippostrongylus brasiliensis* in iron and protein deficient rats, it is known that normal immune mesenteric lymph node cells fail to cause parasite rejection in nutritionally deficient recipients, illustrating how the nutritional status of the host influences lymphocyte function (Cummins et al., 1978). It was not established in those studies, however, whether the iron and protein deficiency influenced lymphocyte migration to the infected gut.

Table 8.4 Comparison between Fe absorption, blood flow, number of IgA-positive cells, and blast cell migration to different segments of small intestine

Segment	Fe absorption*	Blood flow†	IgA-positive cells‡	Blast cell migration†
Duodenum	69.8 ± 6.05	7.7 ± 1.5	1,953 (1,588–2,429)	1.42 ± 0.10
Mid-jejunum	28.6 ± 4.08	5.6 ± 1.1	1,235 (1,005–1,652)	1.46 ± 0.15
Jejunum–ileum	9.2 ± 3.08	3.6 ± 0.6		0.85 ± 0.07
Ileum	2.1 ± 0.64	3.1 ± 0.5	963 (712–1,404)	0.58 ± 0.09

*Data from Duthie (1964), experiments in male Sprague–Dawley rats, 170–220 g weight, % of dose, of 59 Fe injected directly into the bowel.
†Unpublished data from Ottaway and Parrott, experiments in 7–14 week-old mice of the NIH inbred strain.
‡Data from Husband and Gowans (1978), male and female PVG/c rats, weight or age not specified.

Table 8.5 Differences in lymphocyte migration to small intestine and liver in adult sheep and the foetal lamb. Data from Cahill et al. (1979)

Source of lymphocytes infused	Mean % radioactivity in*							Total % radioactivity recovered
	Lung	Liver	Spleen	Small intestine	Mesenteric lymph node	Peripheral lymph nodes	Blood†	
Foetus								
Intestinal lymph	8.4	32.6	12.2	3.0	1.2	1.2	12.1	70.7
Prescapular lymph	9.6	23.7	11.7	2.5	1.6	3.2	12.6	64.9
Adult								
Intestinal lymph	24.0	4.4	20.0	12.9	3.4	2.8	6.8	74.3
Prescapular lymph	28.3	2.8	25.7	1.4	2.2	3.6	6.7	70.7

*Three animals were used in each group.
†Blood volume estimated from foetal age according to Bancroft (1947).

On the assumption that lymphocyte migration to the small intestine is related to iron absorption, differences are to be expected between the lymphocyte migration to the small intestine in foetal and in adult life. In a comparative study of the migration of ^{51}Cr-labelled lymphocytes collected from intestinal duct lymph in adult sheep and the foetal lamb, Cahill and co-workers (Cahill *et al.*, 1979) have found a much higher recovery of radioactivity in the small intestine in the adult (12.9%) than in the foetus (3.0%). The possibility that antigen alone is responsible for these differences is ruled out by the fact that on a weight basis, recirculation of lymphocytes in the foetus is equal to that of the adult, yet lymphocytes in the immunologically virgin foetal lamb develop in the absence of extrinsic antigen (Pearson *et al.*, 1976).

One additional piece of evidence compatible with a possible association between iron accumulation and lymphocyte migration is the finding of significantly higher numbers of labelled lymphocytes in foetal than in adult liver (Table 8.5), since in the foetus the liver is a predominantly haemopoietic organ (Cahill *et al.*, 1979) with a high iron content (Chang, 1973).

Abnormal lymphocyte accumulations have also been described in the mucous membranes of the stomach and intestine in patients with Kaschin-Beck's disease, an epidemic disease attributed to high intake of iron from well water (Hiyeda, 1939). A detailed description of the pathological features of this disease is presented later.

8.2.1.2 Mammary Gland

In ontogeny, exposure of the stomach and small intestine to iron occurs first during lactation. Studies of human breast milk have provided us with a detailed picture of the cellular, protein, and trace element content of milk at different times of lactation (Diaz-Jouanen and Williams, 1974; Parmely *et al.*, 1976; Picciano and Guthrie, 1976; Lonnerdal *et al.*, 1976; Siimes *et al.*, 1979; Ogra and Ogra, 1978; McClelland *et al.*, 1978). Unfortunately, some of these studies were not done in the same species at comparable times during lactation, and therefore it is difficult to draw comparisons between specific associations of trace elements and cells, or trace elements and proteins or immunoglobulins. As far as possible, however, this was done for the changes occurring in lymphocyte numbers and Fe concentration in rat and human breast milk (Fig. 8.1). The most striking changes take place within the first days of lactation and consist in marked declines in numbers of T lymphocytes (10^5/ml on first day of lactation to 10^4/ml on day 5 to 2,000/ml at 50–200 days of lactation, data from Ogra and Ogra, 1978), lactoferrin concentration (1,500 mg/100 ml on day 1, 520 mg/100 ml on day 5, 300 mg/100 ml at 8–28 days of lactation, and 150 at 150 days, data from McClelland *et al.*, 1978), and IgA concentration (1,200 mg/100 ml on day 1, 490 mg/100 ml on day 5, and 151 and 148 mg/100 ml at 8–28 days and 180 days post lactation, data from McClelland *et al.*, 1978). Available data on the changes in iron content of human and rat milk during the first week of lactation (Fabiano,

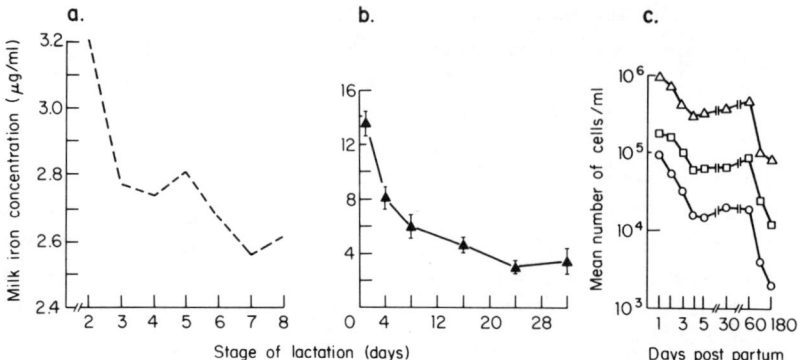

Figure 8.1 Illustration of parallel changes occurring during the first week of lactation in women (a, c) and female rats (b), in milk concentration of iron (a, b) and in concentration of mononuclear cells (Δ), total lymphocytes (□), and T lymphocytes (O). Modified and combined from Fabiano (1956), a; Ezekiel and Morgan (1963), b; Ogra and Ogra (1978), c

1956; Ezekiel and Morgan, 1963) indicate that the changes in iron concentration parallel the changes in lymphocyte concentration (Fig. 8.1). At two weeks the median concentration was 0.56 mg/l in a study of 22 g breast milk samples obtained from 27 mothers during a 6-month period of lactation (Siimes et al., 1979). Thereafter, the value declined gradually and reached a plateau at approximately 0.3 mg/l after 5 months of lactation (Siimes et al., 1979). Data pooled from studies of Zn concentration during lactation indicate that Zn too declines from the first available determinations, from 5.3–3.6 and 5.07 mg/l at 5 days to 3.24 mg/l at the 15th day to 1.63 at the 6th–12th week of lactation (Picciano and Guthrie, 1976). By contrast, little change takes place in the copper content of milk during lactation.

Studies of the mitogenic responses of the cells present in milk have shown consistently a failure of lymphocytes in milk to respond to stimulation by PHA but not to other antigens (Diaz-Jouanen and Williams, 1974; Parmely et al., 1976; Ogra and Ogra, 1978).

Furthermore, cell-free colostrum or milk was found to inhibit the PHA response of peripheral blood or milk lymphocytes (Parmely et al., 1976; Ogra and Ogra, 1978), thus indicating the possible existence of an inhibitor of T cell function in milk. The possibility that iron itself is the inhibitor seems likely in the light of the results of *in vitro* experiments using concentrations of iron similar to those present in breast milk (Bryan et al., 1980; Munn and de Sousa, unpublished data).

8.2.1.3 Spleen and lymph nodes

In phylogeny, the association of iron-containing phagocytes with lymphocytes has been noted in fish spleen. Lymphocytes are seen to aggregate around macrophages containing stainable iron by the Prussian blue stain. In higher vertebrates, the presence of iron in the spleen as detected by histological stains is confined to

Table 8.6 Distribution of iron in control and RA axillary lymph nodes detected by histological staining and spectrophotometry. Data from Muirden (1970)

Group	Total no. studied	Sample	Histological grade					Fe (µg/g) (mean)
			0	+	++	+++	++++	
Control	30	Section	23	4	3	0	0	
		Ashed						35.37
RA (treated)	5	Section	0	1	1	2	1	
		Ashed						139.8
RA (untreated)	6	Section	2	2	2	0	0	
		Ashed						70.5

*Received iron therapy.

the haemosiderin present in red pulp macrophages, although stainable iron is seen occasionally in elongated macrophages in thymus-dependent areas and in the marginal zone.

In normal lymph nodes, the finding of stainable iron by histological stains is rare. Estimations of the iron content of normal human lymph nodes has shown, however, that iron is present in lymph nodes in spite of the failure to stain it (Muirden, 1970).

In a study of the concentration of iron in lymph nodes from 30 control cases from rheumatoid arthritis (RA) patients not treated with iron therapy or blood transfusions and in RA nodes removed from patients who received iron therapy, Muirden found the following mean values for the three groups: control cases = 35.37 µg/g (range 17–131), RA nodes not treated with Fe = 70.5 µg/g, RA nodes treated with Fe = 139.8 µg/g (Table 8.6).

The association of lymph node enlargement with increased iron deposition is perhaps best illustrated by the painful lymphadenopathy reported by Theodoropoulos et al. (1968) in eight female patients following massive infusions of iron dextran. Histological examination of one lymph node removed from one of these patients revealed the presence of iron in hyperplastic reticuloendothelial cells lining the medullary sinuses, but cells containing iron were also seen diffusely in the cortex of the lymph node. Lymph node siderosis has been reported also in Hodgkin's disease (Dumont et al., 1976) and lymph node enlargement is seen frequently in patients with iron overload due to thalassaemia.

8.2.1.4 Synovial fluid

Rheumatoid arthritis is one of the diseases where T lymphocyte maldistribution is well documented. Details of the studies of lymphocyte distribution in peripheral blood and synovial fluid of patients with rheumatoid arthritis and other forms of arthritis were presented in Chapter 6.2. One of the features of the pathology of synovium in rheumatoid arthritis is the presence of large amounts of stainable iron. The other diagnostic features include intimal proliferation, blood vessel proliferation, the appearance of infiltrating lymphocytes, and a generalized increase in fibrous connective tissue. The surface layers of intima cells generally show faint iron staining. Cells containing haemosiderin granules are present in the subintimal region and surrounded by lymphocytes. Haemosiderin staining is also seen in close association with areas of fibrosis. Perivascular macrophages also contain iron, and frequently the giant cells found in RA lesions contain iron too, either distributed evenly within the cytoplasm or as cytoplasmic granules.

The morphological association of iron-containing macrophages and multinuclear giant cells with lymphocyte infiltration of the synovial tissue has also been reported in one case of villonodular synovitis (Muirden and Senator, 1968). By contrast, no lymphocyte infiltration was seen in one case of haemochromatosis – associated arthritis of the knee (Muirden, 1968). In this case, the intima cells were seen to contain iron, and iron-positive material was detected in connective tissue, stroma, lying free in the connective tissue but not in the proximity of blood vessels. In this patient, the serum iron was 200 µg/100 ml, while the synovial fluid iron was 86 µg/100 ml (Muirden and Senator, 1968). If lymphocytes did migrate in iron concentration gradients, they would not be expected to leave the blood compartment towards the synovial fluid compartment in this case. In rheumatoid arthritis patients, however, serum iron levels are low, and lymphocytes would be expected to follow the iron gradient from serum to synovial fluid.

8.2.1.5 Skin

Although metal absorption can take place through the skin and this organ constitutes a favourite site for abnormal lymphocyte migration (see Chapter 6.2), there are no studies analysing simultaneously trace metals and lymphocyte populations in skin. There is, however, one report of an *in vivo* study of trace elements in lepromatous leprous skin, in which diagnostic x-ray spectrometry (DXS) was applied to the analysis of changes in the quantity of three trace metals (iron, zinc, and copper) occurring in leprous skin during periods of disease activity and during remission stage (Sheskin and Zeimer, 1977). The results of the study are summarized in Fig. 8.2. Twenty patients were examined: eight were in the active stage, four in the course of recovery, and eight were arrested cases. Eleven controls were examined. The patients in the active stage showed a significant increase in iron concentration which was related to the lesion; in some cases, the iron level was high even in regions with no detectable lesions. Slightly raised zinc levels were observed only in cases of acute lesion in the active stage. Copper levels did not deviate significantly from normal.

8.2.1.6 Brain

Metallic implants have been applied to the brain particularly for studying mechanisms of epileptogenesis (Chusid and Koeloff, 1967; Hartman *et al.*, 1974; Hirano and Kochen, 1975; Payan, 1967; Willmore *et al.*, 1978). Recently, Levine

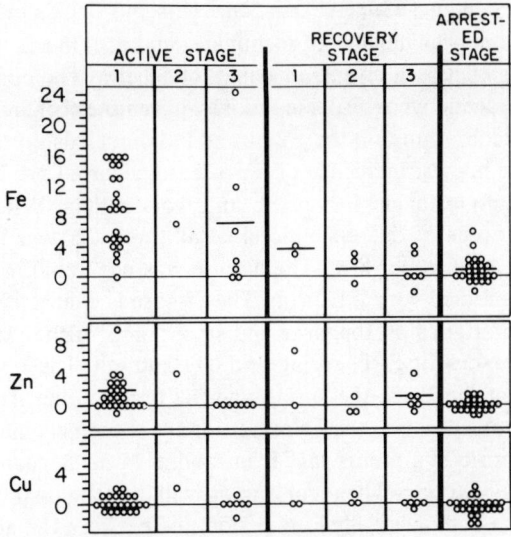

Figure 8.2 Metal content in leprous skin (data from Sheskin and Zeimer, 1977). Zero represents the normal values. The other figures represent the difference between the metallic content of normal subjects and that of patients, expressed in units of standard deviation. Each dot represents one test site in one patient

and Sowinski (1978) analysed the effect of implanting 16 pure metals as pellets of powder or as wires in rat brains on degree of lymphocyte infiltration. From this study, it was found that Al, Be, Cr, Fe, Pb, Sn, and W were relatively innocuous in causing necrosis or lymphocyte infiltration. Mg and Mn produced mild local necrosis, Bi, Cd, Co, Cu, and Ni produced severe necrosis. Viable tissue adjacent to Co and Ni had some necrotic lesions, and some perivascular lymphocytic infiltration associated with cobalt implants had been noted in earlier studies (Payan, 1967, 1971). Of the metals studied by Levine and Sowinski (1978), Zn was the most interesting, since in spite of causing very little necrosis, it gave rise to the appearance of prominent perivascular lymphocyte cuffs. These infiltrates persisted for at least 4 weeks, and disappeared as soon as the zinc was removed.

In the discussion of their observations, Levine and Sowinski suggest the possibility that zinc has a lymphotactic effect *in vivo*. Like iron, zinc binds to transferrin; it competes with iron binding, as shown by the inhibition of iron absorption caused by zinc in tied jejunal loops (Forth and Rummel, 1973) and by the finding of increased zinc absorption in animals maintained on an iron-deficient diet (Pollack *et al.*, 1965).

8.2.1.7 *Kaschin-Beck's disease*

A classical paper on the clinical pathology of this disease was published by

Hiyeda in 1939 (Hiyeda, 1939). At that time, Kaschin-Beck's disease was one of the endemic diseases prevailing in Manchoukuo and also in the border regions of the northern parts of Korea and Transbaikal of Siberia. The communities where the disease was endemic were dispersed mostly in remote corners of mountainous regions. It was seldom found on the plains and it did not exist in the cities. Even in endemic areas, the highest incidence of the disease occurred not in the urban part of the area but among farmers, hunters, and woodcutters. When investigations were made in the wells of one endemic area, all the water was found to contain more than 0.3 mg of iron per litre. The disease was not found in areas where the drinking water contained very little iron. The disease is characterized in the early stages by arthritic attacks on the large and small joints of the extremities, occurring during the seasons of early spring and late autumn. These seasons coincide with the thawing of the ice in the spring and the first autumn frosts. After every attack the pain subsides but the joints gradually become enlarged. The early stages of the arthritic symptoms last from about $1\frac{1}{2}$ to 5 years; thereafter the patient feels occasional pain when working or walking long distances. This condition continues for a comparatively long period and between the ages of 25 and 50 the swelling and deformity of the joints becomes the most remarkable physical feature of the disease. The only remarkable change in the blood picture consists of the finding of an eosinophilia in many cases and of an increase in the amount of serum iron.

The pathology of the joint consists of proliferation of the synovial membrane, ulcers of the joint surface, marginal elevation of the epiphysis, and osteoporosis. The following description of the histopathology of the disease is taken directly from Hiyeda's paper:

> Histologically, there are the infiltrations of lymphocytes and eosinophilous cells in the mucous membrane of the stomach and intestines and proliferation of the fibroblast and new growth of blood capillaries sometimes occur in the wall of the stomach. In the stomach, particularly atrophy of the glands, due to the proliferation of the connective tissue is occasionally visible. There is often saturation of the lymphocytes and the eosinophilous cells in the interstices of the liver and a slight proliferation of the interstices is sometimes seen. Slight proliferation of the fibrous substances or saturation of the lymphocytes is also seen in the spleen, the lymph glands, the circulatory organs, the respiratory organs, the urinary organs and the endocrine organs but there are no marked changes in them.
>
> The deposition of iron pigment can be noticed in all the organs, and very high degrees of it are found in the spleen, the lymph glands, the liver, the kidney, the stomach, the intestines and the bone marrow. The deposition of iron pigment is also sometimes great in the lungs, the mucous membrane of the trachea, the thyroid and the suprarenal glands. This deposition of iron pigment is very interesting. It is found not only in the form of granula in the cytoplasm of cells and along the inner surface of the wall of lymph- and

blood-capillaries, but also in the form of diffuse staining of lymph- and tissue spaces.

Moreover, it is interesting that iron pigment is always found in some of the nuclei of the liver cells. One thing which calls for attention is that the iron pigment deposited in the organs is easily dissolved in the fixative formaline. At the beginning of the investigation the author ignored this fact and was faced with various difficulties, but later it was proved that the deposited iron was easily dissolved by the formic acid contained in the formaline solution.

Having established an association between the high iron intake from the well water and the disease, the author proceeded to the experimental reproduction of the disease in rabbits. The animals were given 0.05–2 g of iron per day and forced to exercise their limbs for 30 minutes a day. After about 10 days of feeding similar changes in the bone and joints were reproduced in the experimental animals and a similar distribution of iron in the organs was observed.

It is of interest to note that both in the patient population and in the experimental animals the following four pathological features concurred: hyperaemia and increase in number of blood capillaries, iron deposition, lymphocyte infiltration, and fibrous tissue.

In conclusion, there seem to be several physiological and pathological situations in which detectable amounts of iron or zinc (but not copper) are found coexisting with the appearance of lymphocytes (summarized in Table 8.7). This does not *per se* constitute evidence that the presence of some metals in one particular site acts as a signal for migration of cells to that site. If, however, the cells are equipped biochemically with proteins capable of binding the metals concerned, or display receptors for such protein–metal complexes, this will provide further evidence for a possible functional connection between the two events. A review of data on the association of iron-binding proteins with selected populations of immune cells is presented in the next section.

Table 8.7 Situations in which an association between lymphocyte migration and the presence of Fe or Zn is documented

Physiological	Absorption in small intestine
	Lactation
	Foetal liver
Pathological	Synovium in rheumatoid arthritis
	Lepromatous skin
	Kaschin-Beck's disease
	Lymph node enlargement after massive iron transfusion
	Siderosis in Hodgkin's disease lymph nodes
	Lymph node enlargement in thalassaemia patients
Experimental	Metallic implants in brain

8.2.2 Aspects and implications of the association of iron-binding proteins with cells of the immune system

8.2.2.1 Biochemistry

A number of extensive detailed reviews of the biochemistry of transferrins and ferritin have been published in recent years (Zschocke and Bezkorovainy, 1974a,b; Morgan, 1974; Harrison, 1977; Drysdale *et al.*, 1977; Munro and Linder, 1978). These reviews will be indispensable to the reader interested in the many well-established biochemical aspects of iron-binding, transport, and storage. Briefly, lactoferrin and transferrin have similar molecular weights, whose estimations vary between 73,000 and 82,000; presently, 76,000 is considered the most acceptable figure (Morgan, 1974). They both have two iron-binding sites and iron-binding is dependent on bicarbonate. Lactoferrin has an amino acid sequence homologous with that of transferrin and ovotransferrin (MacGillivray *et al.*, 1977; Jolles *et al.*, 1976), and it contains two oligosaccharide chains, which are structurally similar to those of transferrin except that additional fucose residues are in $\alpha 1 \rightarrow 3$ linkage with the N-acetylglucosamine residues adjacent to galactose and the chains containing fucose are devoid of sialic acid (Prieels *et al.*, 1978).

The two proteins differ in immunological properties in association constant, in the effect of pH on the reaction with iron, and in tissue distribution. In the presence of citrate as a mediatory agent the association constant for transferrin is approximately $5 \times 23/M$ and in the absence of citrate as high as 10^{36} under physiological conditions (Aasa *et al.*, 1963). The iron–lactoferrin association constant is some 300 times greater than that for transferrin (Masson and Heremans, 1968; Aisen and Leibman, 1972). Lowering the pH results in the release of iron from transferrin at pH 5.0–6.0; lactoferrin retains its iron until the pH is below 4.0 (Groves, 1960; Johansson, 1960).

The liver is the main site of transferrin synthesis in the adult, although a large variety of other tissues have been shown to synthesize transferrin; these include the lactating mammary gland, the yolk sac, the newborn thymus, the foetal lung, the bone marrow, spleen, and peritoneal and lung macrophages (Morgan, 1974). Lactoferrin is secreted by the mammary, lachrymal, bronchial and salivary gland, the mucosa of the endometrium, and seminal vesicles. Thus, lactoferrin is mostly confined to external secretions, whereas transferrin is a major plasma protein, distributed throughout most of the extracellular fluid of the body, with a continuous circulation from plasma to lymph. It has been identified in interstitial fluid, lymph, oedema fluid, cerebrospinal fluid, and urine (Morgan, 1974).

By virtue of their high iron-binding capacity, both proteins in the apoform have been shown to have bacteriostatic properties which diminish with increasing iron saturation (Weinberg, 1978; Bullen *et al.*, 1978; Kochan, 1977). Transferrin is the prime mediator of iron metabolism by delivering iron to reticulocytes which efficiently utilize the metal for haemsynthesis (Moore and Goldberg, 1974). This process is temperature sensitive and the rate of iron uptake increases as the iron concentration is raised up to a certain maximum beyond which no further increase in uptake occurs.

Transferrin also plays a major role in the delivery of iron to the foetus during pregnancy, a process mediated by the presence of transferrin receptors on trophoblast (Faulk and Galbraith, 1979).

Lactoferrin has been shown to control the colony stimulatory activity of macrophages and thus regulate the differentiation of CFU–C into granulocyte colonies *in vitro* (Broxmeyer *et al.*, 1978). This regulatory property is dependent on iron saturation of the protein. It is probable that lactoferrin also acts in the control of granulopoiesis *in vivo*, but the evidence for its *in vivo* action is limited to the reduction of the rebound granulopoiesis that follows administration of cyclophosphamide in mice (Broxmeyer *et al.*, 1978).

Transferrin and lactoferrin will bind other metals, including chromium, manganese, cobalt, cadmium, zinc, nickel, gallium, indium, scandium, and plutonium (Worwood, 1974).

Ferritin is a more complex molecule, whose main function has thus far been thought to be the storage and recycling of iron for synthesis of haem and other proteins, thereby contributing to the sequestration of potentially toxic-free iron (Granick, 1946). Ferritin is a water-soluble macromolecule consisting of an outer shell of protein subunits with an aggregate molecular weight of 450,000 within which up to 4,500 atoms of iron can be stored (Harrison, 1977; Munro and Linder, 1978). Although the gross morphology of most ferritins seems to be similar, i.e. the molecules consist of a roughly spherical protein shell about 130 Å in diameter, enclosing a variable core of up to 80 Å in diameter, further details of shell architecture and estimates of subunit composition are not resolved. Structural and immunological studies of human ferritins have indicated that they are synthesized from two subunits of approximate molecular weights of 21,000 and 19,000 (Drysdale *et al.*, 1977; Arosio *et al.*, 1978). Further isoelectric focusing studies resolved additional subunit bands which could be fractionated on the basis of iron content (Lavoie *et al.*, 1978). According to Lavoie *et al.* (1978), it seems likely that the subunit heterogeneity of ferritin accounts for the microheterogeneity of assembled ferritin molecules, and this in turn has a direct bearing on the question of ferritin tissue and species specificity and variations in ferritin types observed in developing and neoplastic cells.

8.2.2.2 *Iron-binding proteins and cells of the immune system*

A summary of known associations between cells of the immune system and transferrin, lactoferrin, and ferritin is represented diagrammatically in Fig. 8.3. The relevant references to the studies which established those associations are quoted in the legend.

Two distinct aspects must be considered: (1) synthesis and secretion by selected cell sets; (2) binding to selected cell sets. Lactoferrin has been shown to be associated with granulocytes and macrophages; the major protein component of

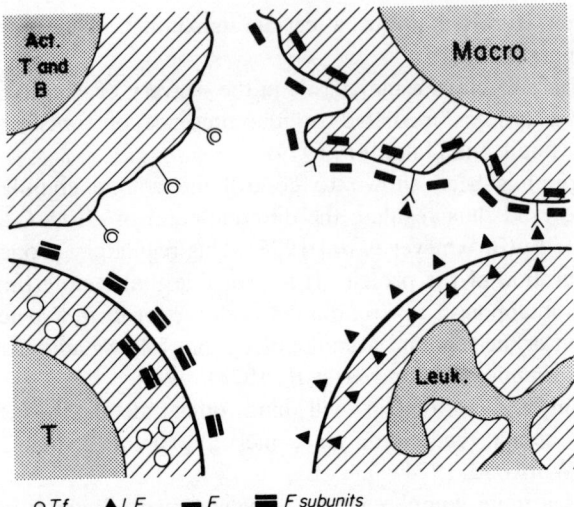

○ Tf   ▲ LF   ▬ F   ≡ F subunits

Figure 8.3 Diagrammatic representation of known associations of transferrin (Tf), lactoferrin (Lf), and ferritin (F) with macrophages (Macro), granulocytes (Leuk.), T lymphocytes (T), and activated T and B lymphocytes (Act. T and B). Macrophages have receptors for Lf (—<) and synthesize F (van Snick and Masson, 1976; Summers et al., 1974; Okhuma et al., 1976). Activated T and B lymphocytes have Tf receptors (—<) (Galbraith et al., 1980; Hamilton et al., 1979; Phillips, 1976). Granulocytes contain and release lactoferrin (Masson et al., 1969). T lymphocytes have been shown by Moroz et al. to have F on their surface in patients with Hodgkin's disease (Moroz et al., 1977) and by Dörner et al. to synthesize and secrete F subunits (Dörner et al., 1980). Transferrin (○) has also been seen in T lymphocytes by immunofluorescence (Nishiya et al., 1980) and identified as a lymphocyte growth promoting factor after PHA stimulation by Tormey et al. (1972)

the specific granules of granulocytes, it is released by granulocytes, and it binds to specific receptors on the surface of macrophages (van Snick and Masson, 1976; Broxmeyer et al., 1980). Lf binding to macrophages is dependent on the iron saturation of the protein. Functionally, binding of fully saturated Lf to macrophages results in inhibition of macrophage colony stimulation activity (Broxmeyer et al., 1978). In a recent study of the association of lactoferrin binding to macrophages and other macrophage surface components, it has been shown that Lf binding can be inhibited by pretreatment of macrophages with specific anti-Ia antiserum (Broxmeyer, 1980).

It has been suggested for some time that peripheral blood lymphocytes synthesize transferrin (Soltys and Brody, 1970). Recent immunofluorescence studies of the association of transferrin with selected lymphocyte populations have indicated that T but not B lymphocytes contain intracytoplasmic transferrin (Nishiya et al., 1980). At the present time, however, it is not known whether the finding of intracytoplasmic Tf in T cells represents *de novo* synthesis of this protein by the cells. After overnight incubation 'halos' of transferrin-positive material were seen, suggesting that the protein had been released from the cells. This observation needs confirmation by more precise biochemical means.

Transferrin receptors have been demonstrated both in mitogen-activated lymphocytes (Phillips, 1976) and in T and B cell lines (Hemmaplardh and Morgan, 1974; Larrick and Cresswell, 1979), but seemingly not in resting lymphocytes (Galbraith et al., 1980). Transferrin receptors, however, have also been identified in numerous other transformed cell lines of different phenotypic cell origin (Hemmaplardh and Morgan, 1974; Hamilton et al., 1979; Galbraith et al., 1980). The transferrin requirement of transformed cells is probably related to its iron transport function, since increased levels of $FeSO_4$ have been shown to substitute for transferrin in cultures of 3T6 Swiss mouse fibroblasts (Rudland et al., 1977) and SV40 transformed 3T3 cells (Young et al., 1979).

Ferritin has been shown both by immunofluorescence and metabolic labelling to be associated with macrophages and T lymphocytes (Okhuma et al., 1976; Dörner et al., 1980). As shown in Plate 21, after metabolic labelling of selected human T and non-T lymphocytes, a much greater amount of radioactivity was found in T cell lysates and supernatants than in non-T lymphoid cells. Moreover, after reduction, more radioactivity was found associated with the acidic ferritin subunit of 21,000 mw than with the 19,000 subunit (Dörner et al., 1980).

8.2.2.3 Significance

The exact significance of the observed associations between iron-binding proteins, granulocytes, macrophages, T lymphocytes, and activated T and B lymphocytes to the presently held view of immune surveillance is not immediately clear. In its most general terms, the immune surveillance theory postulated that tumour cells arise with very high frequency in the normal organism, and that specific immune mechanisms are continuously instrumental in eradicating them. However, the fact that spontaneous tumours fail to immunize syngeneic hosts in contrast to the document immunogenicity of chemically or virally induced tumours (Baldwin, 1966; Prehn, 1976), the numerous instances in which cells of the immune system promote rather than inhibit tumour growth (Prehn, 1976; Naor, 1979), and the basically discouraging clinical results of immunotherapy trials in man (Hewitt, 1979) have led immunologists and non-immunologists alike to question the validity of such a view (Prehn, 1976; Klein and Klein, 1977; Hewitt, 1979). The association of iron-binding proteins with cells of the immune system is highly significant, however, to an alternative view of surveillance, in which the lympho-myeloid system, perhaps with the exception of the highly specific arm of B cell activation and differentiation, is less sensitive in a strict immunological sense of specific antigen recognition, but more effective in a wider biological sense of recognition of and protection from potentially toxic materials and in competition for nutrients used by bacterial and tumour cells. According to this view, it is highly significant that immune cells in general and recirculating lymphocytes or blast cells in particular should be able to synthesize and secrete, or bind, proteins capable of chelating iron and other known toxic metals such as, for instance, cadmium, nickel, and plutonium (Worwood, 1974).

The ability to participate in the binding of iron constitutes a plausible explanation for the detention of circulating lymphocytes in physiological and pathological sites of iron accumulation (Section 8.2.1). In addition, it endows the lymphoid system with an economical biochemical mechanism of control of numerous other major biological systems known to depend on the utilization of iron, such as haem biosynthesis (Moore and Goldberg, 1974), prostaglandin synthesis (Rao *et al.*, 1978), collagen synthesis (Hunt *et al.*, 1979), and corticosteroid synthesis (Williams-Smith and Cammack, 1979).

Iron is also recognized as a determining factor of microbial cell growth *in vitro* (Neilands, 1974; Kochan, 1977; Weinberg, 1978; Bullen *et al.*, 1978) and development of infection *in vivo* (Weinberg, 1978; Bullen *et al.*, 1978; Masawe *et al.*, 1974; Murray *et al.*, 1978). Iron has also been shown to be utilized effectively by certain tumours for their growth *in vivo* (Chandler and Fletcher, 1973; Warner *et al.*, 1978) and by transformed cells *in vitro* (Fernandez-Pol, 1977, 1978; Hamilton *et al.*, 1979; Galbraith *et al.*, 1980), a factor related probably to its requirements in DNA synthesis (Robbins and Pederson, 1970; Hoffbrand *et al.*, 1976). The fact that transferrin receptors have now been identified both in trophoblast (Faulk and Galbraith, 1979) and in numerous transformed cell lines (Hamilton *et al.*, 1979; Galbraith *et al.*, 1980) raises the important question of whether such receptors serve the dual purpose of escaping the surveillance of circulating host cells and providing the 'invading' population with a nutrient indispensable for its own growth and survival. The little publicized finding that certain tumour-association proteins have unique structures remotely related to those of ferredoxins (Bogoch, 1977) is also of interest, since tumours may utilize iron not only for cell division but also for anaerobic respiration. Finally, the fact that transformed cells express receptors for proteins that may be released by T cells, such as Tf, constitutes also a possible explanation for those instances in which the presence of T lymphocytes has been related to promotion of tumour growth (Prehn, 1976; Fiedler *et al.*, 1978; Naor, 1979).

8.3 CONCLUDING REMARKS

In conclusion, the existence of a circulation of lymphocytes between blood and lymph and its importance in the initiation, propagation, and persistence of immunity are undisputed. In spite of the interest that has surrounded the interaction of circulating lymphocytes with high endothelium venules of lymph nodes, its exact significance in the control of normal lymphocyte recirculation and/or lymphocyte recruitment in response to antigen challenge remains to be established, in the light of the fact that both can occur in the absence of such endothelial structures. In my view, more significant progress has been made in the definition of the interaction of asialated lymphocytes with liver cells and thus in illustrating the importance of cell interactions other than lymphocyte-HEV in the overall control of lymphocyte circulation and positioning. This progress was inspired by the purely biochemical work of Ashwell and co-workers on the fate of asialated proteins (Ashwell and Morell, 1974).

The implications of the fact that lymphocytes, as a result of interactions with cells other than HEV, accumulate in the 'wrong places' with concomitant depletions in the peripheral blood have not been fully realized where it truly matters, i.e. in the clinic. It is hoped that the clinical instances reviewed in Chapter 6 will contribute to propagate the awareness that many a T cell deficiency diagnosed in the peripheral blood reflects simply the different mobilizable properties of T and B lymphocytes, and most likely, the different mobilizable properties of subsets within the T cell population.

In the end, we continue basically ignorant of the reasons why lymphocytes go where they go. As reviewed in Chapter 8.2, at least topographically, T lymphocyte migration occurs frequently to physiological and pathological sites of iron deposition. The fact that both macrophages and T lymphocytes can synthesize iron-binding proteins indicates that the association may not represent a pure topographical coincidence, but that cells of the immune system can actively participate in the protection from the toxicity of iron and, probably, other metals. In addition, the ability to participate in the binding of iron would endow the immune system with an economical biochemical basis of control of numerous other major biological systems.

Iron is recognized as a determining factor of microbial cell growth and development of infection. Iron has also been shown to be utilized effectively by certain tumours for their growth *in vivo* and by transformed cells *in vitro*, a factor probably related to its requirement in DNA synthesis and anaerobic respiration. Further major biological systems in which the functional requirement for iron is documented include erythropoiesis, probably granulopoiesis, prostaglandin synthesis, collagen synthesis, and corticosteroid synthesis. Finally, one is tempted to speculate that the recent finding of high superoxide dismutase (SOD) activity in T lymphocytes, and its linkage to H-2 mice (Novak *et al.*, 1980) will have biological implications beyond their significance as disparate pieces of information. Indeed, the biological significance of a circulation of lymphocytes capable of binding Fe and possibly releasing superoxide dismutase could not be doubted by physiologists, biochemists, and immunologists alike. Such a circulation would ensure protection from the potential dangers inherent in the circulation of the blood and in the use of oxygen by cells, i.e. formation of the free radical O_2^- and, in the presence of iron, of the highly toxic oxidant hydroxyl radical (OH) (Fridovich, 1975).

'Let us cease to consider what, perhaps, may never happen, and what, when it happens, will laugh at human speculation.' (Johnson, 1759)

References

Aasa, R., Malmström, B. B., Saltman, P. and Wanngard, T. 1963. The specific binding of iron (III) and copper (II) to transferrin and conalbumin. *Biochem. Biophys. Acta*, **75**, 203.
Abercrombie, M. 1975. The contact behavior of invading cells. In *Cellular Membranes and Tumor Cell Behavior*. Williams & Wilkins, Baltimore, pp. 21–37.
Abercrombie, M. and Gitlin, G. 1965. The locomotory behaviour of small groups of fibroblasts. *Proc. Roy. Soc. London* (B), **162**, 289–302.
Abercrombie, M. and Heaysman, J. E. M. 1954. Observations on the social behaviour of cells in tissue culture. II. 'Monolayering' of fibroblasts. *Exp. Cell Res.*, **13**, 276–91.
Abercrombie, M. and Heaysman, J. E. M. 1976. Invasive behaviour between sarcoma and fibroblast populations in cell culture. *J. Nat. Cancer Inst.*, **56**, 561–70.
Abercrombie, M., Lamont, O. and Stephenson, E. M. 1968. The monolayering in tissue culture of fibroblasts from different sources. *Proc. Roy. Soc. London* (B), **170**, 349–60.
Adams, C. W. 1977. Pathology of multiple sclerosis: progression of the lesion. *Brit. Med. Bull.*, **33**, 15.
Adler, F. L. 1964. Competition of antigens. *Progr. Allergy*, **8**, 41.
Aisen, P. and Brown, E. M. 1977. The iron binding function of transferrin in iron metabolism. *Sem. Hematol.*, **14**, 31.
Aisen, P. and Leibman, A. 1972. Lactoferrin and transferrin: a comparative study. *Biochem. Biophys. Acta*, **257**, 314.
Aisen, P. and Leibman, A. 1973. The role of the anion binding site of transferrin in its interaction with the reticulocytes. *Biochem. Biophys. Acta.*, **304**, 797.
Alario, A., Ortonne, J. P., Schmitt, D. and Thivolet, J. 1978. Lichen planus: study with anti-human T-lymphocyte antigen (anti-HTLA) serum on frozen sections. *Brit. J. Dermatol.*, **98**, 601.
Allardyce, R. A., Shearman, D. J. C., McClelland, P. B. L., Marswick, K., Simpson, A. J. and Laidlow, R. B. 1974. Appearance of specific colostrum antibodies after clinical infection with Salmonella-typhimurium. *Brit. Med. J.*, **3**, 307.
Allwood, G. G. 1975. The migratory behaviour of T blasts to contact sensitivity reactions in actively and passively sensitised mice. *Immunology*, **28**, 681.
Aly, R., Maibach, H. I. and Mandel, A. 1976. Bacterial flora in psoriasis. *Br. J. Dermatol.*, **95**, 603.
Anderson, A. O. 1980. Structure and Physiology of Lymphatic Tissues. In *The Cell Biology of Immunity and Inflammation*, ed. J. Oppenheim. Elsevier/North Holland, in press.
Anderson, A. O. and Anderson, N. D. 1975. Studies on the structure and permeability of the microvasculature in normal rat lymph nodes. *Am. J. Pathol.*, **80**, 387–418.
Anderson, A. O., Anderson, N. D. and White, J. D. 1979. Basic mechanisms of lymphocyte recirculation in the Lewis Rats. *Adv. Exp. Med. Biol.*, **114**, 73.
Anderson, N. D., Anderson, A. O. and Wyllie, R. G. 1976. Specialized structure and

metabolic activities of high endothelial venules in rat lymphatic tissue. *Immunology*, **31**, 455.

Anderson, J., Sjoberg, O. and Moller, G. 1972. Mitogens as probes for immunocyte activition and cellular co-operation. *Transpl. Rev.*, **11**, 131.

Anderson, R. E., Sprent, J. and Miller, J. F. A. P. 1974. Radio-sensitivity of T and B lymphocytes. I. Effect of irradiation on cell migration. *Eur. J. Immunol.*, **4**, 199–203.

Andrews, P., Ford, W. L. and Stoddart, R. W. 1980. Metabolic studies of high-walled endothelium of post capillary venules in rat lymph nodes. Ciba Foundation Symposium No. 71, pp. 211–30.

Arnaud-Battandier, F., Bundy, B. M., O'Neill, M., Bienenstock, J. and Nelson, D. L. 1978. Cytotoxic activities of gut mucosal lymphoid cells in guinea pigs. *J. Immunol.*, **121**, 1059.

Arosio, P., Adelman, T. G. and Drysdale, J. W. 1978. On ferritin heterogeneity. Further evidence for heteropolymers. *J. Biol. Chem.*, **253**, 4451.

Asherson, G. L. 1966. Selective and specific inhibition of 24 hour skin reactions in the guinea pig. II. The mechanism of immune deviation. *Immunology*, **10**, 179.

Asherson, G. L. and Allwood, G. G. 1972. Inflammatory lymphoid cells; cells in immunised lymph nodes that move to sites of inflammation. *Immunology*, **22**, 493.

Asherson, G. L., Allwood, G. G. and Mayhew, B. 1973. Movement of T blast in the draining lymph nodes to sites of inflammation. *Immunology*, **25**, 485.

Ashwell, G. and Morell, A. G. 1974. The role of surface carbohydrates in the hepatic recognition of circulating glycoproteins. *Adv. Enzymol.*, **41**, 99.

Atkins, R. C. and Ford, W. L. 1975. Early cellular events in a systemic graft versus host reaction. I. The migration of donor lymphocytes after intravenous injection. *J. Exp. Med.*, **141**, 664.

Austin, C. M. 1968. Patterns of migration of lymphoid cells. *Aust. J. Exp. Biol. Med. Sci.*, **46**, 581.

Axelrod, R. A. and Rowley, D. A. 1968. Hypersensitivity: specific immunologic suppression of the delayed type. *Science*, **160**, 1465.

Baker, R. D. 1932–33. The cellular content of chyle in relation to lymphoid tissue and fat transportation. *Anat. Rec.*, **55**, 207–19.

Baldwin, R. W. 1966. Tumor-specific immunity against spontaneous rat tumors. *Int. J. Cancer*, **1**, 257.

Balfour, B. M. and Humphrey, J. H. 1966. Localization of labelled antigens in germinal centres and its relationship to the immune response. *Germinal Centres in Immune Responses*. Springer Verlag, Berlin, p. 80.

Balinsky, B. I. 1965. *An Introduction to Embryology*, 2nd edn., Saunders, Philadelphia & London, pp. xvi and 674.

Bancroft, J. 1974. *Researches on Pre-natal life*. Charles C. Thomas, Springfield, 30–72.

Barbera, A. J. 1975. Adhesive recognition between developing retinal cells and the optic tecta of the chick embryo. *Dev. Biol.*, **46**, 167–91.

Barnett, A. J. 1974. Scleroderma (progressive systemic sclerosis). Thomas, Springfield, Ill., p. 14.

Bartlett, P. F. and Edidin, M. 1978. Effect of the H-2 gene complex rates of fibroblast intercellular adhesion. *J. Cell Biol.*, **77**, 377–88.

Basten, A., Sprent, J. and Miller, J. F. A. P. 1972. Receptor for antibody–antigen complexes used to separate T cells from B cells. *Nature New Biol.*, **235**, 178.

Battisto, J. R. and Pappas, F. 1974. Dextran's regulatory effect on Immunoglobulin synthesis is mediated through T cells. *Cell. Immunol.*, **10**, 489.

Bazin, H. 1976. The secretory antibody response. In A. Ferguson and R. N. M. MacSween (eds.). *Immunological Aspects of the Liver and Gastrointestinal Tract*. University Park Press, Baltimore, M.D., p. 33.

Beh, K. J. and Lacelle, A. K. 1974. Class specificity of intracellular and surface immunoglobulin of cells in popliteal and intestine lymph from sheep. *Aust. J. Exp. Bio. Med. Sci.*, **52**, 505.

Bell, R. G. and Lafferty, J. J. 1972. The flow and cellular characteristics of cervical lymph from anaesthetized ducks. *Aust. J. Exp. Biol. Med.*, **50**, 611.

Bell, E. B. and Shand, F. L. 1975. Changes in lymphocyte recirculation and liberation of the adoptive memory response from cellular regulation in irradiated recipients. *European J. Immunol.*, **5**, 1–7.

Bergstrom, K., Franksson, C., Matell, G. and Von Reis, G. 1973. The effect of B_2 thoracic duct lymph drainage in myastenia gravis. *Europe. Neurol.*, **9**, 157.

Berman, V. J., Donnfest, B. S., Handler, E. S. and Handler, E. E. 1972. Microangiographic study of splenic arterial vascularization in normal and leukemic rat spleen. *J. Reticulo-endoth. Soc.*, **12**, 449.

Berne, R. M. and Levey, M. N. 1972. *Cardiovascular Physiology*, 2nd edn. Mosby, St. Louis.

Bernheimer, A. W. 1970. Cytolytic toxins of bacteria. In *Microbial Toxins*, ed. S. J. Aj and S. Kadis. Vol. 1, *Bacterial Protein Toxins*. Academic Press, New York, London, p. 183.

Bernstein, I. M., Webster, K. H., Williams, R. C. and Strickland, R. G. 1974. Reduction in circulating lymphocytes in alcoholic liver disease. *Lancet*, **2**, 488.

Beverley, P. 1977. Lymphocyte heterogeneity. In *B and T Cells in Immune Recognition*, ed. F. Loor and G. E. Roelants. Wiley, Chichester, p. 42.

Bezkorovainy, A. and Zschocke, R. H. 1974a. Structure and function of transferrins. I. Physical, chemical and iron binding properties. *Arzneim Forsch*, **24**, 476.

Bieber, C. P. and Bieber, M. M. 1973. Detection of ferritin as a circulating tumor associated antigen in Hodgkin's disease. *Nat. Cancer Inst. Mono.*, **36**, 147.

Bienenstock, J. 1974. The physiology of the local immune response and the gastrointestinal tract. In *Progress in Immunology* II, Vol. 4, ed. L. Brent and J. Holborow. North Holland, Amsterdam, pp. 197–207.

Bienenstock, J. and Johnston, N. 1976. A morphologic study of rabbit bronchial lymphoid aggregates and lymphoepithelium. *Lab. Invest.*, **35**, 343.

Bienenstock, J., McDermott, M., Befus, A. D. and O'Neill, M. 1978. A common mucosal immunologic system, involving the bronchus, breast and bowel. In *Secretory Immunity and Infection*. Plenum, New York, pp. 53–9.

Bienenstock, J., McDermott, M. and Befus, A. D. 1979. A common mucosal immune system. Proc. Conf. on the Immunology of Breast Milk.

Billingham, R. C., Brent, L. and Medawar, P. B. 1954. Quantitative studies on tissue transplantation immunity. II. The origin, strength and duration of actively and adoptively acquired immunity. *Proc. Roy. Soc. B*, **143**, 58.

Billingham, R. C., Silvers, W. K. and Wilson, D. B. 1962. Adoptive transfer of transplantation immunity by means of blood borne cells. *Lancet*, **i**, 512.

Billingham, R. E., Silvers, W. K. and Wilson, D. B. 1963. Further studies of adoptive transfer of sensitivity to skin homografts. *J. Exp. Med.*, **118**, 397.

Binns, R. M. 1980. *Pig Lymphocytes – Behaviour, Distribution and Classification*. Monographs in Allergy. Karger, Basel.

Binns, R. M. and Hall, J. G. 1966. The paucity of lymphocytes in the lymph of unanaesthetised pigs. *Brit. J. Exp. Path.*, **47**, 275.

Binns, R. M., McFarlin, D. E. and Sugar, J. R. 1972. Lymphoid depletion and immunosuppression after thymectomy in the young pig. *Nature New Biol.*, **238**, 181.

Bjerke, J. R. and Krogh, H. H. 1978. Identification of mononuclear cells *in situ* in skin lesions of lichen planus. *Brit. J. Dermatol.*, **98**, 605.

Bockman, D. E. and Cooper, M. D. 1973. Pinocytosis by epithelium associated with lymphoid follicles in the bursa of Fabricus, appendix and Peyer's patches: an electron microscope study. *Am. J. Anat.*, **136**, 455.

Bodmer, W. F. 1972. Evolutionary significance of the HL-A system. *Nature*, **237**, 139–45.
Bogoch, S. 1977. Astrocytin and malignin: two polypeptide fragments (recognins) related to brain tumor. *Nat. Cancer Inst. Monograph*, **46**, p. 133.
Bonomini, V., Mioli, V., Albertazzi, A. and Vangelista, A. 1970. Immunosuppressive drugs and lymphatic depletion by thoracic duct fistula in adult progressive glomerulonephritis. *Nephron*, **7**, 389.
Boyse, E. A. and Bennett, D. 1974. Differentiation and the cell surface: illustrations from work with T cells and sperm. In *Cellular Selection and Regulation of the Immune Response*, ed. G. Edelman. Raven Press, New York.
Boyse, E. A., Miyazawa, M., Aoki, T. and Old, L. J. 1968. Ly-A and Ly-B: two systems of lymphocyte isoantigens in the mouse. *Proc. Roy. Soc. B.*, **170**, 175.
Bradfield, J. W. B. and Born, G. V. R. 1974. Lymphocytosis produced by heparin and other sulphated polysaccharides in mice and rats. *Cell. Immunol.*, **14**, 22.
Brahim, F. and Osmond, D. G. 1970. Migration of bone marrow lymphocytes demonstrated by selective bone marrow labelling with thymidine-H3. *Anat. Rec.*, **168**, 139.
Brahim, F. and Osmond, D. G. 1973. The migration of lymphocytes from bone marrow to popliteal lymph nodes demonstrated by selective bone marrow labelling with ³H-thymidine *in vivo. Anat. Rec.*, **175**, 737.
Brandtzaeg, P. and Baklien, K. 1976. Immunoglobulin-producing cells in the intestine in health and disease. *Clin. Gastroenterol.*, **5** (No. 2), 251.
Brenner, A. I., Scheinberg, M. A. and Cathcart, E. S. 1975. Surface characteristics of synovial fluid and peripheral blood lymphocytes in inflammatory arthritis. *Arthr. and Rheum.*, **18**, 297.
Bremer, K., Fliedner, T. M. and Schick, P. 1973. Kinetic differences of autotransfused (³H)-cytidine labelled blood lymphocytes in leukemic and non-leukemic lymphoma patients. *Eur. J. Cancer*, **9**, 113.
Bremer, K., Wack, O. and Schick, P. 1973. Impaired recirculation of autotransfused blood lymphocytes via thoracic duct lymph in patients with chronic lymphoid leukemia. *Biomedicine*, **18**, 393.
Broder, S., Edelson, R. L., Lutzner, M. A., Nelson, D. L., MacDermott, R. P., Durm, M., Goldman, C. K., Meade, B. D. and Waldman, T. A. 1976. The Sezary syndrome: a malignant proliferation of helper T cells. *J. Clin. Invest.*, **58**, 1297.
Broxmeyer, H. 1980. Lactoferrin acts on Ia-like antigen-positive subpopulations of human monocytes to inhibit production of colony stimulatory activity *in vitro. J. Clin. Invest.*, **64**, 1717.
Broxmeyer, H., de Sousa, M., Smithyman, A., Ralph, P., Hamilton, J., Kurland, J. I. and Bognacki, J. J. 1980. Specificity and modulation of the action of lactoferrin, a negative feedback regulator of myelopoiesis. *Blood*, **55**, 324.
Broxmeyer, H. E., Smithyman, A., Eger, R. R., Meyers, P. A. and de Sousa, M. 1978. Identification of lactoferrin as the granulocyte-derived inhibitor of colony stimulating activity production. *J. Exp. Med.*, **148**, 1052–67.
Brown, W. R., Borthistle, B. K. and Chen. S. T. 1975. Immunoglobulin E and IgE-containing cells in human gastrointestinal fluids and tissues. *Clin. Exp. Immunol.*, **20**, 227.
Bryan, C. F., Nishiya, K., Pollack, M., DuPont, B. and de Sousa, M. 1980. Differential inhibition of the MLR by iron: association with HLA phenotype. *Immunogenetics*.
Bull, D. M. and Bockman, M. A. 1977. Isolation and functional characterisation of human intestinal mucosal lymphoid cells. *J. Clin. Invest.*, **59**, 966–74.
Bullen, J. J., Rogers, H. J. and Griffiths, E. 1978. Role of iron in infection. *Curr. Topics Microbiol. & Immunol.*, **80**, 1.
Bullock, W. E. 1976a. Perturbation of lymphocyte circulation in experimental murine leprosy. I. Description of the defect. *J. Immunol.*, **117**, 1164.

Bullock, W. E. 1976b. Perturbation of lymphocyte circulation in experimental murine leprosy. II. Nature of the defect. *J. Immunol.*, **117**, 1171.

Burke, J. S. and Simon, G. T. 1970. Electron microscopy of the spleen. I. Anatomy and microcirculation. *Am. J. Pathol.*, **58**, 127.

Burnet, F. M., McCrea, J. F. and Stone, J. D. 1946. Modification of human red cells by virus action; receptor gradient for virus action in human red cells. *Br. J. Exp. Pathol.*, **27**, 228.

Butcher, E. Scollay, R. and Weissman, I. 1979. Lymphocyte–high endothelial venule interactions: examination of species specificity. *Adv. Exp. Med. Biol.*, **114**, 65.

Buultjens, T. E. J. and Edwards, J. G. 1977. Adhesive selectivity as exhibited *in vitro* by cells from adherent tissues of the embryonic chick retina. *J. Cell Sci.*, **23**, 101–16.

Caffrey, R. H., Rieke, W. O. and Everett, N. B. 1962. Radioautographic studies of small lymphocytes in the thoracic duct of the rat. *Acta. Haematol.* (Basel), **28**, 145.

Cahill, R. N. P., Frost, H. and Trnka, Z. 1976. The effects of antigen on the migration of recirculating lymphocyte through single lymph nodes. *J. Exp. Med.*, **143**, 870.

Cahill, R. N. P., Poskitt, D. C., Frost, H. and Trnka, Z. 1977. Two distinct pools of recirculating T lymphocytes: migrating characteristics of nodal and intestinal lymphocytes. *J. Exp. Med.*, **145**, 420.

Cahill, R. N. P., Poskitt, D. C., Hay, J. B., Heron, I. and Trnka, Z. 1979. The migration of lymphocytes in the fetal lamb. *Eur. J. Immunol.*, **9**, 251–3.

Cahill, R. N. P. and Trnka, Z. 1980. Growth and development of recirculating lymphocytes in the sheep fetus. *Monographs in Allergy*, **16**, 38.

Campbell, P. A. and Cooper, M. R. 1975. Irradiation-resistant primed T cell function. *Cell. Immunol.*, **17**, 74.

Cantor, H. and Boyse, E. A. 1975. Functional subclasses of T lymphocytes bearing different Ly antigens. *J. Exp. Med.*, **141**, 1376.

Cantor, H., McVay-Boudreau, L., Hugenberger, J., Naidorf, K., Shen, F. W. and Gershon, R. K. 1978. Immunoregulatory circuit among T cell sets. II. Physiologic role of feedback inhibition *in vivo*: absence of NZB mice. *J. Exp. Med.*, **147**, 1116.

Carter, T. C., Lyon, M. and Phillips, R. F. S. 1955. Gene-tagged chromosome translocations in eleven stocks of mice. *J. Genetics*, **53**, 154.

Case, D. C., Jr., Hansen, J. A., Corrales, E., Yonng, C. W., Dupont, B., Pinsky, C. M. and Good, R. A. 1976. Comparison of multiple *in vivo* and *in vitro* parameters in untreated patients with Hodgkin's disease. *Cancer*, **38**, 1807.

Casley Smith, J. R. 1970. In *Progress in Lymphology* II, ed. M. Viamonte *et al.* Thienie, Stuttgart, pp. 51–4, 122–4, 255–60.

Casley Smith, J. R. 1971. The fine structure of the vascular system of amphioxus: Implications in the development of lymphatics and fenestrated blood capillaries. *Lymphology*, **4**, 79–94.

Casley Smith, J. R. 1973. The lymphatic system in inflammation. In *The Inflammatory Process*, Vol. II, ed. B. W. Zweifach, L. Grant and R. T. McCluskey. Academic Press, New York, p. 161.

Cebra, J. J., Kamat, R., Gearhart, P., Robertson, S. M. and Tseng, J. 1977. The secretory IgA system of the gut. In Ciba Foundation Symposium No. 46, 'Immunology of the Gut', p. 5.

Celada, F. 1966. Quantitative studies of the adoptive immunological memory in mice. *J. Exp. Med.*, **124**, 1.

Chanana, H. D., Joel, D. D., Schadeli, J., Hess, M. W. and Cottier, H. 1973. Thymus cell migration: ^{3}HTdR labeled and theta-positive cells in peripheral lymphoid tissues of newborn mice. *Adv. Exp. Med. Biol.*, **29**, 79.

Chandler, F. W. and Fletcher, O. J. 1973. Radioiron incorporation by a transplantable lymphoid tumor. *Cancer Res.*, **33**, 342.

Chang, L. L. 1973. Storage of iron in foetal livers. *Acta Paediat. Scand.*, **62**, 173.

Cheers, C., Sprent, J. and Miller, J. F. A. P. 1974. Interaction of thymus lymphocytes with histoincompatible cells. IV. Mixed lymphocyte reaction of activated thymus lymphocytes. *Cell. Immunol.*, **10**, 57.

Chisari, F. V. and Eddington, T. S. 1975. Lymphocyte E rosette inhibitory factor: a regulatory serum lipoprotein. *J. Exp. Med.*, **142**, 1092.

Chu, A. C. and MacDonald, D. 1979. Identification *in situ* of T lymphocytes in the dermal and epidermal infiltrates of mycosis fungoides. *Brit. J. Dermatol.*, **100**, 177.

Chusid, J. G. and Koeloff, L. M. 1967. Epileptogenic effects of metal powder implants in motor cortex of monkeys. *Intl. J. Neuropsych.*, **3**, 24–8.

Claesson, M. H., Jorgensen, O. and Topke, C. 1971. Light and electron microscopic studies of the paracortical post-capillary high entothelial venules. *Z. Zellforsch. Mikrosk. Anat.*, **119**, 195.

Cochrane, A. M., Moussouros, M. G., Thomson, A. D., Eddleston, A. L. and Williams, R. 1976. Antibody-dependent cell-mediated (K cell) cytotoxicity against isolated hepatocytes in chronic active hepatitis. *Lancet*, **1**, 441.

Cole, L. J. and Ellis, M. 1954. Studies on the chemical nature of the radiation protection factor in mouse spleen. *Radiation Research*, **1**, 347.

Cole, L. J., Fishler, M. C. and Bond, V. P. 1953. Subcellular fractionation of mouse spleen radiation protection activity. *Proc. Nat. Acad. Sci.*, **39**, 759.

Cornes, J. S. 1965. Number, size and distribution of Peyer's patches in the human small intestine. Part II. The effect of age on Peyer's patches. *Gut*, **6**, 230.

Cottier, H., Hess, M. W. and Keller, H. U. 1980. Structural basis for lymphoid tissue functions: established and disputable sites of antigen-cell and cell-to-cell interactions *in vivo*. *Monographs in Allergy*, **16**, 50–71.

Coutinho, A., Möller, G. and Richeter, W. 1974. Molecular basis of B cell activation. *Scand. J. Immunol.*, **3**, 321.

Crabbe, P. A. and Heremans, J. F. 1966. The distribution of immunoglobulin containing cells along the human gastrointestinal tract. *Gastroenterology*, **51**, 305.

Crabbe, P. A., Nash, D. R., Bazin, H., Eyssen, H. and Heremans, J. F. 1970. Immunohistochemical observations on lymphoid tissues from conventional and germ-free mice. *Lab. Invest.*, **22**, 448.

Craig, S. W. and Cebra, J. J. 1971. Peyer's patches: an enriched source of precursors for IgA producing immunocytes in the rabbit. *J. Exp. Med.*, **134**, 188.

Craig, S. W. and Cebra, J. J. 1975. Rabbit Peyer's patches, appendix and popliteal lymph node B lymphocytes: a comparative analysis of their membrane immunoglobulin components and plasma cell precursor potential. *J. Immunol.*, **114**, 492.

Crandall, M. 1978. Mating-type interactions in yeasts. *Symp. Soc. Exp. Biol.*, **32**, 105–19.

Crick, F. 1970. Diffusion in embryogenesis. *Nature*, **225**, 420–2.

Cuatrecasas, P. and Hollenberg, M. D. 1976. Membrane receptors and hormone action. *Adv. Protein Chem.*, **30**, 252–451.

Cummins, A. G., Duncombe, V. M., Bolin, T. D., Davis, A. E. and Kelly, J. D. 1978. Suppression of rejection of Nippostrongylus brasiliensis in iron and protein deficient rats: effect of syngeneic lymphocyte transfer. *Gut*, **19**, 823.

Curran, R. C. and Jones, E. L. 1977. Immunoglobulin-containing cells in human tonsils demonstrated by immunohistochemistry. *Clin. Exp. Immunol.*, **28**, 103.

Curry, J. L. and Trentin, J. J. 1967. Hemopoietic spleen colony studies. I. Growth and differentiation. *Dev. Biol.*, **15**, 395–413.

Curry, J. L., Trentin, J. J. and Wolf, N. S. 1967. Hemopoietic spleen colony studies. II. Erythropoiesis. *J. Exp. Med.*, **125**, 703.

Curtis, A. S. G. 1960. Cell contacts: some considerations. *Am. Nat.*, **94**, 37–56.

Curtis, A. S. G. 1962. Cell contact and adhesion. *Biol. Rev.*, **37**, 82–129.

Curtis, A. S. G. 1967. *The Cell Surface: Its Molecular Role in Morphogenesis*. Logos Press, London, pp. ix and 399.

Curtis, A. S. G. 1970a. Problems and some solutions in the study of cellular aggregation. *Symp. Zool. Soc. London*, **25**, 335–52.
Curtis, A. S. G. 1970b. On the occurrence of specific adhesion between cells. *J. Embryol. Exp. Morph.*, **23**, 253–72.
Curtis, A. S. G. 1973. Cell adhesion. *Progr. Biophys. Mol. Biol.*, **27**, 315.
Curtis, A. S. G. 1974. The specific control of cell positioning. *Arch. Biol.*, **85**, 105–21.
Curtis, A. S. G. 1976. Le positionnement cellulaire et la morphogenèse. *Bull. Soc. Zool. de France*, **1**, 9–21.
Curtis, A. S. G. 1978a. Cell positioning, *Receptors and Recognition*, Series B, **4**, 159–90.
Curtis, A. S. G. 1978b. Cell–cell recognition: positioning and patterning systems. *Symp. Soc. Exp. Biol.*, **32**, 51–82.
Curtis, A. S. G. 1979a. Cell recognition and intercellular adhesion. In *Biochemistry of Cellular Recognition*, Vol. 4, *The Cell Surface*, ed. P. Knox. CRC Press, Cleveland, Ohio.
Curtis, A. S. G. 1979b. Individuality and graft rejection in sponges. In Systematics Association Special Vol. No. 11, *Biology and Systematics of Colonial Organisms*, Ed. G. Larwood and B. R. Rosen, 1978. Academic Press, London, New York, pp. 39–48.
Curtis, A. S. G. 1979c. The H-2 histocompatibility system and lymphocyte adhesion: interaction modulation factor involvement. *J. Immunogenetics* (in press).
Curtis, A. S. G., Campbell, J. and Shaw, F. M. 1975. Cell surface lipids and adhesion. I. The effects of lysophosphatidyl compounds, Phospholipase A_2 and Aggregation-inhibiting protein. *J. Cell. Sci.*, **18**, 347.
Curtis, A. S. G. and de Sousa, M. 1973. Factors influencing adhesion of lymphoid cells. *Nature New Biol.*, **244**, 45–7.
Curtis, A. S. G. and de Sousa, M. 1975. Lymphocyte interactions and positioning. 1. Adhesive interactions. *Cell. Immunol.*, **19**, 282–97.
Curtis, A. S. G., Miles, D. and Wilkinson, P. C. W. 1978. New evidence on control mechanisms in lymphocyte traffic. *Adv. Exp. Med. Biol.*, **114**, 93.
Curtis, A. S. G. and Van de Vyver, G. 1971. The control of cell adhesion in morphogenetic systems. *J. Embryol. Exp. Morph.*, **26**, 295–312.
Dahl, M. V., Lindross, W. E. and Nelson, R. D. 1978. Chemokinetic and chemotactic factors in psoriasis scale extracts. *J. Invest. Dermatol.*, **71**, 402.
Daniele, R. P., Beacham, C. H. and Gorenberg, D. J. 1977. The bronchoalveolar lymphocyte studies on the life history and lymphocyte traffic from blood to the lung. *Cell. Immunol.*, **31**, 48–54.
De Horatius, R. J., Stickland, R. G. and Williams, R. C. 1974. T and B lymphocytes in acute and chronic hepatitis. *Clin. Immunol. Immunopathol.*, **2**, 353.
De Kruyff, R. H., Durkin, H. G., Gilmour, D. G. and Thornbecke, G. J. 1975. Migratory patterns of B lymphocytes. II. Fate of cells from control lymphoid organs in the chicken. *Cell. Immunol.*, **16**, 301–14.
de Kruyff, V. H., Ponzio, N. M. and Thornbecke, J. 1977. Evaluation of the possible role of B cell receptors in the tendency of B cells to migrate into follicles in mice and chickens. *Eur. J. Immunol.*, **7**, 237.
de Sousa, M. A. B. 1969. Reticulum arrangement related to the behaviour of cell populations in the mouse lymph node. In *Lymphatic Tissue and Germinal Centers in Immune Response*. Plenum Press, New York, p. 49.
de Sousa, M. 1971. Kinetics of the distribution of thymus and bone marrow cells in the peripheral organs of the mouse: ecotaxis. *Clin. Exp. Immunol.*, **9**, 371.
de Sousa, M. 1973. The ecology of thymus-dependency. In *Contemporary Topics in Immunobiology*. Plenum Press, New York, p. 119.
de Sousa, M. 1976. Cell traffic. In *Receptors and Recognition*, Series A, Vol. 2, ed. P. Cuatrecases and M. F. Greaves. Chapman and Hall, London, p. 105.
de Sousa, M. 1978a. Ecotaxis, ecotaxopathy and lymphoid malignancy. In

Immunopathology of Lymph Neoplasms, ed. R. A. Good and J. Twomey. Plenum Press, New York, p. 325.
de Sousa, M. 1978b. Lymphoid cell positioning: a new proposal for the mechanism of control of lymphoid cell migration. *Symp. Soc. Exp. Biol.*, **32**, 393.
de Sousa, M. and Anderson, J. M. 1970. A study of human lymph node biopsies. In *The Biology and Surgery of Tissue Transplantation*, ed. J. M. Anderson. Blackwell, Oxford, Edinburgh, p. 175.
de Sousa, M., Ferguson, A. and Parrott, D. M. V. 1973. Ecotaxis of B cells in the mouse. *Adv. Exp. Med. Biol.*, **29**, 55.
de Sousa, M., Freitas, A., Huber, B., Cantor, H. and Boyse, E. A. 1979. Migratory patterns of the Ly subsets of T lymphocytes in the mouse. *Adv. Exp. Med. Biol.*, **114**, 51.
de Sousa, M. and Good, R. A. 1978. T and B cell populations in gut and gut associated lymphoid organs: arrangement, migration, and function. In *Gastrointestinal Tract Cancer*, ed. M. Lipkin and R. A. Good. Plenum Publishing Corporation, New York.
de Sousa, M., Humphrey, J. H. and Balfour, J. H. 1971. The side effects of high zone tolerance. *Adv. Exp. Med. Biol.*, **12**, 235.
de Sousa, M. and Parrott, D. M. V. 1967. Definition of a germinal center area as distinct from the thymus-dependent area in the lymphoid tissue of the mouse. In *Germinal Centers in Immune Responses*, ed. H. Cottier and Odartchenko. Springer Verlag, New York, p. 361.
de Sousa, M. A. B. and Parrott, D. M. V. 1969. Induction and recall in contact sensitivity. *J. Exp. Med.*, **130**, 671.
de Sousa, M. and Pritchard, H. 1974. The cellular basis of immunological recovery in nude mice after thymus grafting. *Immunology*, **26**, 769.
de Sousa, M. A. B., Parrott, D. M. V. and Pantelouris, E. M. 1969. The lymphoid tissues in mice with congenital aplasia of the thymus. *Clin. Exp. Immunol.*, **4**, 637.
de Sousa, M., Smithyman, A. M. and Tan, C. T. C. 1978. Suggested models of ecotaxopathy in lymphoreticular malignancy. *Am. J. of Pathol.*, **90**, 497.
de Sousa, M., Tan, C. T. C., Siegal, F. P., Fillipa, D. A. and Good, R. A. 1978. Immunologic parameters in childhood Hodgkin's disease. II. T and B lymphocytes in the peripheral blood of normal children and in the spleen and peripheral blood of children with Hodgkin's disease. *Ped. Res.*, **12**, 143.
de Sousa, M., Yang, M., Lopes-Corrales, E., Tan, C., Hansen, J. A., Dupont, B. and Good, R. A. 1977. Ecotaxis: the principle and its application to the study of Hodgkin's disease. *Clin. Exp. Immunol.*, **27**, 143.
Diamanstein, T., Meinhold, H. and Wagner, B. 1971. Stimulation of humoral antibody formation by polyanions. V. Relationship between enhancement of sheep red blood cell uptake by the spleen and adjuvant action of dextran sulphate. *Eur. J. Immunol.*, **1**, 429.
Diamanstein, T., Vogt, W., Ruhl, H. and Bechet, G. 1973. Stimulation of DNA synthesis in mouse lymphoid cells by polyanions *in vitro*. *Eur. J. Immunol.*, **3**, 488.
Diamanstein, T. and Wagner, B. 1973. The use of polyanions to break immunological tolerance. *Nature New Biol.*, **241**, 117.
Diamanstein, T., Wagner, B., Beyse, L., Odenwald, M. V. and Schulz, G. Stimulation of humoral antibody formation by polyanions. 1971. II. The influence of sulfate esters of polymers on the immune response in mice. *Eur. J. Immunol.*, **1**, 340.
Diaz-Jouanen and Williams, R. C., Jr. 1974. T and B lymphocytes in human colostrum. *Clin. Immunol. Immunopath.*, **3**, 248.
Dierich, M. P., Wilhelmi, D. and Till, G. 1977. Essential role of surface-bound chemoattractant in leucocyte migration. *Nature*, **270**, 351–2.
Dineen, J. K. and Adams, D. B. 1970. The effect of long term lymphatic drainage on the lymphomyeloid system in the guinea pig. *Immunology*, **19**, 11.

Doherty, P. C. and Zinkernagel, R. M. 1974. T cell-mediated immunopathology in viral infections. *Transplant. Rev.*, **19**, 89.

Dorey, H. M., Magnusson, B. J., Gulaskharan, J. and Pearson, J. E. 1965. The properties of phospholipase enzymes in staphylococcal toxins. *J. Gen. Microbiol.*, **40**, 208.

Dörner, M., Silverstone, A. E., Nishiya, K., de Sostoa, A., Munn, G. and de Sousa, M. 1980. Ferritin synthesis by human T lymphocytes. *Science*, **209**, 1019.

Douglas, A. P., Weetman, A. P. and Haggith, J. W. 1976. The distribution and enteric loss of ^{51}Cr-labelled lymphocytes in normal subjects and in patients with coeliac disease and other disorders of the small intestine. *Digestion*, **14**, 29–43.

Dresser, D. 1961. A study of the adoptive secondary response to a protein antigen in mice. *Proc. Roy. Soc.*, **154**, 398.

Dresser, D. W., Taub, R. N. and Krantz, A. R. 1970. The effect of localized injection of adjuvant material on the draining lymph node. II. Circulating lymphocytes. *Immunology*, **18**, 663.

Drysdale, J. W., Adelman, T. G., Arosio, P., Casareale, D., Fitzpatrick, P., Hazard, J. T. and Yakota, M. 1977. Human isoferritins in normal and disease states. *Sem. Hematol.*, **14**, 71–88.

Dubreuil, A. E., Herman, P. G., Tilney, N. L. and Mellins, H. Z. 1975. Microangiography of the white pulp of the spleen. *Am. J. Roent.*, **123**, 427.

Dumont, A. E., Ford, R. J. and Becker, F. F. 1976. Siderosis of lymph nodes in patients with Hodgkin's disease. *Cancer*, **38**, 1274.

Dunn, G. A. 1971. Mutual contact inhibition of extension of chick sensory nerve fibers *in vitro*. *J. Comp. Neurol.*, **143**, 491–508.

Durkin, H. G., Caporale, L. and Thornbecke, G. J. 1975. Migratory patterns of B lymphocytes. I. Fate of cells from central and peripheral lymphoid organs in the rabbit and its selective alteration by anti-immunoglobulin. *Cell. Immunol.*, **16**, 285.

Durkin, H. G., Carboni, J. M. and Waksman, B. H. 1978. Antigen induced increase in migration of large cortical thymocytes (regulatory cells?) to the marginal zone and red pulp of the spleen. *J. Immunol.*, **121**, 1075.

Duthie, H. L. 1964. The relative importance of the duodenum in the intestinal absorption of iron. *Brit. J. Haematol.*, **10**, 59–68.

East, J., de Sousa, M. A. B. and Parrott, D. M. V. 1965. Immunopathology of New Zealand Black Mice. *Transplantation*, **3**, 711.

Ebendal, T. 1976. The relative roles of contact inhibition and contact guidance in orientation of axons extending on aligned collagen fibrils *in vitro*. *Exp. Cell Res.*, **98**, 159–69.

Edelson, R. L., Smith, R. W., Frank, M. M. and Green, I. 1973. Identification of subpopulations of mononuclear cells in cutaneous infiltrates. *J. Invest. Dermatol.*, **61**, 82.

Edelstein, B. B. 1971. Cell specific diffusion model of morphogenesis. *J. Theoret. Biol.*, **30**, 515–23.

Ellis, A. E. and de Sousa, M. 1974. Phylogeny of the lymphoid system. I. A study of the fate of circulating lymphocytes in plack. *Eur. J. Immunol.*, **4**, 338.

Elton, R. A. and Tickle, C. A. 1971. The analysis of spatial distributions in mixed cell populations: a statistical method for detecting sorting out. *J. Embryol. Exp. Morph.*, **26**, 135–56.

Emeson, E. E. 1978. Migratory behaviour of lymphocytes with specific reactivity to alloantigens. II. Selective recruitment to lymphoid cell allografts and their draining lymph nodes. *J. Exp. Med.*, **147**, 13.

Engeset, A., Froland, S. S. and Bremer, K. 1974. Studies of human peripheral lymph II. Low lymphocyte count and few B-lymphocytes in peripheral lymph of patients with chronic lymphocytic leukemia. *Scand. J. Haematol.*, **13**, 93.

Erickson, C. A. 1978. Contact behaviour and pattern formation of BHK and polyoma virus-transformed BHK fibroblasts in culture. *J. Cell. Sci.*, **33**, 53–84.

Eshhar, Z., Order, S. E. and Katz, D. H. 1974. Ferritin, a Hodgkin's disease associated antigen. *Proc. Natl. Acad. Sci.*, **71**, 3956.
Eyre, H. J., Rosen, P. J. and Perry, S. 1970. Relative labelling of leukocytes, erythrocytes and platelets in human blood by ^{51}Chromium. *Blood*, **36**, 250.
Ezekiel, E. and Morgan, E. H. 1963. Milk iron and its metabolism in the lactating rat. *J. Physiol.*, **165**, 336.
Fabiano, A. 1956. Valori siderimetrici del latte materno e trattamento marziale. *Ann. Obstr. Ginecologia*, **78**, 1043.
Fagraeus, A. 1948. The plasma cellular reactions and its relation to the formation of antibodies *in vitro*. *J. Immunol.*, **58**, 1.
Fahy, V. A., Gerber, H. A., Morris, B., Trevella, W. and Zukoski, C. F. 1980. The function of lymph nodes in the formation of lymph. In *Essays in the Anatomy and Physiology of Lymphoid Tissues*, Monographs in Allergy, ed. Z. Trnka. Karger, Basel.
Faulk, W. P. and Galbraith, G. M. P. 1979. Trophoblast transferrin and transferrin receptors in the host–parasite relationship of human pregnancy. *Proc. Roy. Soc. Lond.*, B, **204**, 83–97.
Faulk, W. P., McCormick, M. N., Goodman, J. R., Yoffey, J. M. and Fudenberg, H. H. 1971. Peyer's patches. Morphologic studies. *Cell. Immunol.*, **1**, 500.
Fell, H. B. 1939. Origin and developmental mechanics of the avian sternum. *Phil. Trans. Roy. Soc. London*, B, **229**, 407–63.
Ferguson, A. 1977. Intraepithelial lymphocytes of the small intestine. *Gut*, **18**, 921.
Ferguson, A. and Parrott, D. M. V. 1972a. The effect of antigen deprivation on thymus-dependent and thymus-independent lymphocytes in the small intestine of the mouse. *Clin. Exp. Immunol.*, **12**, 477.
Ferguson, A. and Parrott, D. M. V. 1972b. Growth and development of antigen-free grafts of foetal mouse intestine. *J. Pathol.*, **106**, 95.
Fernandez, H. N., Henson, P. M., Otani, A. and Hugli, T. E. 1978. Chemotactic response to human C3a and C5a anaphylatoxins: I. Evaluation of C3a and C5a leukotaxis *in vitro* and under simulated *in vivo* conditions. *J. Immunol.*, **120**, 109.
Fernandez-Pol, J. A. 1977. Transition metal irons induce cell growth in NRK cell synchronized in G_1 by picolinic acid. *Biochem. Biophys. Res. Comm.*, **76**, 413.
Fernandez-Pol, J. A. 1978. Isolation and characterisation of a siderophore like growth factor from mutants of SV-40 transformed cells adapted to picolinic acid. *Cell*, **14**, 489.
Fichtelius, K. E. 1953. On the fate of the lymphocyte. *Acta Anat. Suppl.*, **19**, 1.
Fichtelius, K. E. 1964. A factor in the liver scattering aggregates of lymphoid cells in artificially prepared suspensions. *Acta Path. et Microbiol. Scandinavia*, **62**, 47–52.
Fiedler, I. J., Gerstein, D. M. and Hart, I. R. 1978. The biology of cancer invasion and metastasis. *Adv. Cancer Res.*, **28**, 150.
Fischer, H., Ferber, E., Haupt, I., Kohlschutter, A., Modelell, M., Munder, P. G. and Sonak, R. 1967. Lysophosphatides and cell membranes. *Protides Biol. Fluids. Proc. Colloq.*, **15**, 175.
Flad, H. D., Huber, C., Bremer, K., Menne, H. D. and Huber, H. 1973. Impaired recirculation of B lymphocytes in chronic lymphocytic leukemia. *Eur. J. Immunol.*, **3**, 688.
Fleischmajer, R., Damiano, V. and Nedwich, A. 1972. Alteration of subcutaneous tissue in systemic scleroderma. *Arch. Dermatol.*, **105**, 59.
Florey, H. W. and Gowans, J. L. 1958. The reticulo-endothelial system. The omentum–lymphatic drainage. In *The Lymphocyte in General Pathology*, ed. H. Florey. Lloyd-Luke (Medical books), London, p. 98.
Ford, C. E., Hamerton, J. L., Barnes, D. W. H. and Loutit, J. F. 1956. Cytological identification of radiation chimeras. *Nature*, **177**, 452.

Ford, W. L. 1968. Duration of the inductive effect of sheep erythrocytes on the recruitment of lymphocytes in the rat spleen. *Brit. J. Exp. Pathol.*, **49**, 502.

Ford, W. L. 1969. The kinetics of lymphocyte recirculation within the rat spleen. *Cell Tissue Kinet.*, **2**, 171.

Ford, W. L. 1975. Lymphocyte migration and immune responses. *Progress in allergy*, **19**, 1.

Ford, W. L., Andrews, P. and Smith, M. E. 1978. Lymphocyte migration in relation to the pathophysiology of inflammatory rheumatic disease. In *Research into Rheumatoid Arthritis and Allied Diseases*, ed. D. C. Dumonde and R. N. Maini, M. T. P., Lancaster (in press).

Ford, W. L. and Atkins, R. C. 1971. Specific unresponsiveness of recirculating lymphocytes after exposure to histocompatibility antigens in F_1 hybrid rats. *Nature New Biol.*, **234**, 178.

Ford, W. L. and Atkins, R. C. 1973. The proportion of lymphocytes capable of recognizing strong transplantation antigens *in vivo*. *Adv. Exp. Med. Biol.*, **29**, 255.

Ford, W. L. and Gowans, J. L. 1969. The traffic of lymphocytes. *Sem. Haematol.*, **6**, 67.

Ford, W. L. and Hunt, S. V. 1973. In *Handbook of Experimental Immunology*, ed. D. M. Weir. Blackwell, Oxford and Edinburgh, Chapter 23, pp. 1–27.

Ford, W. L., Sedgley, M., Sparshott, S. M. and Smith, M. E. 1976. The migration of lymphocytes across specialized vascular endothelium. II. The contrasting consequences of treating lymphocytes with trypsin or neuraminidase. *Cell and Tissue Kinetics*, **9**, 351–61.

Ford, W. L., Smith, M. E. and Andrews, P. 1978. Possible clues to the mechanism underlying the selective migration of lymphocytes from the blood. *Symp. Soc. Exp. Biol.*, **32**, 359.

Forth, W. and Rummel, W. 1973. Iron absorption. *Physiol. Rev.*, **53**, 724.

Fossum, S., Bell, E. B., Smith, M. E. and Ford, W. L. 1980. The architecture of rat lymph nodes. 3). The lymph nodes and lymph borne cells of the athymic, nude rat. *Scand. J. Immunol.* (in press).

Franksson, C. F. and Blomstrand, R. 1968. Drainage of the thoracic drainage lymph duct during homologous transplantation in man. *Kidney Tranpl.*, **51**.

Franksson, C., Lundgren, G., Magnusson, G. and Rineden, O. 1976. Drainage of thoracic duct lymph in renal transplant patients. *Transplantation*, **21**, 133.

Freitas, A. A. 1976. Control mechanisms of lymphocyte traffic. Ph.D. thesis. Glasgow University.

Freitas, A. A. and Bognaki, J. J. 1979. The role of cell locomotion in lymphocyte migration. *Immunology*, **36**, 247.

Freitas, A. A. and de Sousa, M. A. B. 1975. Control mechanisms of lymphocyte traffic. Modification of the traffic of ^{51}Cr-labelled mouse lymph node cells by treatment with plant lectins in intact and splenectomized mice. *Eur. J. Immunol.*, **5**, 831–8.

Freitas, A. A. and de Sousa, M. A. B. 1976a. The role of cell interactions in the control of lymphocyte traffic. *Cellular Immunol.*, **22**, 345–50.

Freitas, A. A. and de Sousa, M. A. B. 1976b. Control mechanisms of lymphocyte traffic. Altered distribution of ^{51}Cr-labelled mouse lymph-node cells pretreated *in vitro* with lipopolysaccharide. *Eur. J. Immunol.*, **6**, 269–73.

Freitas, A. A. and de Sousa, M. A. B. 1976c. Control mechanisms of lymphocyte traffic. Altered migration of ^{51}Cr-labelled mouse lymph-node cells pretreated *in vitro* with phospholipases. *Eur. J. Immunol.*, **6**, 703–11.

Freitas, A. A. and de Sousa, M. A. B. 1977. Control mechanisms of lymphocyte traffic. A study of the action of two sulphate polysaccharides on the distribution of ^{51}Cr and (^{3}H)-adenosine-labelled mouse lymph node cells. *Cellular Immunol.*, **31**, 62–77.

Freitas, A. A., Rocha, B., Chiao, J. W. and de Sousa, M. 1978. Divergent actions of monomeric, dimeric and tetrameric concanavalin A on lymphocyte traffic. *Cell. Immunol.*, **35**, 59.

Freitas, A. A., Rose, M. L. and Parrott, D. M. V. 1977. Murine mesenteric and peripheral lymph nodes: a common pool of small T cells. *Nature (London)*, **270**, 731.

Freitas, A. A., Rose, M. L., and Rocha, B. 1980. Random migration of small T lymphocytes from mouse thoracic duct. *Lymph. Cell. Immunol.* (in press).

Fridovich, I. 1975. Superoxide dismutases. *Ann. Rev. Biochem.*, **44**, 147.

Froland, S. S., Natvig, J. B. and Husby, G. 1973. Immunological characterization of lymphocytes in synovial fluid from patients with rheumatoid arthritis. *Scand. J. Immunol.*, **2**, 67.

Frost, H., Cahill, R. N. P. and Trnka, Z. 1975. The migration of recirculating autologous and allogeneic lymphocytes through single lymph nodes. *Eur. J. Immunol.*, **5**, 839.

Frost, P. and Lance, E. M. 1974. The relation of lymphocyte trapping to the mode of action of adjuvants. In *Immunopotentiation*, Ciba Found, Symp. No. 18 (new series), p. 29.

Frydén, A. 1977. B and T lymphocytes in blood and cerebrospinal fluid in acute aseptic meningitis. *Scand. J. Immunol.*, **6**, 1283.

Galbraith, G. M. P., Galbraith, R. M. and Faulk, W. P. 1980. Transferrin binding by human lymphoblastoid cell lines and other transformed cells. *Cell. Immunol.*, **49**, 215–22.

Galili, U., Rosenthal, L., Galili, N. and Klein, E. 1979. Activated T cells in the synovial fluid of arthritic patients: characterization and comparison with *in vitro* activated human and murine T cells in cooperation with monocytes in cytotoxicity. *J. Immunol.*, **122**, 878.

Garrod, D. R., Swan, A. P., Nicol, A. and Forman, D. 1978. Cellular recognition in slime mould development. *Symp. Soc. Exp. Biol.*, **32**, 173–202.

Gershon, R. K. 1974. T cell control of antibody production. In *Cont. Topics in Immunobiology*, Vol. 3, ed. M. D. Cooper and N. L. Warren. Plenum Press, New York.

Gershon, R. K., Askenase, R. W. and Gershon, M. D. 1975. Requirement for vasoactive amines for production of delayed type hypersensitivity reactions. *J. Exp. Med.*, **142**, 732.

Gesner, B. M. 1966. Cell surface sugars as sites of cellular reactions: possible role in physiological processes. *Ann. N.Y. Acad. Sci.*, **129**, 758.

Gesner, B. M. and Ginsburg, V. 1964. Effect of glycosidases on the fate of transfused lymphocytes. *Proc. Nat. Acad. Sci.*, **52**, 750.

Gillette, R. W. 1975. Homing of labelled lymphoid cells in athymic mice: evidence for additional immunologic defects. *Cell. Immunol.*, **17**, 374.

Gillette, R. W., McKenzie, G. O. and Swanson, M. H. 1973. Effect of concanavalin A on the homing of labelled T lymphocytes. *J. Immunol.*, **111**, 1902.

Girardet, R. E. and Benninghoff, D. L. 1977. Long term physiologic study of thoracic duct lymph and lymphocytes in rat and man. *Lymphology*, **10**, 36.

Goldblum, R. M., Ahlstedt, S., Carlsson, B., Hanson, L. A., Jodai, U., Lidin-Janson, G. and Sohl-Akerhund, A. 1975. Antibody-forming cells in human colostrum after oral immunization. *Nature*, **257**, 797.

Goldschneider, I. and McGregor, D. D. 1968a. Migration of lymphocytes and thymocytes in the rat. I. The route of migration from blood to spleen and lymph nodes. *J. Exp. Med.*, **127**, 155.

Goldschneider, I. and McGregor, D. D. 1968b. Migration of lymphocytes and thymocytes in the rat. II. Circulation of lymphocytes and thymocytes from blood to lymph. *Lab. Invest.*, **18**, 397.

Good, R. A. and Gabrielson, A. 1964. *The Thymus in Immunobiology*. Harper and Row, New York.

Goos, M. and Kaiserling, H. K. 1975. Dermatopathic lymphadenitis – an alteration of the T-lymphocyte areas in skin-related lymph nodes. 2nd Eur. Meeting on Electron Microscopy Applied to Cutaneous Pathology, Milano, Jan. 17–18.

Goos, M., Kaiserling, E. and Lennert, K. 1976. Mycosis fungoides: model for T-lymphocyte homing to skin? *Brit. J. Dermatol.*, **94**, 221.

Gowans, J. L. 1957. The effect of the continuous re-infusion of lymph and lymphocytes on the output of lymphocytes from the thoracic duct in unanaesthetized rats. *Brit. J. Exp. Pathol.*, **38**, 67.

Gowans, J. L. 1959. The recirculation of lymphocytes from blood to lymph in the rat. *J. Physiol.*, **146**, 54.

Gowans, J. L. 1962. The fate of parental strain lymphocytes in F_1 hybrid rats. *Ann. N.Y. Acad. Sci.*, **99**, 335.

Gowans, J. L. and Knight, E. J. 1964. The route of recirculation of lymphocytes in the rat. *Proc. Roy. Soc. B.*, **159**, 257.

Gowans, J. L., McGregor, D. D. and Cowen, D. M. 1963. The role of small lymphocytes in the rejection of homografts of skin. In *The Immunologically Competent Cell*. Ciba Found. Study Group, No. 16, p. 20.

Graham, R. C. and Shannon, S. L. 1972. Peroxidase arthritis II Lymphoid cell–endothelial interactions during a developing immunologic inflammatory response, *Am. J. Pathol.*, **69**, 7.

Granick, S. 1946. Ferritin: Its properties and significance for iron metabolism. *Chem. Rev.*, **38**, 379.

Grant, L. 1973. The sticking and emigration of white blood cells in inflammation. In *The Inflammatory Process*, Vol. II, ed. B. W. Zweifach, L. Grant and R. T. McCluskey. Academic Press, New York, p. 205.

Greaves, M. F., Owen, J. J. T. and Raff, M. C. 1974. T and B lymphocytes. *Excerpta Medica*, North Holland, Amsterdam.

Griscelli, C., Vassalli, P. and McCluskey, R. J. 1969. The distribution of large dividing lymph node cells in syngeneic recipient rats after intravenous transfer. *J. Exp. Med.*, **130**, 1427.

Groves, M. L. 1960. The isolation of a red protein from milk. *J. Am. Chem. Soc.*, **82**, 3345.

Guillou, P. J., Brennan, T. G. and Giles, G. R. 1973. Lymphocyte transformation in the mesenteric lymph nodes of patients with Crohn's disease. *Gut*, **14**, 20.

Gupta, S. and Good, R. A. 1977. Subpopulations of human T lymphocytes. II. Effect of thymopoietin, corticosteroids and irradiation. *Cell. Immunol.*, **34**, 10–18.

Gupta, S. and Tan, C. T. C. 1980. Subpopulations of human T lymphocytes XIV Abnormality of T cell locomotion and of distribution of subpopulations of T and B lymphocytes in peripheral blood and spleen from children with untreated Hodgkin's disease. *Clin. Immunol. Immunopathol.*, **15**, 133.

Gutman, G. A. and Weissman, I. L. 1972. Lymphoid tissue architecture. Experimental analysis of the origin and distribution of T cells and B cells. *Immunology*, **23**, 465.

Gutman, G. A. and Weissman, I. L. 1973. Homing properties of thymus-independent follicular lymphocytes. *Transplan.*, **16**, 621.

Guy-Grand, D., Griscelli, C. and Vassalli, P. 1974. The gut associated lymphoid system: nature and properties of the large dividing cells. *Europ. J. Immunol.*, **4**, 435.

Guy-Grand, D., Griscelli, C. and Vassalli, P. 1978. The mouse gut T lymphocyte, a novel type of T cell: nature, origin, and traffic in mice, in normal and gvh conditions. *J. Exp. Med.*, **148**, 1661–77.

Hadden, J. W., Johnson, E. M., Hadden, E. M., Goffey, R. G. and Johnson, L. D. 1975. Cyclic GMP and lymphocyte activation. In *Immune recognition*, ed. A. S. Rosenthal, Academic Press, New York, p. 359.

Hales, J. R. S. 1973. Radioactive microsphere measurement of cardiac output and regional tissue blood flow in the sheep. *Pfugers Anch. Eur. J. Physiol.*, **344**, 119.

Hall, J. G. 1967. Studies of the cells in the afferent and efferent lymph of lymph nodes draining the site of skin homografts. *J. Exp. Med.*, **125**, 737–54.

Hall, J. G. 1980. The effect of skin painting with oxazolone on the local extravasation of mononuclear cells in sheep. *Ciba Found. Symp.*, No. 71, pp. 197–209.
Hall, J. G., Hopkins, J. and Orlans, E. 1977. Studies on the lymphocytes of sheep. III. Destination of lymph-borne immunoblasts in relation to their tissue of origin. *Europ. J. Immunol.*, **7**, 30.
Hall, J. G. and Morris, B. 1962. The output of cells in lymph from the popliteal node of the sheep. *Quant. J. Exp. Physiol.*, **47**, 360.
Hall, J. G. and Morris, B. 1963. The lymph borne cells of the immune response. *Q.J. Exp. Physiol.*, **48**, 255.
Hall, J. G. and Morris, B. 1964. Effect of X-irradiation of the popliteal lymph node on its output of lymphocytes and immunological unresponsiveness. *Lancet*, **i**, 1077.
Hall, J. G. and Morris, B. 1965. The origin of the cells in the efferent lymph from a single lymph node. *J. Exp. Med.*, **121**, 901.
Hall, J. G., Morris, B., Moreno, G. D. and Bessis, M. C. 1967. The ultrastructure and function of the cell, in lymph following antigenic stimulation. *J. Exp. Med.*, **125**, 91.
Hall, J. G., Parry, D. M. and Smith, M. E. 1972. The distribution and differentiation of lymph borne immunoblasts after intravenous injection into syngeneic recipients. *Cell Tissue Kinet.*, **5**, 269.
Hall, J. G., Scollay, R. and Smith, M. 1976. Recirculation of lymphocytes through peripheral lymph nodes and tissues. *Eur. J. Immunol.*, **6**, 117.
Hall, J. G. and Smith, M. G. 1971. Studies on the afferent and efferent lymph of lymph nodes draining the site of fluorodinitrobenzene. *Immunology*, **21**, 69.
Halstead, T. E. and Hall, J. G. 1972. The homing of lymph-borne immunoblasts to the small gut of neonatal rats. *Transplantation*, **14**, 339.
Ham, A. W. 1979. *Histology*. J. B. Lippincott Company.
Hamilton, T. A., Wada, H. G. and Sussman, H. H. 1979. Identification of transferrin receptors on the surface of human cultured cells. *Proc. Natl. Acad. Sci.*, **76**, 6406–10.
Hamilton, M. E. and Winfield, J. B. 1979. T cells in systemic lupus erythematosus. Variation with disease cavity. *Arth. & Rheum.*, **22**, 1.
Hansen, J. A. and Good, R. A. 1974. Malignant disease of the lymphoid system in immunological perspective. *Hum. Pathology*, **5**, 568.
Hapel, A. and Gardner, I. 1974. Appearance of cytotoxic T cells in cerebrospinal fluid of mice with ectromelia virus-induced meningitis. *Scand. J. Immunol.*, **3**, 311.
Harris, A. K. 1976. Is cell sorting caused by differences in the work of intercellular adhesion? A critique of the Steinberg hypotheses. *J. Theor. Biol.*, **61**, 267–85.
Harris, H. 1961. Chemotaxis. *Exp. Cell. Res. Suppl.*, **8**, 199–208.
Harrison, P. M. 1977. Ferritin: An iron storage molecule. *Sem. Hematol.*, **14**, 55.
Hartman, E. R., Colasanti, B. K. and Craig, C. R. 1974. Epileptogenic properties of cobalt and related metals applied directly to cerebral cortex of rats. *Epilepsia*, **15**, 121–9.
Haston, W. S. 1979. A study of lymphocyte behavior in cultures of fibroblast-like lymphoreticular cells. *Cell. Immunol.*, **45**, 74.
Hay, I. B., Murphy, M. J., Morris, B. and Bessis, M. C. 1972. Quantitative studies on the proliferation and differentiation of antibody-forming cells in lymph. *Amer. J. Path.*, **66**, 1.
Hay, J. B., Cahill, R. S. and Trnka, Z. 1975. The kinetics of antigen reactive cells during lymphocyte recruitment. *Cell. Immunol.*, **10**, 145.
Hay, J. B. and Hobbs, B. B. 1977. The flow of blood to lymph nodes and its relation to lymphocyte traffic and the immune response. *J. Exp. Med.*, **145**, 31.
Hay, J. B., Hobbs, B. B., Johnston, M. G. and Movat, H. Z. 1977. The role of hyperemia in cellular hypersensitivity reactions. *Int. Arch. Allergy and Appl. Immunol.*, **55**, 324.
Hay, J. B., Lachman, P. J. and Trnka, Z. 1973. The appearance of migration inhibition factor and a mitogen in lymph draining tuberculin reactions. *Eur. J. Immunol.*, **3**, 127–31.

Head, J. R. 1977. Immunobiology of lactation. *Seminars in Perinatology*, **1**, 195.
Hemmaplardh, D. and Morgan, E. H. 1974. Transferrin and iron uptake by human cells in culture. *Exp. Cell. Res.*, **87**, 207.
Hendriks, H. R. 1978. Occlusion of the lymph flow to rat popliteal lymph nodes for protracted periods. *Z. Versuchstierk Bd. Z.*, **5**, 105.
Herman, P. G., Utsunomiya, R. and Hessel, S. J. 1979. Arteriovenous shunting in the lymph node before and after antigenic stimulus. *Immunology*, **36**, 793.
Herman, P. G., Yamamoto, I. and Mellins, H. Z. 1972. Blood micro-circulation in the lymph node during the primary immune response. *J. Exp. Med.*, **136**, 697.
Hersey, P. 1971. The separation and ^{51}Chromium labeling of human lymphocytes with *in vivo* studies of survival and migration. *Blood*, **38**, 360.
Hewitt, H. B. 1979. A critical examination of the foundations of immunotherapy for cancer. *Clin. Radiol.*, **30**, 361.
Heyman, M. A., Payne, B. D., Hoffman, J. I. E. and Rudolph, H. M. 1977. Blood flow measurements with radionuclide labelled particles. *Prog. Cardiovasc. Dis.*, **20**, 55.
Hill, W. C. 1969. The influence of the cellular infiltrate on the evolution and intensity of delayed hypersensitivity reactions. *J. Exp. Med.*, **129**, 363.
Hirano, A. and Kochen, J. A. 1975. Some effects of intracerebral lead implantation in the rat. *Acta. Neuropath.*, **33**, 307–15.
Hiyeda, K. 1939. The cause of Kaschin-Beck's disease. *Jap. J. Med. Sci.*, **4**, 91–106.
Hoefsmit, E. C. M., Balfour, B. M., Kamperdigk, E. W. A. and Cvetano, J. 1979. Cells containing Birbeck granules in the lymph and the lymph node. *Adv. Exp. Med. Biol.*, **114**, 389.
Hoffbrand, A. V., Ganeshaguru, K., Hooton, J. W. L. and Tattersall, M. H. N. 1976. Effect of iron deficiency and desferrioxamine on DNA synthesis in human cells. *Brit. J. Haematol.*, **33**, 517.
Hoover, R. L. 1978. Modulations of the cell surface and the effects on cellular interactions. *Symp. Soc. Exp. Biol.*, **32**, 221–40.
Hopkins, J. and Hall, J. G. 1976. Selective entry of immunoblasts in gut from intestinal lymph. *Nature*, **259**, 308.
Horder, T. J. and Martin, K. A. 1978. Morphogenetics as an alternative to chemospecificity in the formation of nerve connections. *Symp. Soc. Exp. Biol.*, **32**, 275.
Howard, J. C. 1972. The life-span and recirculation of marrow derived small lymphocytes from the rat thoracic duct. *J. Exp. Med.*, **135**, 185.
Howard, J. C., Hunt, S. V. and Gowans, J. L. 1972. Identification of marrow-derived and thymus-derived small lymphocytes in the lymphoid tissue and thoracic duct lymph of normal rats. *J. Exp. Med.*, **135**, 200.
Howard, J. C. and Wilson, B. K. 1974. Specific positive selection of lymphocytes reactive to strong histocompatibility antigens. *J. Exp. Med.*, **140**, 660.
Humphrey, J. H. 1964. The fate of antigen and its relationship to the immune response. The complexity of antigens. *Antibiotica et Chemoterapia*, **15**, 7.
Humphrey, J. H. 1980. Macrophages and differential migration of lymphocytes. *Ciba Found. Symp.*, **71**, 287. Excerpta Medica, Elsevier, North Holland, Amsterdam.
Humphrey, J. C., Parrott, D. M. V. and East, J. 1964. Studies on globulin and antibody production in mice thymectomized at birth. *Immunology*, **7**, 419.
Hunninghake, G. W. and Fauci, A. S. 1976. Immunological reactivity of the lung. II. Cytotoxic effector functions of pulmonary mononuclear cell subpopulations. *Cell. Immunol.*, **26**, 98–104.
Hunt, J., Richards, R. J., Worwood, R. and Jacobs, A. 1979. The effect of desferrioxamine on fibroblasts and collagen formation in cell cultures. *British Journal of Haematology*, **41**, 69.
Husband, A. J., Beh, K. J. and Lascelles, A. K. 1979. IgA containing cells in the ruminant intestine following intraperitoneal and local immunization. *Immunology*, **37**, 597–601.

Husband, A. J. and Gowans, J. L. 1978. The origin and antigen-dependent distribution of IgA containing cells in the intestine. *J. Exp. Med.*, **148**, 1146–60.
Husband, A. J., Monie, H. J. and Gowans, J. L. 1977. The natural history of the cells producing IgA in the gut. *Ciba Found. Symp.*, **46**, 29.
Husby, G., Hoagland, P. M., Strickland, R. G. and Williams, R. C., 1976. Tissue T and B cell infiltration of Primary and Metastatic Cancer. *J. Clin. Inv.*, **57**, 1471.
Husby, G., Strickland, R. G., Caldwell, J. L. and Williams, R. C. 1975. Localization of T and B cells and alpha fetoprotein in hepatic biopsies from patients with liver disease. *J. Clin. Invest.*, **56**, 1198–209.
Inchley, C. J., Micklem, H. S., Barrett, J., Hunter, J. and Minty, C. 1976. Age related changes in localization of injected radio-labelled lymphocytes in the lymph nodes of antigen stimulated mice. *Clin. Exp. Immunol.*, **26**, 286.
Jacobson, L. O., Simmons, E. L., Marks, E. O., Gaston, B. S., Robson, M. J. and Eldredge, B. S. 1951. Further studies on recovery from radiation injury. *J. Lab. and Clin. Med.*, **37**, 683.
Jansen, C. R., Cronkite, E. P., Mather, G. C., Nielsen, N. O., Rai, K., Adamik, E. R. and Sipi, C. R. 1962. Studies on lymphocytes. II. The production of lymphocytosis by intravenous heparin in calves. *Blood*, **20**, 443.
Joel, D. D., Hess, M. W. and Cottier, H. 1972. Magnitude and pattern of thymic lymphocyte migration in neonatal mice. *J. Exp. Med.*, **135**, 907.
Johansson, B. G. 1960. Isolation of an iron-containing red protein from human milk. *Acta Chem. Scand.*, **14**, 510.
Johnson, R. L. and Ziff, M. 1976. Lymphokine stimulation of collagen accumulation. *J. Clin. Invest.*, **56**, 240.
Johnson, S. 1759. *The History of Rasselas, Prince of Abyssinia*. The Folio Society, London, 1975, p. 79.
Jolles, J., Mazurier, J., Boutigue, M. H., Spik, G., Montreiul, J. and Jolles, P. 1976. The N-terminal sequence of human lactotransferrin: its close homology with the amino terminal regions of other transferrins. *FEBS Lett.*, **69**, 27.
Jondal, M., Holm, G. and Wigzell, H. 1972. Surface markers on human T and B lymphocytes. I. A large population of lymphocytes forming non-immune rosettes with sheep red blood cells. *J. Exp. Med.*, **136**, 207.
Jondal, M. and Klein, G. 1975. Classification of lymphocytes in nasopharyngeal carcinoma (NPC) biopsies. *Biomedicine*, **23**, 163.
Jones, G. E. 1977. Cell disposition and adhesiveness in the developing chick neural retina. *J. Embryol. Exp. Morph.*, **40**, 253.
Jones, J. V., Housley, J., Ashurst, P. M. and Hawkins, C. F. 1969. Development of delayed hypersensitivity to dinitrochlorobenzene in patients with Chron's disease. *Gut*, **10**, 52.
Jordon, R. E., Deheer, D., Schroeter, H. and Winkelmann, R. K. 1971. Antinuclear antibodies: their significance in scleroderma. *Mayo Clin. Proc.*, **46**, 111.
Joyner, M. V., Patrice-Cassuto, J., Dujardin, P., Barety, M., Duplay, H. and Audoly, P. 1979. Cutaneous T-cell lymphoma in association with a monoclonal gammopathy. *Arch. Dermatol.*, **115**, 326.
Jungi, T. W. and McGregor, D. D. 1978. Activated lymphocytes trigger lymphoblast extravasation. *Cell. Immunol.*, **38**, 78–83.
Jungi, T. W. and McGregor, D. D. 1979. Role of complement in the expression of delayed-type hypersensitivity in rats. Studies with cobra venom factor. *Infection and Immunity*, **23**, 633–43.
Kabat, E. A., Freedman, D. A., Murray, J. P. and Knaub, V. 1950. A study of the chrystalline albumin, gammaglobulin and total protein in the cerebrospinal fluid of 100 cases of multiple sclerosis and in other diseases. *Amer. J. Med. Sci.*, **219**, 55.
Kam-Hansen, S. 1979. Reduced number of active T cells in cerebrospinal fluid in multiple sclerosis. *Neurology*, **29**, 897.

Kam-Hansen, S., Frydén, A. and Link, H. 1978. B and T lymphocytes in cerebrospinal fluid and blood in multiple sclerosis, optic neuritis and mumps meningitis. *Acta Neurol. Scand.*, **58**, 95.
Kapadia, A., de Sousa, M., Markenson, A. L., Miller, D. R., Good, R. A. and Gupta, S. 1980. Lymphoid cell sets and serum immunoglobulins in patients with thalassemia intermedia: relationship to serum iron and splenectomy. *Brit. J. Haematol.*, **45**, 405.
Kaplan, H. S. 1976. Hodgkin's disease and other human malignant lymphomas: advances & prospects. *Cancer Res.*, **36**, 3863.
Kaur, J., Catovsky, D., Spiers, A. S. D. and Galton, D. A. G. 1974. Increase of T lymphocytes in the spleen of Hodgkin's disease. *Lancet*, **1**, 834.
Kelly, R. H., Balfour, B. M., Armstrong, J. A. and Griffiths, S. 1978. Functional anatomy of lymph nodes: peripheral lymph borne mononuclear cells. *Anat. Rec.*, **190**, 5.
Kelly, R. H., Wolstencroft, R., Dumonde, D. and Balfour, B. H. 1972. Role of lymphocyte activation products (LAP) in cell-mediated immunity. *Clin. Exp. Immunol.*, **10**, 49–65.
Keren, D. F., Holt, P. S., Collins, H. H., Gemski, P. and Formal, S. B. 1978. The role of Peyer's patches in the local immune response of rabbit ileum to live bacteria. *J. Immunol.*, **120**, 1892–6.
Klein, G. and Klein, G. 1977. Rejectability of virus-induced tumours and non-rejectability of spontaneous tumors – a lesson in contrasts. *Transpl. Proc.*, **9**, 1095.
Knisley, M. H. 1936. Spleen studies. I. Microscopic observations of circulation system of living unstimulated mammalian spleens. *Anat. Rec.*, **65**, 25.
Kobayashi, Y., Okahata, B., Sakano, T., Tanake, K. and Usui, T. 1979. Superoxide dismutase activity of T lymphocytes and non-T lymphocytes. *FEBS Lett.*, **98**, 391.
Kochan, I. 1977. Role of siderophores in nutritional immunity and bacterial parasitism, pp. 251–89. In E. D. Weinberg (ed.) *Microorganisms and Minerals*. M. Dekker, Inc., New York.
Koike, T., Kobayashi, S., Yoshiki, T., Itoh, T. and Shirai, T. 1979. Differential sensitivity of functional subsets of T cells to the cytotoxicity of natural T-lymphocytotoxic autoantibody of systemic lupus erythematosus. *Arthr. Rheum.*, **22**, 123.
Kolb, H. and Kolb-Bachofen, V. 1978. A lectin-like receptor on mammalian macrophages. *Biochem. Biophys. Res. Commun.*, **85**, 678.
Kolb, H., Schudt, C., Kolb-Bachofen, V. and Kolb, H. A. 1978. Cellular recognition by rat liver cells of neuraminidase-treated erythrocytes. *Exp. Cell. Res.*, **113**, 319.
Kolb, H., Kriese, A., Kolb-Bachofen, V. and Kolb, H. A. 1978. Possible mechanism of entrapment of neuraminidase treated lymphocytes in the liver. *Cell. Immunol.*, **40**, 457.
Kolb, H., Schudt, C., Kolf-Bachofen, V. and Kolb, H. A. 1978. Cellular recognition by rat liver cells of neuraminidase treated erythrocytes. *Exp. Cell Res.*, **113**, 319.
Kolb-Bachofen, V. and Kolb, H. 1979. Autoimmune reactions against liver cells by syngeneic neuraminidase treated lymphocytes. *J. Immunol.*, **123**, 2830.
Kondo, H., Rabin, B. S. and Rodnan, G. P. 1976. Cutaneous antigen stimulating lymphokine production by lymphocytes of patients with progressive systemic sclerosis (scleroderma). *J. Clin. Invest.*, **58**, 1388.
Kopriwa, B. M. and Leblond, C. P. 1962. Improvements in the coating technique of radioautography. *J. Histochem. Cytochem.*, **10**, 269.
Kornfeld, R. and Kornfeld, S. 1974. Structure of membrane receptors for plant lectins. *Ann. N.Y. Acad. Sci.*, **234**, 276.
Kornfeld, S. and Kornfeld, R. 1971. Cell surface receptors: structure and function. *Prog. Hematol.*, **7**, 161.
Kruyt, H. R. 1952. Irreversible systems. In *Colloid Science*, ed. H. R. Kruyt. Elsevier, Amsterdam, pp. xx and 389.
Kuttner, B. and Woodruff, J. 1979. Selective adherence of lymphocytes to myelinated areas of rat brain. *J. Immunol.*, **122**, 1666–71.

Laissue, J. A., Chanana, A. D., Cottier, H., Cronkite, E. P. and Joel, D. D. 1976. The fate of thymic radioactivity after local labelling with ^{125}Iododeoxyuridine. *Blood*, **47**, 21.
Lampert, I. A., Pizzolo, G., Thomas, A. and Janossy, G. 1979. Immunohistochemical characterization of cells involved in dermatopathic lymphadenopathy. *J. Pathol.* (in press), quoted in Humphrey, 1980.
Langhof, H. and Muller, H. 1966. Leukotaktische Eigenschaften von psoriasschuppen. *Hautartz*, **17**, 101.
Larner, B. J. 1973. Redistribution of mixed lymphocyte culture-reactive cells after antigen administration. *Transplantation*, **16**, 134.
Larrick, J. W. and Cresswell, P. 1979. Transferrin receptors on human B and T lymphoblastoid cell lines. *Biochem. Biophys. Acta*, **583**, 483.
Lavender, J. P., Goldman, J. M., Arnot, R. N. and Thakur, M. L. 1977. Kinetics of indium-111 labelled lymphocytes in normal subjects and patients with Hodgkin's disease. *Brit. Med. J.*, **2**, 797.
Lavoie, D. J., Ishikawa, K. and Listowsky, I. 1978. Correlations between subunit distribution, microheterogeneity, and Iron content of human liver ferritin. *Biochemistry*, **17**, 5448.
Lazarus, G. S., Yost, F. J. and Thomas, C. A. 1977. Polymorphonuclear leukocytes. Possible mechanisms of accumulation in psoriasis. *Science*, **198**, 1162.
Lehman, H. E. and Youngs, L. M. 1959. Extrinsic and intrinsic factors influencing amphibian pigment pattern formation. In *Pigment Cell Biology*, ed. M. Gordon. Academic Press, New York, pp. 1–36.
Lemaitre-Coelho, I., Jackson, G. D. F. and Veerman, J. P. 1978. High levels of secretory IgA and free secretory component in the serum of rats with bile duct obstruction. *J. Exp. Med.*, **147**, 934–9.
Lennert, K., Kaiserling, E. and Muller-Hermelink, H. K. 1978. Malignant lymphomas: Models of differentiation and co-operation of lymphoreticular cells. In *Differentiation of Hormonal and Neoplastic Hematopoietic Cells*. Cold Spring Harbor Symposium, p. 897.
Levine, S. and Sowinski, R. 1978. Lymphocytic inflammation produced by intracerebral implantation of zinc and other metals. *J. Neuropath. Exp. Neurol.*, **37**, 471–8.
Lindsley, D. L., Odell, T. T. and Lausche, F. G. 1955. Implantation of functional erythropoietic elements following total body irradiation. *Proc. Soc. Exp. Biol. and Med.*, **90**, 512.
Link, H., 1967. Immunoglobulin and low molecular weight proteins in human cerebrospinal fluid. Chemical and immunological characterization with special reference to multiple sclerosis. *Acta. Neurol. Scand.*, **43** (Suppl. 28), 1.
Link, H. 1972. Oligoclonal Immunoglobulin G in multiple sclerosis brains. *J. Neurol. Sci.*, **16**, 103.
Lis, H. and Sharon, N. 1973. The biochemistry of plant lectins (phytohemagglutinins). *Ann. Rev. Biochem.*, **42**, 541.
Lomnitzer, R., Rabson, A. R. and Koornhof, H. J. 1976. Leucocyte capillary migration: an adherence dependent phenomenon. *Clinical and Experimental Immunol.*, **25**, 303–10.
Lonnerdal, B. Forsum, E., Gebra-Medhin, M. and Hambraues, L. 1976. Breast milk composition in Ethiopian and Swedish mothers. II. Lactose nitrogen and protein contents. *Am. J. Clin. Nut.*, **29**, 1134–41.
Lorenz, E., Uphoff, D., Reed, T. R. and Shelton, E. 1951. Modification of irradiation injury in mice and guinea pigs by bone marrow injections. *J. Nat. Cancer Inst.*, **12**, 197.
Love, R. J. and Ogilvie, B. M. 1977. *Nippostrongylus brasiliensis* and *Trichinella spiralis*: localization of lymphoblasts in the small intestine of parasitized rats. *Exp. Parisitol.*, **41**, 124.

Lutzner, M., Edelson, R., Schein, P., Green, I. Kirkpatrick, C. and Ahmed, A. 1975. Cutaneous T cell lymphomas: The Sézary syndrome, mycosis fungoides and related disorders. *Ann. Int. Med.*, **83**, 534.

MacDonald, T. T. and Ferguson, A. 1978. Small intestinal epithelial cell kinetics and protozoal infection in mice. *Gastroenterology*, **74**, 496.

MacGillivray, R. T. A., Mendez, E. and Brew, K. 1977. *Structure and Evolution of Serum Transferrin in Proteins of Iron Metabolism*, ed. E. B. Brown, P. Aisen, J. Fielding and R. R. Crichton. Grune and Stratton, New York, pp. 133–41.

MacKie, R., Sless, F. R., Cochran, R. and de Sousa, M. 1976. Lymphocyte abnormalities in mycosis fungoides. *Brit. J. Dermatol.*, **94**, 173.

MacNeal, W. J. 1929. Circulation of blood through spleen pulp. *Arch. Path.*, **7**, 215.

MacPherson, G. G. and Steer, H. W. 1979. Properties of phagocytes derived from the small intestine wall of rats. *Adv. Exp. Med. Biol.*, **114**, 433–38.

Main, J. M. and Prehn, R. 1955. Successful skin homografts after the administration of high dosage X radiation and homologous bone marrow. *J. Nat. Cancer Inst.*, **15**, 1023.

Makëla, O. and Michison, N. A. 1965. The role of cell number and source of adoptive immunity. *Immunology*, **8**, 539.

Malpighi, M. 1686. *Marcelli Malpighi opera Omnia*. Londini.

Manconi, P. E., Fadden, M. F., Cadoni, A., Cornaglia, P., Zacches, D. and Grifoni, V. 1978. Subpopulations of T lymphocytes in human extravascular fluids. *Int. Arch. Allergy Appl. Immunol.*, **56**, 385.

Mann, J. D. and Higgins, G. M. 1950. Lymphocytes in thoracic duct, intestinal and hepatic lymph. *Blood*, **5**, 177.

Manson-Smith, D., Bruce, R. G. and Parrott, D. M. V. 1979. Villous atrophy and expulsion of intestinal Trichinella Spiralis are mediated by T cells. *Cell Immunol.*, **47**, 285.

Manson-Smith, D. F., Bruce, R. G., Rose, M. L. and Parrott, D. M. V. 1979. Migration of lymphoblasts to the small intestine III. Strain differences and relationships to distribution and duration of trichinella spiralis infection. *Clin. Exp. Immunol.*, **38**, 475.

Marchase, R. B. 1977. Biochemical investigations of retinotectal adhesive specificity. *J. Cell. Biol.*, **75**, 237–57.

Marchesi, V. T. and Gowans, J. L. 1964. The migration of lymphocytes through the endothelium of venules in lymph nodes: an electron microscope study. *Proc. Roy. Soc.*, Series B, **159**, 283.

Marples, R. R., Heaton, C. L. and Kligman, A. M. 1973. Staphylococcus aureus in psoriasis. *Arch. Dermatol.*, **107**, 568.

Marsh, M. D. 1975a. Studies of intestinal lymphoid tissue. I. Electron microscopic evidence of 'blast transformation' in epithelial lymphocytes of mouse small intestinal mucosa. *Gut*, **16**, 665.

Marsh, M. D. 1975b. Studies of intestinal lymphoid tissue. II. Aspects of proliferation and migration of epithelial lymphocytes in the small intestine of mice. *Gut*, **16**, 674.

Martin, W. J. 1969. Assay for the immunosuppressive capacity of antilymphocyte serum. I. Evidence for opsonization. *J. Immunol.*, **103**, 974.

Martineau, R. S. and Johnson, J. S. 1978. Normal mouse serum immunosuppressive activity: Action on adherent cells. *J. Immunol.*, **120**, 1550–3.

Masawe, A. C., Muindi, J. M. and Swai, G. B. R. 1974. Infections in iron deficiency and other types of anemia in the tropics. *Lancet*, **ii**, 314.

Masson, P. L. and Heremans, J. F. 1968. Metal combining properties of human lactoferrin (red milk protein) I. The involvement of bicarbonate in the reaction. *Eur. J. Biochem.*, **6**, 579.

Masson, P. L., Heremans, J. F. and Schonne, E. 1969. Lactoferrin, and iron-binding protein in neutrophilic leukocytes. *Journal of Experimental Medicine*, **130**, 643.

Matchett, K. M., Huang, A. T. and Kremer, W. B. 1973. Impaired lymphocyte transformation in Hodgkin's disease. *J. Clin. Invest.*, **52**, 1908.

Mattioli, C. A. and Tomasi, T. B. 1973. The life span of IgA plasma cells from the mouse intestine. *J. Exp. Med.*, **138**, 452.
McClay, D. R. 1971. An autoradiographic analysis of species specificity during sponge cell reaggregation. *Biol. Bull.*, **141**, 319–30.
McClay, D. R. and Gooding, L. R. 1978. Involvement of histocompatibility antigens in embryonic cell recognition events. *Nature*, **274**, 367–8.
McClay, D. R. and Hausman, R. C. 1975. Specificity of cell adhesion: differences between normal and hybrid sea urchin cells. *Dev. Biol.*, **47**, 454–60.
McClelland, D. B., McGrath, J. and Samson, R. R. 1978. Antimicrobial factors in human milk. *Acta. Scand. Suppl.* 271, Edinburgh.
McCord, J. M. and Fridovich, I. 1969. Superoxide dismutase. An enzymatic function for erythrocuprein (hemocuprein). *J. Biol. Chem.*, **244**, 6049.
McFarland, W., Heilman, D. H. and Moorhead, J. F. 1966. Functional anatomy of the lymphocytes in immunologic reactions *in vitro*. *J. Exp. Med.*, **124**, 851.
McFarlin, D. E. and Binns, R. M. 1973. Lymph node function and lymphocyte circulation in the pig. In *Microenvironmental Aspects of Immunity*, 4th Int. Conf. on Lymph Tissue and Germinal Centers in Immune Reactions, ed. B. D. Jancokvic and K. Isakovic, p. 87.
McGregor, D. D. and Gowans, J. L. 1963. The antibody response of rats depleted of lymphocytes by chronic drainage from the thoracic duct. *J. Exp. Med.*, **117**, 303.
McGregor, D. D. and Logie, P. S. 1974. The mediator of cellular immunity. VII. Localization of sensitized lymphocytes in inflammatory exudates. *J. Exp. Med.*, **139**, 1415.
McGregor, D. D., McCullagh, P. J. and Gowans, J. L. 1967. The role of lymphocytes in antibody formation. I. Restoration of the haemolysin response in x-irradiated rats with lymphocytes from normal and immunologically tolerant donors. *Proc. Roy. Soc.*, **168**, 229.
McGuire, E. J. and Burdick, C. L. 1976. Intercellular adhesive selectivity. I. An improved assay for the measurement of embryonic chick intercellular adhesion (liver and other tissues). *J. Cell. Biol.*, **68**, 80–9.
McKenzie, D. W., Jr., Whipple, A. O. and Wintersteiner, M. P. 1951. Studies on microscopic anatomy and physiology of living transilluminated mammalian spleens. *Am. J. Anat.*, **68**, 397.
McWilliams, M., Phillips-Quagliata, J. M. and Lamm, M. E. 1975. Characteristics of mesenteric lymph node cells homing to gut-associated lymphoid tissue in syngeneic mice. *J. Immunol.*, **115**, 54.
Meader, R. D. and Landers, D. F. 1967. Electron and light microscopic observations on relationships between lymphocytes and intestinal epithelium. *Am. J. Anat.*, **121**, 763–74.
Mehrishi, J. 1973. Molecular aspects of the mammalian cell surface. *Prog. Biophys. Mol. Biol.*, **25**, 1.
Merritt, J. A., Coco, F. V. and Desforges, J. F. 1969. Blood and organ studies of circulating lymphocytes in humans with normal leucocyte counts. *Am. J. Med. Sci.*, **258**, 237.
Mestecky, J., McGhee, J. R., Arnold, R. R., Michalek, S. M., Prince, S. J. and Babb, J. L. 1978. Selective induction of an immune response in human external secretions by ingestion of bacterial antigen. *J. Clin. Invest.*, **61**, 731–7.
Meuwissen, S. G. M., Feltkamp-Vroom, T. M., Brutel de La Riviere. A., Von Dem Borne, A. E. G. Kr. and Tytgat, G. N. 1976. Analysis of the lympho-plasmacytic infiltrate in Chron's disease with special reference to identification of lymphocyte subpopulations. *Gut*, **17**, 770.
Meyer, D. B. 1964. The migration of primordial germ cells in the chick embryo. *Develop. Biol.*, **10**, 154–90.
Micklem, H. S., Ford, C. E., Evans, E. P. and Gray, J. 1966. Interrelationships of myeloid

and lymphoid cells: studies with chromosome-marked cells transfused into lethally irradiated mice. *Proc. Roy. Soc. Lond.* (B), **165**, 78.

Middleton, A. A. 1973. The control of epithelial cell locomotion in tissue culture. In *Locomotion of Tissue Cells*. Ciba Found. Symp., 14 (new ser.). Elsevier, Amsterdam, pp. 250–70.

Mikata, A. and Niki, R. 1971. Permeability of postcapillary venules of the lymph nodes. An electron microscopic study. *Exp. Mol. Pathol.*, **14**, 209.

Mikata, A., Niki, R. and Watanabe, S. 1968. Reticuloendothelial system of the lymph node parenchyma, with special reference to post-capillary venules and granuloma formation. *Rec. Advances, R.E.S. Res.*, **8**, 143.

Miller, H. R. P. 1971. Immune reactions in mucous membranes. II. The differentiation of intestinal mast cells during helminth expulsion in the rat. *Lab. Invest.*, **24**, 339–47.

Miller, H. R. P. and Adams, E. P. 1977. Reassortment of lymphocytes in lymph from normal and allografted sheep. *Amer. J. Path.*, **87**, 59–80.

Milne, R. W., Bienenstock, J. and Perey, D. Y. E. 1975. The influence of antigenic stimulation on the ontogeny of lymphoid aggregates and immunoglobulin-containing cells in mouse bronchial and intestinal mucosa. *J. Reticuloendothel. Soc.*, **17**, 361–9.

Mitchell, J. 1972. Antigens in immunity. XVII. The migration of antigen-binding, bone marrow-derived and thymus derived spleen cells in mice. *Immunol.*, **22**, 231.

Montgomery, P. C., Connelly, K. M. and Skandera, C. A. 1978. Remote-site stimulation of secretory IgA antibodies following bronchial and gastric stimulation; in secretory immunity and infection. *Adv. Exp. Med. Biol.* Plenum, New York, pp. 113–22.

Montgomery, P. C., Khaled, S. A., Goudswaard, J. and Virella, G. 1977. Selective transport of an oligomenic IgA into canine saliva. *Immunol. Comm.*, **6**, 633.

Moore, A. R. and Hall, J. 1972. Evidence for a primary association between immunoblasts and the small gut. *Nature (Lond.)*, **239**, 161.

Moore, A. R. and Hall, J. G. 1973. Nonspecific entry of thoracic duct immunoblasts into intradermal foci of antigen. *Cell. Immunol.*, **8**, 112.

Moore, M. R. and Goldberg, A. 1974. Normal and abnormal haem biosynthesis. In *Iron in Biochemistry and Medicine*, ed. A. Jacobs and M. Worwood. Academic Press, New York, p. 115.

Morell, A. G., Gregoriadis, G., Scheinberg, I. H., Mickman, J. and Ashwell, G. 1971. The role of sialic acid in determining the survival of glycoproteins in the circulation. *J. Biol. Chem.*, **246**, 1461.

Moretta, L., Ferrarini, M., Mingari, M. C., Moretta, A. and Webb, S. R. 1976. Subpopulations of human T cells identified by receptors for immunoglobulins and mitogen responsiveness. *J. Immunol.*, **117**, 2171.

Moretta, L., Webb, S. R., Grossi, C. E., Ludyard, P. M. and Cooper, M. D. 1977. Functional analysis of two human T cell subpopulations: help and suppression of B cell responses by T cells bearing receptors for IgM or IgG. *J. Exp. Med.*, **146**, 184.

Morgan, E. H. 1974. Transferrin and transferrin iron. In *Iron in Biochemistry and Medicine*, ed. A. Jacobs and M. Worwood. Academic Press, New York, pp. 29–71.

Moroz, C., Lahat, N., Biniaminov, M. and Ramot, B. 1977. Ferritin on the surface of lymphocytes in Hodgkin's disease patients. *Clin. Exp. Immunol.*, **29**, 30.

Morris, B. and Sass, M. D. 1966. The formation of lymph in the ovary. *Proc. Roy. Soc. B.*, **164**, 577.

Morse, S. I. 1964. Studies on the lymphocytosis induced in mice by Bordetella pertussis. *J. Exp. Med.*, **121**, 49.

Morse, S. I. and Barron, B. A. 1970. Studies on the leukocytosis and lymphocytosis induced by Bordetella pertussis. III. The distribution of transfused lymphocytes in pertussis treated and normal mice. *J. Exp. Med.*, **132**, 663.

Morse, S. I. and Bray, K. K. 1969. The occurrence and properties of leukocytosis and lymphocytosis stimulating material in the supernatant fluids of Bordetella pertussis cultures. *J. Exp. Med.*, **129**, 523.

Morse, S. I. and Riester, S. K. 1967a. Studies on the leukocytosis and lymphocytosis induced by Bordetella pertussis. I. Radioautographic analysis of the circulating cells in mice undergoing pertussis-induced hyperleukocytosis. *J. Exp. Med.*, **125**, 401.
Morse, S. I. and Riester, S. K. 1967b. Studies on the leukocytosis and lymphocytosis induced by Bordetella pertussis. II. The effect of pertussis vaccine on the thoracic duct lymph and lymphocytes of mice. *J. Exp. Med.*, **125**, 619.
Moscona, A. A. 1962. Analysis of cell recombinations in experimental synthesis of tissues in vitro. *J. Cell. & Comp. Physiol.*, Suppl. 1, **60**, 65–80.
Mowatt, A. M. 1975. The intraepithelial lymphocyte – its nature and function. Project report for BSc, Glasgow University.
Muirden, K. D. 1970. Lymph node iron in rheumatoid arthritis. *Ann. Rheum. Dis.*, **29**, 81–8.
Muirden, K. D. and Senator, G. B. 1968. Iron in the synovial membrane in rheumatoid arthritis and other joint diseases. *Ann. Rheum. Dis.*, **27**, 38–48.
Müller-Hermelink, H. K. 1974. Characterization of the B cell and T cell regions of human lymphatic tissue through enzyme histochemical demonstration of ATPase or 5'-nucleotidase activities. *Virchows Arch. B Cell Pathol.*, **16**, 371.
Müller-Hermelink, H. K., Heusermann, U., Kaiserling, E. and Stutte, H. J. 1976. Human lymphatic microecology specificity, characterization and ontogeny of different reticulum cells in the B cell and T cell regions. In *Immune Reactivity of Lymphocytes. Adv. Exp. Biol. Med.*, **66**, 177. Plenum Press, New York, London.
Munn, G., Markenson, A. J., Kapadia, A. and de Sousa, M. 1980. Mitogen responses in patients with thalassemia intermedia. *The Thymus* (submitted).
Munro, H. N. and Linder, M. C. 1978. Ferritin: structure, biosynthesis and role in iron metabolism. *Phys. Rev.*, **58**, 317–96.
Murray, M. J., Murray, A. B., Murray, M. B. and Murray, C. J. 1978. The adverse effect of iron repletion on the course of certain infections. *Brit. Med. Journal*, **2**, 1113–15.
Naor, D. 1979. Suppressor cells: permitters and promoters of malignancy. *Adv. Cancer Res.*, **29**, 45.
Navaratnam, V. 1975. *The Human Heart and Circulation*. Academic Press, New York.
Neilands, J. B. 1974. Iron and its role in microbial physiology. In *Microbial Iron Metabolism*, ed. J. B. Neilands. Academic Press, New York, p. 4.
Newby, T. J. and Bourne, F. J. 1976. Nature of the local immune system in bovine small intestine. *Immunol.*, **31**, 475.
Niewenhuis, P. 1971. On the origin and fate of immunologically competent cells. Doctoral thesis, Groningen University, Groningen, Germany.
Niewenhuis, P. and Ford, W. L. 1976. Comparative migration of B and T lymphocytes in the rat spleen and lymph nodes. *Cell. Immunol.*, **23**, 254.
Nishiya, K., Chiao, J. W. and de Sousa, M. 1980. Iron-binding proteins in selected human peripheral blood cell sets: Immunofluorescence. *Brit. J. Haematol.*, **46**, (in press).
Noden, D. M. 1978. Interactions directing the migration and cytodifferentiation of avian neural crest cells. In *Receptors and Recognition*, Ser. B, vol. 4, *Specificity of Embryological Interactions*, ed. D. R. Garrod, Chapman and Hall, London, pp. 3–50.
Nordqvist, B. C. and Kinney, J. P. 1976. T and B cells and cell-mediated immunity in mycosis fungoides. *Cancer*, **37**, 714–18.
Novak, R., Boszd, Z., Matkovics, B. and Fachet, J. 1980. Gene affecting superoxide dismutase activity linked to the histocompatibility complex in H-2 congenic mice. *Science*, **207**, 86.
Novogrodsky, A. and Ashwell, G. 1977. Lymphocyte mitogenesis induced by a mammalian liver protein that specifically binds desialylated glycoproteins. *Proc. Natl. Acad. Sci.*, **74**, 676.
Novogrodsky, A. and Katchalski, E. 1971. Induction of lymphocyte transformation by periodate. *FEBS Lett.*, **12**, 297.

Nyman, K., Bangert, R., Machleder, H. and Paulus, H. E. 1977. Thoracic duct drainage in SLE with cutaneous vasculitis. A case report. *Arth. Rheum.*, **20**, 1129–34.

Ogra, P. L., 1971. Effect of tonsillectomy and adenoidectomy on nasopharyngeal antibody response to polio virus. *N. Eng. J. Med.*, **284**, 59–64.

Ogra, S. S. and Ogra, P. L. 1978. Immunologic aspects of human colostrum and milk. II. *J. Pediatrics*, **92**, 550.

Okhuma, S., Noguchi, H., Amano, F., Mizuno, D. and Yasuda, T. 1976. Synthesis of apoferritin in mouse peritoneal macrophages. Characterization of 20S particles. *J. Biochem.*, **79**, 1365.

Old, L. J., Boyse, E. A. and Stockert, E. 1963. Antigenic properties of experimental leukemias. I. Serological studies *in vitro* with spontaneous and radiation induced leukemias. *J. Nat. Cancer Inst.*, **31**, 977.

Ormai, S., Hagenbeck, A., Palkovits, M. and van Bekkum, D. W. 1973. Changes of lymphocyte kinetics in the normal rat, induced by the lymphocyte mobilizing agent polymethacrylic acid. *Cell Tissue Kinet.*, **6**, 407.

O'Toole, C. M. and Davies, A. J. S. 1971. Pre-emption in immunity. *Nature*, **230**, 187.

Ottaway, C. A. and Parrott, D. M. V. 1979. Regional blood flow and its relationship to lymphocyte and lymphoblast traffic during a primary immune reaction. *J. Exp. Med.*, **150**, 218–30.

Ottaway, C., Rose, M. L. and Parrott, D. M. V. 1979. The gut as an immunological system. *Int. Rev. of Physiol. Gastrointestinal Physiology* III, Vol. 19, ed. R. K. Crane. University Park Press, Baltimore, p. 323.

Owen, R. L. 1977. Sequential uptake of horseradish peroxidase by lymphoid follicle epithelium of Peyer's patches in the normal unobstructed mouse intestine: an ultrastructural study. *Gastroenterology*, **72**, 440.

Owen, R. L. and Jones, A. L. 1974. Epithelial cell specialization within Peyer's patches: an ultrastructural study of intestinal lymphoid follicles. *Gastroenterology*, **66**, 189.

Owen, R. L. and Nemanic, P. 1978. Antigen processing of the mammalian intestinal tract: An SEM study of lymphoepithelial organs. *Scanning Electron Microscopy*, **II**, 367.

Owen, R. L., Nemanic, P. C. and Stevens, D. P. 1979. Ultrastructural observations on giardisis in a murine model. I. Intestinal distribution attachment and relationship to the immune system of Giardia muris. *Gastroenterology*, **76**, 757.

Pabst, R., Munz, D. and Trepel, F. 1977. Splenic lymphocytopoiesis and migration patterns of splenic lymphocytes. *Cell. Immunol.*, **33**, 44.

Pauluska, O. J. and Hamilton, L. H. 1963. Effect of heparin on leukocyte response to hydrocortisone injections. *Amer. J. Physiol.*, **204**, 1103.

Papamichail, M., Gutierrez, C., Embling, P., Johnson, P., Holborow, E. J. and Pepys, M. B. 1975. Complement dependence of localization of aggregated IgG in germinal centres. *Scand. J. Immunol.*, **4**, 343.

Parent, K., Barrett, J. and Wilson, I. D. 1971. Investigation of the pathogenic mechanisms in regional enteritis with *in vitro* lymphocyte cultures. *Gastroenterology*, **61**, 431.

Parker, J. W., O'Brien, R. L., Lukes, R. J. and Steiner, J. 1972. Transformation of human lymphocytes by sodium periodate. *Lancet*, **1**, 103.

Parkinson, E. K. and Edwards, J. G. 1978. Non-reciprocal contact inhibition of locomotion of chick embryonic choroid fibroblasts by pigmented retina epithelial cells. *J. Cell Sci.*, **33**, 103–20.

Parmely, J. J., Beer, A. E. and Billingham, R. E. 1976. *In vitro* studies on the T-lymphocyte population of human milk. *J. Exp. Med.*, **144**, 358–70.

Parmely, M. J. and Williams, S. B. 1979. The selective expression of immunocompetence in human colostrum: Preliminary evidence for the control of cytotoxic T lymphocytes including those specific for paternal alloantigens. In *Immunology of Breast Milk*, ed. P. L. Ogra and D. Dayton. Raven Press, New York.

Parrott, D. M. V. 1967. The response of draining lymph nodes to immunological stimulation in intact and thymectomized animals. *Symp. Tissue Org. Transplant. J. Clin. Pathol. Suppl.*, **20**, 456.
Parrott, D. M. V. 1976a. The gut as a lymphoid organ. *Clin. Gastroenterol.*, **5**, 211.
Parrott, D. M. V. 1976b. The gut-associated lymphoid tissues and gastrointestinal immunity. In A. Ferguson and R. N. M. McSween (eds.) *Immunological Aspects of the Liver and Gastrointestinal Tract*. University Park Press, Baltimore, p. 1.
Parrott, D. M. V. and de Sousa, M. A. B. 1967. The persistence of donor-derived cells in thymus grafts, lymph nodes and spleens of recipient mice. *Immunol.*, **13**, 193.
Parrott, D. M. V. and de Sousa, M. A. B. 1971. Thymus-dependent and thymus-independent populations: origin, migratory patterns and lifespan. *Clin. Exp. Immunol.*, **8**, 663.
Parrott, D. M. V. and de Sousa, M. A. B. 1974. B cell stimulation in nude (nunu) mice. In *Proceedings of the First International Workshop on Nude Mice*, ed. J. Rygaard and C. O. Povlsen. Stuttgart, Gustav Fischer, p. 61.
Parrott, D. M. V., de Sousa, M. A. B. and East, J. 1966. Thymus dependent areas in the lymphoid organs of neonatally thymectomized mice. *J. Exp. Med.*, **123**, 191.
Parrott, D. M. V. and East, J. 1964. Studies on a fatal wasting syndrome of mice thymectomized at birth in *The Thymus and Immunobiology*. Harper & Row, New York, p. 532.
Parrott, D. M. V. and Ferguson, A. 1974. Selective migration of lymphocytes within the mouse small intestine. *Immunol.*, **26**, 571.
Parrott, D. M. V. and Ottaway, C. A. 1980. The control of lymphoblast migration to the small intestine. In *Mucosal Immune System in Health and Disease*, The Eighty First Ross Conference on Pediatric Research, ed. P. L. Ogra and J. Bienenstock.
Parrott, D. M. V. and Rose, M. L. 1978. Migration pathways of T lymphocytes in the gut mucosa. In J. R. McGhee and J. Mestecky (eds.) *The Secretory Immune System and Caries Immunity*. Plenum, New York.
Parrott, D. M. V., Tilney, N. L. and Sless, F. 1975. The different migratory characteristics of lymphocyte populations from a whole spleen transplant. *Clin. Exp. Immunol.*, **19**, 459.
Parrott, D. M. V. and Wilkinson, P. C. 1981. Lymphocyte locomotion and migration. *Progress in Allergy* (in press).
Paulus, H. E., Machleder, H. I., Bangert, R., Stratton, J. A., Goldberg, L., Whitehouse, M. W., Yu, D. and Pearson, C. M. 1973. A case report: Thoracic duct lymphocyte drainage in rheumatoid arthritis. *Clin. Immunol. Immunopathol.*, **1**, 173.
Payan, H. M. 1967. Cerebral lesions produced in rats by various implants: epileptogenic effect of cobalt. *J. Neurosurg.*, **27**, 146, 152.
Payan, H. M. 1971. Morphology of cobalt experimental epilepsy in rats. *Exp. Molec. Pathol.*, **150**, 312–19.
Payne, S. V., Jones, D. B., Haegert, D. G., Smith, J. C. and Wright, D. H. 1976. T and B lymphocytes and Reed-Sternberg cells in Hodgkin's disease lymph nodes and spleens. *Clin. Exp. Immunol.*, **24**, 280.
Pearson, L. D., Simpson-Morgan, M. W. and Morris, B. 1976. Lymphopoiesis and lymphocyte circulation in the sheep fetus. *J. Exp. Med.*, **143**, 167.
Peck, H. N. and Hoerr, N. L. 1951. Intermediary circulation in red pulp of mouse spleen. *Anat. Rec.*, **109**, 447.
Pederson, N. C. and Morris, B. 1970. The role of the lymphatic system in the rejection of homografts: a study of lymph from renal transplants. *J. Exp. Med.*, **131**, 936–69.
Pepys, M. B. 1975. Studies *in vitro* of cobra factor and murine C3. *Immunology*, **28**, 369.
Petterson, T., Klockars, M., Hellstrom, P-E., Riska, H. and Wangel, A. 1978. T and B lymphocytes in pleural effusions. *Chest*, **73**, 49–51.
Phillips, H. M. 1969. Equilibrium measurements of embryonic cell adhesiveness: physical formulation and testing of the differential adhesion hypothesis. Doctoral dissertation. The Johns Hopkins University.

Phillips, J. L. 1976. Specific binding of zinc transferrin to human lymphocytes. *Biochem. Biophys. Res. Commun.*, **72**, 634.
Phillips, J. L. 1978. Uptake of transferrin bound zinc by human lymphocytes. *Cell Immunol.*, **35**, 318.
Phillips, H. M., Wiseman, L. L. and Steinberg, M. S. 1977. Self vs. nonself in tissue assembly. Correlated changes in recognition behavior and tissue cohesiveness. *Dev. Biol.*, **57**, 150–9.
Picciano, M. F. and Guthrie, H. A. 1976. Copper, iron and zinc contents of mature human milk. *Am. J. Clin. Nutr.*, **29**, 242–54.
Pierce, N. F. and Gowans, J. L. 1975. Cellular kinetics of the intestinal immune response to cholera toxoid in rats. *J. Exp. Med.*, **142**, 1550.
Pollack, S., George, J. N., Reba, R. C., Kaufman, R. M. and Crosby, W. H. 1965. The absorption of nonferrous metals in iron deficiency. *J. Clin. Invest.*, **44**, 147.
Porter, P., Noakes, D. E. and Allen, W. D. 1972. Intestinal secretion of immunoglobulins in the pre-ruminant calf. *Immunol.*, **23**, 299.
Potvin, C., Tarpley, J. L. and Chreten, B. 1975. Thymus-derived lymphocytes in patients with solid malignancies. *Clin. Immunol. Immunopathol.*, **3**, 476.
Prehn, R. 1976. Tumor progression and homeostasis. *Adv. Cancer Res.*, **23**, 203.
Prieels, J. P., Pizzo, S. V., Glasgon, L. R., Paulson, J. C. and Hill, R. L. 1978. Hepatic receptor that specifically binds oligosaccharides containing fucosyl α 1 → 3 N. acetylglucosamine linkages. *Proc. Nat. Acad. Sci., USA*, **75**, 2215–19.
Projan, A. and Tanneberger, S. 1973. Some findings on movement and contact of human normal and tumor cells *in vitro*. *Eur. J. Canc.*, **9**, 703–8.
Rannie, G. H. and Donald, K. J. 1977. Estimation of the migration of thoracic duct lymphocytes to non-lymphoid tissues. *Cell. Tissue Kinet.*, **10**, 523.
Rannie, G. H., Smith, M. E. and Ford, W. L. 1977. Lymphocyte migration into cell-mediated immune lesions is inhibited by trypsin. *Nature*, **267**, 520–2.
Rannie, G. H., Thakur, M. L. and Ford, W. L. 1977. An experimental comparison of radioactive labels with potential application to lymphocyte migration studies in patients. *Clin. Exp. Immunol.*, **29**, 509.
Rao, G. H. R., Gerrard, J. M., Eaton, J. W. and White, J. G. 1978. The role of iron in prostaglandin synthesis: ferrous iron mediated oxidation of arachidonic acid. *Prostaglandins and Medicine*, **1**, 55–70.
Rausch, E., Kaiserling, E. and Goos, M. 1977. Langerhans cells and interdigitating reticulum cells in the thymus-dependent region in human dermatopathic lymphadenitis. *Virchows Arch. B Cell Pathol.*, **25**, 327.
Ravnskov, U., Dahlback, O. and Messeter, L. 1977. Treatment of glomerulonephritis with drainage of the thoracic duct and plasmapheresis. *Acta Med. Scand.*, **202**, 489.
Reich, E., Rifkin, D. B. and Shaw, E. 1975. Proteases and biological control. Cold Spring Harbor Conferences on Cell Proliferation, Vol. 2, pp. ix and 1011.
Revillard, J. P., Brochier, J., Durix, A., Bernardt, J., Bryon, P. A., Archimand, J. P., Fries, D. and Traeger, J. 1968. Drainage du canal thoracique avant transplantation chez de malades atteints d'insuffisance rénale chronique. *Nouv. Rev. Francaise d'Hematol.*, **8**, 58–602.
Reynolds, J. 1980. Gut-associated lymphoid tissues in lambs before and after birth. *Monographs in Allergy*, **16**, 187–202.
Rhodin, J. A. G. 1973. Ultrastructure of the microvascular bed. In *The Microcirculation in Clinical Medicine*, ed. R. Wells. Academic Press, New York, p. 13.
Robbins, E. and Pederson, T. 1970. Iron: its intracellular localization and possible role in cell division. *Proc. Nat. Acad. Sci.*, **66**, 1244.
Rodnan, G. P. 1972. Progressive systemic sclerosis (scleroderma) In *Arthritis and Allied Conditions*, 8th edition, ed. J. L. Hollander and J. D. McCarty, Jr. Lea & Febiger, Philadelphia, p. 962.

Rodnan, G. P. and Medsger, T. A. 1966. Musculo-skeletal involvement in progressive systemic sclerosis (scleroderma). *Bull. Rheum. Dis.*, **17**, 419.
Roitt, I. M. 1977. *Essential Immunology*. Blackwell Scientific Publications.
Romagnani, S., Maggi, E., Biagiotti, R., Giudizi, M. G., Anadori, A. and Ricci, M. 1978. Altered proportion of Tµ and Tγ-cell subpopulations in patients with Hodgkin's disease. *Scand. J. Immunol.*, **7**, 511.
Rose, M. L. and Parrott, D. M. V. 1977. Vascular permeability and lymphoblast extravasation into inflamed skin are not related. *Cell Immunol.*, **33**, 62.
Rose, M. L., Parrott, D. M. V. and Bruce, R. G. 1976a. Migration of lymphoblasts to the small intestine. II. Divergent migration of mesenteric and peripheral immunoblasts to sites of inflammation in the mouse. *Cell. Immunol.*, **27**, 36.
Rose, M. L., Parrott, D. M. V. and Bruce, R. G. 1976b. Migration of lymphoblasts to the small intestine. I. Effect of Trichinella spiralis infection on the migration of mesenteric lymphoblasts and mesenteric T lymphoblasts in syngeneic mice. *Immunol.*, **31**, 723.
Rose, M. L., Parrott, D. M. V. and Bruce, R. G. 1978. The accumulation of immunoblasts in extravascular tissues including mammary gland, peritoneal cavity, gut and skin. *Immunology*, **35**, 415.
Rosenquist, G. C. 1970. Location and movements of cardiogenic cells in the chick embryo: the heart forming portion of the primitive streak. *Dev. Biol.*, **22**, 461–75.
Roth, S., McGuire, E. J. and Roseman, S. 1971. An assay for intercellular adhesive specificity. *J. Cell Biol.*, **51**, 525–35.
Roth, S. A. and Weston, J. A. 1967. The measurement of intercellular adhesion. *Proc. Nat. Acad. Sci U.S.A.*, **58**, 974.
Rothfield, N. F. and Rodnan, G. P. 1968. Serum antinuclear antibodies in progressive systemic sclerosis (scleroderma). *Arthritis Rheum.*, **11**, 607.
Roux, M. E., McWilliams, M., Phillips-Quaqliata, J. M., Wiess Carrington, P. W. and Lamm, M. E. 1977. Origin of IgA secretory plasma cells in the mammary glands. *J. Exp. Med.*, **146**, 1311.
Rowley, D. A., Gowans, J. L., Atkins, R. C., Ford, W. L. and Smith, N. G. 1972. The specific selection of recirculating lymphocytes by antigen in normal and preimmunized rats. *J. Exp. Med.*, **136**, 499.
Rudland, P. S., Durbin, H., Clingan, D. and Jimenez de Asua, L. 1977. Iron salts and transferrin are specifically required for cell division of cultured 3T6 cells. *Biochem. Biophys. Res. Comm.*, **75**, 556.
Rudzik, O. and Bienenstock, J. 1974. Isolation and characteristics of gut mucosal lymphocytes. *Lab. Invest.*, **30**, 260.
Rudzik, O., Clancy, R. L., Perey, D. Y. E., Bienenstock, J. and Singal, D. P. 1975. The distribution of a rabbit thymic antigen and membrane immunoglobulins in lymphoid tissue, with special reference to mucosal lymphocytes. *J. of Immunology*, **114**, 1.
Russell, R. J., Wilkinson, P. C., Sless, F. and Parrott, D. M. V. 1975. Chemotaxis of lymphoblasts. *Nature*, **256**, 646.
Russell, S. W., Doe, W. F., Hoskins, R. G. and Cochrane, C. G. 1976a. Inflammatory cells in solid murine neoplasms I. Tumor disaggregation and identification of constituent inflammatory cells. *Int. J. Cancer*, **18**, 322.
Russell, S. W., Gillespie, G. Y., Hansen, C. B. and Cochrane, C. G. 1976b. Inflammatory cells in solid murine neoplasms. II. Cell types found throughout the course of Moloney sarcoma regression or progression. *Int. J. Cancer*, **18**, 331.
Rydgren, L., Norberg, B., Hakansson, C. H., Mecklenberg, C. and Soderstrom, N. 1976. Lymphoblasts locomotion I. The initiation, velocity, pattern and path of locomotion *in vitro*. *Lymphology*, **9**, 89.
Sachar, D. B., Taub, R. N., Brown, S. M., Present, D. H., Korelitz, B. I. and Janowitz, H. D. 1973. Impaired lymphocyte responsiveness in inflammatory bowel disease. *Gastroenterology*, **64**, 203.

Sainte-Marie, G. 1975. A critical analysis of the validity of the experimental basis of current concept of the mode of lymphocyte recirculation. *Bull. Inst. Pasteur*, **73**, 255.

Sanchez-Tapias, J., Thomas, H. C. and Sherlock, S. 1977. Lymphocyte populations in liver biopsy specimens from patients with chronic liver disease. *Gut*, **18**, 472–475.

Sandberg-Wollheim, M. 1974. Immunoglobulin synthesis *in vitro* by cerebrospinal fluid cells in patients with multiple sclerosis. *Scand. J. Immunol.*, **5**, 717.

Sandberg-Wollheim, M. and Turesson, I. 1975. Lymphocyte subpopulations in the cerebrospinal fluid and periphral blood of patients with multiple sclerosis. *Scand. J. Immunol.*, **4**, 831.

Sarles, H. E., Remmers, A. R., Fish, J. C., Canales, C. O., Thomas, F. D., Tyson, D. R. T., Beathard, G. A. and Ritzmann, S. E. 1970. Depletion of lymphocytes for the protection of renal allografts. *Arch. Int. Med.*, **125**, 443.

Sasaki, S. 1967. Production of lymphocytosis by Polysaccharide polysulphates (heparinoids). *Nature*, **214**, 1041.

Saunders, J. W., Jr. 1966. Death in embryonic systems. *Science*, **154**, 604–12.

Scheinberg, M. A. and Cathcart, E. S. 1974. B and T cell lymphopenia in systemic lupus erythematosus. *Cell. Immunol.*, **12**, 309.

Schlesinger, M. and Israel, E. 1974. The effect of lectins on the migration of lymphocytes *in vivo*. *Cell. Immunol.*, **14**, 66.

Schlossman, S. F., Levin, H. A., Rocklin, R. E. and David, J. R. 1971. The compartmentalization of antigen-reactive lymphocytes in desensitized guinea pigs. *J. Exp. Med.*, **134**, 741.

Schmitt, D., Alario, A. and Thivolet, J. 1979. In situ characterization of tissue cells of cutaneous infiltrates using specific membrane antigens. *Clin. Exp. Dermatol.*, **4**, 161.

Schmitt, D., Alario, A., Touraine, J. L., Claudy, A. L., Perrot, H. and Thivolet, J. 1977. Specific surface antigen of human B and T lymphocytes: the use in the ultrastructural identification of cells extracted from cutaneous infiltrations. *J. Cutaneous Pathol.*, **4**, 211.

Schmitt, D., Viac, J., Brochier, J. and Thivolet, J. 1976. Thymus derived origin of Sezary cells demonstrated by peroxidase conjugated anti-HTLA serum. *Acta Dermatovenereologica*, **56**, 489.

Schoefl, G. I. and Miles, R. E. 1972. The migration of lymphocytes across the vascular endothelium in lymphoid tissue. *J. Exp. Med.*, **136**, 568.

Scholley, J. C. and Kelly, S. 1964. Influence of the thymus on the output of thoracic duct lymphocytes. In *The Thymus in Immunobiology*, ed. R. A. Good and A. E. Gabrielsen. Harper and Row, New York, p. 236.

Scollay, R., Hall, J. G. and Orlans, E. 1976. Studies on the lymphocytes of sheep. II. Some properties of cells in various compartments of the recirculating lymphocyte pool. *Eur. J. Immunol.*, **6**, 121.

Scollay, R., Kochen, M., Butcher, E. and Weissman, I. 1979. Ly+ markers on thymus cell migrants. *Nature*, **275**, 79.

Sheldon, P. J. and Holborow, E. J. 1975. H-rossette formation in T cell proliferative diseases. *Brit. Med. J.*, **4**, 381.

Sheldon, P. J., Pappamichail, M. and Holborow, E. J. 1974. Studies on synovial fluid lymphocytes on rheumatoid arthritis. *Ann. Rheum. Dis.*, **33**, 509.

Sheskin, J. and Zeimer, R. 1977. *In vitro* study of trace elements in leprous skin. *Dermatol.*, **16**, 745–7.

Siegal, F. P. and Siegal, M. 1977. Enhancement by irradiated T cells of human plasma cell production: dissection of helper and suppressor functions. *J. Immunol.*, **118**, 642.

Siimes, M. A., Vuori, E. and Kuitunen, P. 1979. Breast milk iron in a declining concentration during the course of lactation. *Act. Paed. Scand.*, **68**, 29–31.

Silverstone, A. E., Rosenberg, N., Baltimore, D., Sato, V. L., Scheid, M. P. and Boyse, E. A. 1978. Correlating terminal deoxynucleotidyl transferase and cell surface markers

in the pathway of lymphocyte ontogeny in differentiation of normal and neoplastic hematopoietic cells. Cold Spring Harbor Laboratory, pp. 433–53.
Simic, M. M. and Petrovic, M. Z. 1970. Cell interaction during the production of hemolysin-releasing cells from circulating lymphocytes. In *Developmental Aspects of Antibody Formation and Strucuture*. Academic Press, New York. p. 585.
Simic, M. M., Sljivic, V. S., Petrovic, M. Z. and Cinkovic, D. M. 1965. *Bull. Boris Kidric Inst. Nucl. Sci. Belgrade*, **16**, suppl. 1.
Skinner, J. M. and Whitehead, R. 1974. The plasma cells in inflammatory disease of the colon: a quantitative study. *J. Clin. Pathol.*, **27**, 643.
Smith, J. B., Cunningham, A. J., Lafferty, K. J. and Morris, B. 1970. The role of the lymphatic system and lymphoid cells in the establishment of immunological memory. *Aust. J. Exp. Biol. Med. Sci.*, **48**, 57.
Smith, C. W. and Goldman, A. S. 1968. The cells of human colostrum. I. *In vitro* studies of morphology and functions. *Pediatric Res.*, **2**, 103.
Smith, C. and Henon, B. K. 1959. Histological and histochemical study of high endothelium of post-capillary veins of the lymph node. *Anat. Rec.*, **135**, 207.
Smith, J. B., McIntosh, G. H. and Morris, B. 1970a. The traffic of cells through tissues: a study of peripheral lymph in sheep. *J. Anan.*, **107**, 87–100.
Smith, J. B., McIntosh, G. H. and Morris, B. 1970b. The migration of cells through chronically inflamed tissues. *J. Pathol.*, **100**, 21.
Smith, R. P. C., Lackie, J. M. and Wilkinson, P. C. 1979. The effect of chemotactic factors on the adhesiveness of rabbit neutrophil granulocytes. *Exp. Cell Res.*, **122**, 169.
Snook, T. 1946. Deep lymphatics of the spleen. *Anat. Rec.*, **94**, 43–56.
Soderstrom, N. 1967. Post-capillary venules as basic structural units in the development of lymphoglandular tissue. *Scand. J. Haematol.*, **4**, 411.
Soeberg, B., Sumerska, T. and Balfour, B. M. 1979. The role of afferent lymph in the induction of contact sensitivities. *Am. Exp. Med. Biol.*, **66**, 191–6.
Soltys, H. D. and Brody, J. I. 1970. Synthesis of transferrin by human peripheral blood lymphocytes. *Journal of Laboratory Clinical Medicine*, **75**, 250–7.
Sordat, B., Hess, M. W. and Cottier, H. 1971. IgG immunoglobin in the wall of post-capillary venules: possible relationship to lymphocyte recirculation. *Immunology*, **20**, 115.
Sprent, J. 1973. Circulating T and B lymphocytes of the mouse. I. Migratory properties. *Cell. Immunol.*, **7**, 10.
Sprent, J. 1976. Fate of H2 activated T lymphocytes in syngeneic hosts 1. Fate in lymphoid tissues and intestines traced with ^{3}H-thymidine, ^{125}I-dioxyuridine, and ^{51}Chromium. *Cell Immunol.*, **21**, 278.
Sprent, J. 1977. Recirculating lymphocytes. In *The Lymphocyte: Structure and Function*, ed. J. J. Marchalonis, pp. 43–111. Marcel Dekker, New York.
Sprent, J., Anderson, R. E. and Miller, J. F. A. P. 1974. Radiosensitivity of T and B lymphocytes. II. Effect of irradiation on response of T cells to alloantigens. *Eur. J. Immunol.*, **4**, 204–10.
Sprent, J. and Basten, A. 1973. Circulating T and B lymphocytes of the mouse. II. Lifespan. *Cell. Immunol.*, **7**, 40.
Sprent, J. and Lefkovits, I. 1976. Effect of recent antigen priming on adoptive immune responses. IV. Antigen-induced selective recruitment of recirculating lymphocytes to the spleen demonstrable with microculture system. *J. Exp. Med.*, **143**, 1289.
Sprent, J. and Miller, J. F. A. P. 1972a. Interaction of thymus lymphocytes with histoincompatible cells. I. Quantitation of the proliferative response of thymus cells. *Cell. Immunol.*, **3**, 361.
Sprent, J. and Miller, J. F. A. P. 1972b. Interaction of thymus lymphocytes with histoincompatible cells. II. Recirculating lymphocytes derived from antigen activated thymus cells. *Cell. Immunol.*, **3**, 385.

Sprent, J. and Miller, J. F. A. P. 1972c. Interaction of thymus lymphocytes with histoincompatible cells. III. Immunological characteristics of recirculating lymphocytes derived from activated thymus cells. *Cell. Immunol.*, **3**, 213.

Sprent, J. and Miller, J. F. A. P. 1974. Effect of recent antigen priming on adoptive immune responses. II. Specific unresponsiveness of circulating lymphocytes from mice primed with heterologous erythrocytes. *J. Exp. Med.*, **139**, 1.

Sprent, J. and Miller, J. F. A. P. 1976. Fate of H2-activated T lymphocytes in syngeneic hosts. III. Differentiation into long-lived recirculating memory cells. *Cell. Immunol.*, **21**, 314.

Sprent, J., Miller, J. F. A P. and Mitchell, G. F. 1971. Antigen induced selective recruitment of recirculating lymphocytes. *Cell. Immunol.*, **2**, 171.

Spry, C. J. 1972. Inhibition of lymphocyte recirculation by stress and corticotropin. *Cell. Immunol.*, **4**, 86.

Spry, C. J. F., Lane, J. T. and Vyakarnam, A. 1977. The effects of complement activation by Cobra venom factor on the migration of T and B lymphocytes, into rat thoracic duct lymph. *Immunology*, **32**, 947.

Stamper, H. B. and Woodruff, J. J. 1976. Lymphocyte homing into lymph nodes: *in vitro* demonstration of the selective affinity of recirculatory lymphocytes for high-endothelial venules. *J. Exp. Med.*, **144**, 828.

Stamper, H. B., Jr. and Woodruff, J. J. 1977. An *in vitro* model of lymphocyte homing. I. Characterization of the interaction between thoracic duct lymphocytes and specialized high-endothelial venules of lymph nodes. *J. Immunol.*, **119**, 772–80.

Steinberg, M. S. 1962. On the mechanism of tissue reconstruction by dissociated cells. I. Population kinetics, differential adhesiveness and the absence of directed migration. *Proc. Nat. Acad. Wash.*, **48**, 1577–82.

Steinberg, M. S. 1963. On the mechanism of tissue reconstruction by dissociated cells. II. Time course of events. *Science*, **137**, 762–3.

Steinberg, M. S. 1964. The problem of adhesive selectivity in cellular interactions. In *Cellular Membranes in Development*, ed. M. Locke. Academic Press, New York, pp. 321–66.

Steinberg, M. S. 1970. Does differential adhesion govern self-assembly processes in histogenesis? Equilibrium configurations and the emergence of a hierarchy among populations of embryonic cells. *J. Exp. Zool.*, **173**, 395–434.

Steinberg, M. S. 1975. Adhesion-guided multicellular assembly: a commentary upon the postulates, real and imagined, of the differential adhesion hypothesis, with special attention to computer simulations of cell sorting. *J. Theor. Biol.*, **55**, 431–43.

Steinberg, M. S. 1978a. Specific cell ligands and the differential adhesion hypothesis: How do they fit together? In *Receptors and Recognition*, Ser. B, Vol. 4, *Specificity of Embryological Interactions*, ed. D. R. Garrod. Chapman and Hall, New York, pp. 99–130.

Steinberg, M. S. 1978b. Cell–cell recognition in multicellular assembly: levels of specificity. *Symp. Soc. Exp. Biol.*, **32**, 25–49.

Stephenson, E. M. and Stephenson, N. G. 1978. Invasive locomotory behaviour between malignant human melanoma cells and normal fibroblasts filmed *in vitro*. *J. Cell Sci.*, **32**, 389–418.

Strelkauskas, A. J., Callery, R. T., Borel, Y. and Schlossman, S. F. 1979. Functional characteristics of human T-lymphocyte subsets identified by sera from patients with systemic lupus erythematosus. *Clin. Immunol. and Immunopathol.*, **14**, 47.

Strickland, R. G., Husby, G., Black, W. C. and Williams, R. C. 1975. Peripheral blood and intestinal lymphocyte subpopulations in Crohn's disease. *Gut*, **16**, 847–53.

Strober, S. 1968. Initiation of primary antibody responses of both circulating and non-circulating lymphocytes. *Nature*, **219**, 649.

Strober, S. 1969. Initiation of antibody responses by different classes of lymphocytes. I.

Types of thoracic duct lymphocytes involved in primary antibody responses of rats. *J. Exp. Med.*, **130**, 895.
Strober, S. 1970. Initiation of antibody responses by different classes of lymphocytes. II. Differences in tissue distribution of lymphocytes involved in primary and secondary antibody responses. *J. Immunol.*, **105**, 730.
Strober, S. 1972. Initiation of antibody responses by different classes of lymphocytes. V. Fundamental changes in the physiological characteristics of virgin thymus-independent (B) lymphocytes and 'B' memory cells. *J. Exp. Med.*, **136**, 85.
Strober, S. and Dilley, J. 1973. Biological characteristics of T and B memory lymphocytes in the rat. *J. Exp. Med.*, **137**, 1275.
Strober, S. and Dilley, J. 1975. Migration of B lymphocytes in the rat. I. Migration pattern, tissue distribution and turnover rate of unprimed and primed B lymphocytes involved in the adoptive antidinitrophenyl response. *J. Exp. Med.*, **138**, 1331.
Sugimura, M. 1964. Fine structure of post-capillary venules in mouse lymph nodes. *Jap. J. Vet. Res.*, **12**, 83.
Strickmans, P. A., Chanana, A. D. Cronkite, E. P., Greenberg, M. L. and Schiffer, L. M. 1968. Studies on lymphocytes. IX. The survival of autotransfused labeled lymphocytes in chronic lymphocytic leukemia. *Eur. J. Cancer*, **4**, 241.
Stück, B., Boyse, E. A., Old, L. D. and Carswell, E. A. 1964. ML: A new antigen found in leukaemias and mammary tumours of the mouse. *Nature (Lond.)*, **203**, 1033.
Summers, M., White, G. and Jacobs, A. 1974. Ferritin synthesis in lymphocytes, polymorphs and monocytes. *British Journal of Haematology*, **30**, 425.
Tagami, H. and Ofugi, S. 1976. Leukotactic properties of soluble substances in psoriasis scale. *Br. J. Dermatol.*, **95**, 1.
Tan, C. T. C., de Sousa, M., Tan, R., Hansen, J. A. and Good, R. A. 1978. Immunological parameters in childhood Hodgkin's disease. A study of lymphocyte transformation *in vitro* in response to stimulation by mitogens and antigens. *Cancer Res.*, **38**, 886.
Tan, R. S., Byron, N. A. and Hayes, J. P. 1975. A method of liberating living cells from the dermal infiltrate. Studies on skin reticuloses and lichen planus. *Brit. J. Dermatol.*, **93**, 271.
Taub, R. N. 1974. Effects of concanavilin-A on the migration of radioactively labelled lymphoid cells. *Cell. Immunol.*, **12**, 263.
Taub, R. N., Rosett, W., Adler, A. and Morse, S. I. 1972. Distribution of labelled lymph node cells in mice during the lymphocytosis induced by Bordetella pertussis. *J. Exp. Med.*, **136**, 1581.
Taylor, H. E. and Culling, C. F. A. 1966. Cytopathic effect of sensitized spleen cells in fibroblasts. *Lab. Invest.*, **15**, 1960.
Theodoropoulos, G., Maklous, A. and Constantoulakis, M. 1968. Lymph node enlargement after a single massive infusion of iron dextran. *J. Clin. Path.*, **21**, 492–4.
Thomas, H. C., Fremi, M., Sanchez-Tapias, J., DeVilliers, D., Jain, S. and Sherlock, S. 1976. Peripheral blood lymphocytes populations in chronic liver disease. *Clin. Exp. Immunol.*, **26**, 222.
Tillmanns, H., Ikeda, S., Hansen, H., Sarne, J. S. M., Fourel, J. M. and Bing, R. J. 1974. Microcirculation in the ventricle of the dog and turtle. *Circulation Res.*, **34**, 561.
Tilney, N. L. and Ford, W. F. 1974. The migration of rat lymphoid cells into skin grafts. Some sensitized cells localize preferentially in specific allografts. *Transpl.*, **17**, 12.
Tilney, N. L. and Murray, J. E. 1968. Chronic thoracic duct fistula: Operative technique and physiologic effect in man. *Ann. Surg.*, **167**, 1.
Tilney, N. L., Atkinson, J. C. and Murray, J. E. 1970. The immunosuppressive effect of thoracic duct drainage in human kidney transplantation. *Ann. Intern. Med.*, **72**, 59–64.
Tomasi, T. B. and Bienenstock, J. 1968. Secretory immunoglobulins. *Adv. Immunol.*, **9**, 1.

Tormey, D. C., Imrie, R. C. and Muller, G. C. 1972. Identification of transferrin as a lymphocyte growth promotor in human serum. *Exp. Cell. Res.*, **74**, 163.
Townes, P. L. and Holtfreter, J. 1955. Directed movements and selective adhesion of embryonic amphibian cells. *J. Exp. Zool.*, **128**, 53–120.
Trentin, J. J., McGarry, M. P., Jenkins, V. K., Gallagher, M. T., Speirs, R. S. and Wolf, N. S. 1971. Role of inductive microenvironments of haemopoietic (and lymphoid?) differentiation, and role of thymic cells in the eosinophilic granulocyte response to antigen. *Adv. Exp. Med. Biol.*, **12**, 289.
Trowell, D. A. 1958. The lymphocyte. *Internat. Rev. Cytol.*, **7**, 235.
Turbitt, M. and Curtis, A. S. G. 1974. Are there differences in contact inhibition of movement between normal and malignant cells. *Nature*, **249**, 453–4.
Turk, J. L. 1973. Morphological changes in the thymus-dependent lymphoid system associated with pathological conditions in animals and man: their functional significance. *Cont. Topics Immunobiol.*, **2**, 137.
Twitty, V. C. 1944. Chromatophore migration as a response to mutual influences of the developing pigment cells. *J. Exp. Zool.*, **95**, 259–90.
Twitty, V. C. 1949. Developmental analysis of amphibian pigmentation. *Growth, Symposium*, **9**, 133–61.
Twitty, V. C. and Niu, M. C. 1948. Causal analysis of chromatophore migration. *J. Exp. Zool.*, **108**, 405–38.
Twitty, V. C. and Niu, M. C. 1954. the motivation of cell migration, studied by isolation of embryonic pigment cells singly and in small groups *in vitro*. *J. Exp. Zool.*, **125**, 541–73.
Uhr, J. W. 1966. Delayed hypersensitivity. *Physiol. Rev.*, **46**, 359.
Utsinger, P. D. 1975. Synovial fluid lymphocytes in rheumatoid arthritis. *Arthr. and Rheum.*, **18**, 595.
Utsinger, P. 1976. Relationship of lymphocytotoxic antibodies to lymphopenia and parameters of disease activity in systemic lupus erythematosus. *J. Rheumatol.*, **3**, 175.
Vachek, H. and Kölskh, E. 1975. Dextran sulfate stimulates the induction but inhibits the effector phase in T-cell-mediated cytotoxicity. *Transplantation*, **19**, 183.
Van Deurs, B. and Ropke, C. 1975. The postnatal development of high-endothelial venules in lymph nodes of mice. *Anat. Rec.*, **181**, 659.
Van Epps, D. and William, S. R. C. 1976. Suppression of leukocyte chemotaxis by human IgA myeloma components. *J. Exp. Med.*, **144**, 1227.
van Ewijk, W., Brons, H. H. C. and Rozing, J. 1975. Scanning electron microscopy of homing and recirculating lymphocyte populations. *Cellular Immunology*, **19**, 245–61.
van Ewijk, W., Verzijden, J. H. M., van der Kwast, Th.H. and Luijexmeijer, S. W. M. 1974. Reconstruction of the thymus-dependent area in the spleen of lethally irradiated mice. *Cell Tissue Res.*, **149**, 43–60.
Van Lenten, L. and Ashwell, G. 1971. Studies on the chemical and enzymatic modification of glycoproteins. *J. Biol. Chem.*, **246**, 1889.
van de Putte, L. B. A., Meijer, C. J. L. M., Lafeber, G. J. M., Kleinjan, R. and Cats, A. 1976. Lymphocytes in rheumatoid and non-rheumatoid synovial fluids. *Ann. Rheum. Dis.*, **35**, 451.
Van Rooisen, N. 1972. Vascular pathways in white pulp of rabbit spleen. *Acta. Morphol. Nerrl. Scand.*, **10**, 351.
Van Snick, J. L. and Masson, P. 1976. The binding of human lactoferrin to mouse macrophages. *J. Exp. Med.*, **144**, 1568.
Veerman, A. J. P. 1974. On the interdigitating cells in the thymus-dependent area of the rat spleen: A relation between the mononuclear phagocyte system and T lymphocytes. *Cell. Tissue Res.*, **148**, 247.
Veldman, J. E. 1970. *Histophysiology and Electron Microscopy of the Immune Response*. Akad. Proefschrift, Groningen, N.V. Boekdrukkenij Dijkstra. Niemeyer.

Vernon-Roberts, B., Currey, H. L. F. and Perrin, J. 1974. T and B cells in the blood and synovial fluid of rheumatoid patients. *Ann. Rheum. Dis.*, **33**, 430.

Vesely, P. and Weiss, R. A. 1973. Cell locomotion and contact inhibition of normal and neoplastic rat cells. *Inst. J. Cancer*, **11**, 64–76.

Virchow, R. 1858. Lecture IX. Pyemia and leucocytosis. In *Cellular Pathology*, 1860. Churchill, London.

Vuori, E. and Kuitunen, P. 1979. The concentration of copper in human milk. *Act. Ped. Scand.*, **68**, 32–7.

Wack, J. P. and Wyatt, J. P. 1959. Studies on ferrodynamics I. Gastrointestinal absorption of Fe^{59} in the rat under differing dietary states. *Arch. Path.*, **67**, 237.

Waksman, B. H. 1973. The homing pattern of thymus-derived lymphocytes in calf and neonatal mouse Peyer's patches. *J. Immunol.*, **111**, 878.

Waksman, B. H., Arnason, B. G. and Jankovic, B. D. 1962. Role of the thymus in immune reactions in rats. III. Changes in the lymphoid organs of thymectomized rats. *J. Exp. Med.*, **116**, 187.

Waksman, B. H. Ozer, H. and Blythman, H. E. 1973. Appendix and antibody formation. VI. The functional anatomy of the rabbit appendix. *Lab. Invest.*, **28**, 614.

Waldman, R. H. and Henney, C. S. 1971. Cell mediated immunity and antibody responses in the respiratory tract after local and systemic immunization. *J. Exp. Med.*, **134**, 482.

Walther, B. T., Ohman, R. and Roseman, S. 1973. A quantitative assay for intercellular adhesion. *Proc. Nat. Acad. Sci.*, USA, **70**, 1569–73.

Warner, F. W., Stjernholm, R. and Cohn, I. 1978. Electron paramagnetic resonance investigation of high spin Fe(III) in cancer. *Med. Phys.*, **5**, 100.

Warnke, R. A., Slavin, S., Coffman, R. L. Butcher, E. C., Kanpp, M. R., Strober, S. and Weissman, I. 1979. The pathology and homing of a transplantable murine B cell leukemia (BCL_1). *J. Immunol.*, **123**, 1181.

Wegelius, O., Laine, V., Lindstrom, B. and Klochan, M. 1970. Fistula of the thoracic duct as immunosuppressive treatment of rheumatoid arthritis. *Acta Med. Scand.*, **187**, 539–44.

Weinberg, E. D. 1974. Iron and susceptibility to infectious disease. *Science*, **184**, 952.

Weinberg, E. D. 1978. Iron and infection. *Microbiol. Rev.*, **42**, 45.

Weiss, L. 1965. Structure of normal spleen. *Seminars in Haematol.*, **2**, 205.

Weiss, L. 1972. The cells and tissues of the immune system. Structure, functions and interactions. *Foundations of Immunology Series*. Prentice-Hall, Englewood Cliffs, New Jersey.

Weiss, P. 1941. Nerve patterns: the mechanics of nerve growth. *Growth. Suppl.*, **5**, 163–203.

Weiss, P. 1958. Cell contact. *Internat. Rev. Cytol.*, **7**, 391–423.

Weiss, P. 1961. Guiding principles in cell locomotion and cell aggregation. *Exp. Cell Res.*, Suppl. 8, 260.

Weissman, I. L. 1967. Thymus cell migration. *J. Exp. Med.*, **126**, 291.

Weissman, I. 1975. Development and distribution of immunoglobulin bearing cells in mice. *Transplant. Rev.*, **24**, 159.

Weissman, I. 1976. T cell maturation and the ontogeny of splenic lymphoid architecture. In J. R. Battisto (ed.) *Immuno Aspects of the Spleen*. North-Holland, Amsterdam.

Weissman, I. L., Gutman, G. A. and Friedberg, S. H. 1974. Tissue localization of lymphoid cells. *Sem. Haematol.*, **7**, 482.

Weissman, I., Warnke, R., Butcher, E., Rouse, R. and Levy, R. 1978. The lymphoid system: Its normal architecture and the potential for understanding the system through the study of lympho-proliferative diseases. *Human Pathol.*, **9**, 25.

Wenk, E. J., Orlic, D., Reith, E. J. and Rhodin, J. A. G. 1974. The ultrastructure of mouse

lymph node venules and the passage of lymphocytes across their walls. *J. Ultrastruct. Res.*, **47**, 214.
Weston, J. A. 1963. A radioautographic analysis of the migration and localization of trunk neural crest cells in the chick. *Develop. Biol.*, **6**, 279–310.
Wheby, M. S. 1970. Site of iron absorption in man. *Scand. J. Hematol.*, **1**, 57–62.
White, R. G., Henderson, D. C., Eslami, M. B. and Nielsen, K. H. 1975. Localization of a protein antigen in the chicken spleen. *Immunology*, **28**, 1.
Wiese, L. and Wiese, W. 1978. Sex cell contact in Chlamydomonas: a model for cell recognition. *Symp. Soc. Exp. Biol.*, **32**, 83–103.
Wilkinson, P. C. and Curtis, A. S. G. quoted in Parrott and Wilkinson (1981).
Wilkinson, P. C., Parrott, D. M. V., Russell, R. J. and Sless, F. 1977. Antigen induced locomotor responses in lymphocytes. *J. Exp. Med.*, **145**, 1158.
Wilkinson, P. C., Roberts, J. C., Russell, R. J. and McLoughlin, M. 1976. Chemotaxis of mitogen activated human lymphocytes and the effects of membrane active enzymes. *Clin. Exp. Immunol.*, **25**, 280.
Williams, R. C., Jr., DeBord, J. R., Mellbye, O. J., Messner, R. P. and Lindstrom, F. D. 1973. Studies of T and B lymphocytes in patients with connective tissue diseases. *J. Clin. Invest.*, **52**, 283.
Williams, W. J. 1965. A study of Chron's syndrome using tissue extracts and the kveim and Mantoux tests. *Gut*, **6**, 503.
Williams-Smith, D. L. and Cammack, R. 1977. Oxidation-reduction potentials of cytochromes p. 450 and ferredoxin in the bovine adrenal: their modification by substrates and inhibitors. *Biochimica et Biophysica Acta*, **499**, 432–42.
Willis, R. A. 1952. *The Spread of Tumors in the Human Body*. Butterworth, London, pp. ix and 447.
Willmore, L. J., Syrert, G. W., Munson, J. B. and Hurd, R. W. 1978. Chronic focal epileptiform discharges induced by injection of iron into rat and cat cortex. *Science*, **200**, 1501–3.
Wilson, D. B. and Howell, P. C. 1971. Quantitative studies on the mixed lymphocyte interaction of rats. V. Tempo and specificity of the proliferative response and the number of reactive cells from immunized donors. *J. Exp. Med.*, **133**, 442.
Winchester, R., Siegal, F. P., Bentwich, Z. and Kunkel, H. 1973. Alteration in the proportion of B and T lymphocytes in rheumatoid arthritis joint fluids with low complement and increased complexes. *Arthritis and Rheumatism*, **16**, 138.
Winchester, R. J., Winfield, J. B., Siegal, F., Wernet, P., Bentwich, Z. and Kunkel, H. G. 1974. Analysis of lymphocytes from patients with rheumatoid arthritis and systemic lupus erythematosus. Occurrence of interfering cold-reactive anti-lymphocyte antibodies. *J. Clin. Invest.*, **54**, 1082.
Winfield, J. B., Winchester, R. J. and Kunkel, H. G. 1975. Association of cold-reactive antilymphocyte antibodies with lymphopenia in systemic lupus erythematosus. *Arthritis and Rheumat.*, **18**, 587.
Winzler, R. J. 1970. Carbohydrates in cell surfaces. *Int. Rev. Cytol.*, **29**, 77.
Wiseman, L. L., Steinberg, M. S. and Phillips, H. M. 1972. Experimental modulation of intercellular cohesiveness: reversal of tissue assembly patterns. *Dev. Biol.*, **28**, 498–517.
Wolf, N. S. and Trentin, J. J. 1968. Haemopoietic colony studies. V. Effect of haemopoietic organ stroma on differentiation of pluripotent stem cells. *J. Exp. Med.*, **127**, 205.
Wolpert, L. 1969. Positional information and the spatial pattern of cellular differentiation. *J. Theoret. Biol.*, **25**, 1–47.
Wood, S. 1964. Experimental studies of the intravascular dissemination of ascitic V2 carcinoma cells in the rabbit, with special reference to fibrinogen and fibrinolytic agents. *Bull. Swiss Acad. Med. Sci.*, **20**, 92–121.

Woodruff, J. 1974. Role of lymphocyte surface determinants in lymph node homing. *Cell. Immunol.*, **13**, 378.
Woodruff, J. J. and Gesner, B. M. 1968. Lymphocytes: Circulation altered by trypsin. *Science*, **161**, 176.
Woodruff, J. and Gesner, B. M. 1969. The effect of neuraminidase on the fate of transfused lymphocytes. *J. Exp. Med.*, **129**, 551.
Woodruff, J. and Gesner, B. M. 1969. The effect of neuraminidase on the fate of transfused lymphocytes. *J. Exp. Med.*, **129**, 361.
Woodruff, J. J., Katz, I. M., Lucas, L. E. and Stamper, H. B. 1977. An *in vitro* model of lymphocyte homing. Membrane and cytoplasmic events involved in lymphocyte adherence to specialized high-endothelial venules of lymph nodes. *J. Immunol.*, **119**, 1603.
Woodruff, J. J. and Rasmussen, R. A. 1979. *In vitro* adherence of lymphocytes to unfixed and fixed high endothelial cells of lymph nodes. *J. Immunol.*, **123**, 2369.
Woodruff, J. J. and Woodruff, J. F. 1972. Virus induced alterations of lymphoid tissues. III. Fate of radiolabelled thoracic duct lymphocytes in rats inoculated with Newcastle Disease Virus. *Cell. Immunol.*, **5** 307.
Woodruff, J. J. and Woodruff, J. F. 1976a. Influenza A virus interaction with murine lymphocytes. I. The influence of influenza virus A/Japan 305 (H2N2) on the pattern of migration of recirculating lymphocytes. *J. Immunol.*, **117**, 852.
Woodruff, J. J. and Woodruff, J. F. 1976b. Influenza A virus interaction with murine lymphocytes. II. Changes in lymphocyte surface properties induced by influenza virus A/Japan 305 (H2N2). *J. Immunol.*, **117**, 859.
Worwood, M. 1974. Iron and the trace metals. In Jacobs, A. and Worwood, M. (eds.). *Iron in Biochemistry and Medicine*. Academic Press, London and New York, p. 335.
Wourms, J. P. 1972. The developmental biology of annual fishes. II. Naturally occurring dispersion and reaggregation of blastomeres during the development of annual fish eggs. *J. Exp. Zool.*, **182**, 169–200.
Wu, C. Y. and Cinader, B. 1971. Antigenic promotion. Increase in hapten-specific plaque forming cells after preinjection with structurally unrelated macromolecules. *J. Exp. Med.*, **134**, 693.
Wybran, J. and Fudenberg, H. 1973. Thymus-derived rosette forming cells in various human disease states: cancer, lymphoma, bacteria, and viral infections and other diseases. *J. Clin. Invest.*, **52**, 1026.
Yoffey, J. M. 1960. *Quantitative Cellular Haematology*. Charles C. Thomas, Springfield, Ill.
Yoshida, Y. and Osmond, D. G. 1978. Homing of bone marrow lymphoid cells: localization and fate of newly formed cells in lymphocyte-rich marrow fractions injected into lethally irradiated recipients. *Transplantation*, **25**, 246.
Young, D. V., Cox III, F. W., Chipman, S. and Hartman, S. C. 1979. The growth of stimulation of SV3T3 cells by transferrin and its dependence on biotin.
Young, R. C., Corder, M. P., Haynes, H. H. and de Vita, V. T. 1972. Delayed hypersensitivity in Hodgkin's Disease. A study of 103 untreated patients. *Am. J. Med.*, **52**, 63.
Zatz, M. M., Goldstein, D. L., Blumenfeld, O. O. and White, A. 1972. Regulation of normal and leukaemic lymphocyte transformation and recirculation by sodium periodate oxidation and sodium borohydride reaction. *Nature, New Biol.*, **240**, 252.
Zatz, M. M. and Lance, E. M. 1971. The distribution of ^{51}Cr labelled lymphocytes in antigen stimulated mice. Lymphocyte trapping. *J. Exp. Med.*, **134**, 224.
Zatz, M. M., Mellors, R. C. and Lance, E. M. 1971. Changes in lymphoid populations of ageing CBA and NZB mice. *Clin. Exp. Immunol.*, **8**, 494–500.
Zatz, M. M., White, A. and Goldstein, A. L. 1973. Alterations in lymphocyte populations in tumorigenesis. I. Lymphocyte trapping. *J. Immunol.*, **111**, 706.

Zeidman, I. 1961. The state of circulating tumor cells. I. Passage of cells through capillaries. *Cancer Res.*, **21**, 38.

Zelený V., Matousek, V. and Lengerova, A. 1978. Intercellular adhesiveness of H-2 identical and H-2 disparate cells. *J. Immunogenet*, **5**, 41.

Zinkernagel, R. M. and Doherty, P. C. 1974. Activity of sensitized thymus derived lymphocytes in lymphocytic choriomeningitis reflects immunological surveillance against altered self-components. *Nature* (Lond.), **251**, 547.

Zschoke, R. H. and Bezkorovainy, A. 1974. Structure and function of transferrins. II. Transferrin and iron metabolism. *Arzneim. Forsch.*, **24**, 726.

Index

Absorption, small intestine, iron, 203
ACTH, effect of stress on lymphocyte recirculation in the rat, 94
Adhesion, differential adhesion hypothesis, 180
   hypothetical models of cell, 165
   of T and B lymphocytes to HEV, 200
   selectivity of cell, 177
   specific cell, 177, 178
Adjuvants, alum particles, 58
   Bordetella pertussis, 60, 95
Afferent lymph, infusion with ^{3}H-thymidine, 40, 41
   lymphocytes in, 99, 101, 103
   macrophages in, 100, 102
   polymorphs in, 99
   T:B lymphocyte ratios in, 102
   veiled cells in, 33, 102
Age, 77–78
   influence of donor age on bursa cell migration in the chicken, 77
   influence of recipient age, 78
Ageing, effect on lymphocyte migration:
   in mice, 77, 78
   in NZB mice, 77
   in response to antigen stimulation, 78
Aggregation, 175
   methods for study of cell, 175
Albumin, chemokinetic agent to lymphocytes, *in vitro*, 104
Antibodies, anti-lymphocyte antibodies and lymphopenia in SLE, 146, 147
   class of, in SLE, 146
Antibody, effect of anti-immunoglobulin on migration of appendix cells in the rabbit, 79
   effect of anti-lymphocyte antiserum on lymphocyte migration in the mouse, 79
Antigen,
   changes occurring after antigen stimulation:
      in blood flow to the lymph node in the rabbit, 12
      in blood flow to the lymph node in sheep, 11
      in cell output from efferent lymphatics, 57
      in cell output from the spleen, 58, 59
      in lymph node microvasculature, 10
      in lymphocyte recovery from organs draining the site of injection, 59–65
   compartmentalization of antigen-reactive cells, 66
   competition, 66
   immune deviation, 66
   preemption, caused by, 65
Antigen-reactive cells,
   compartmentalization of in the guinea pig, 66
   specific recruitment of, 66–69
Appendix, 35, 114
Aseptic meningitis, 151, 152
   B cells in CSF, 152
   B cells in peripheral blood, 151
   T cells in CSF, 152
   T cells in peripheral blood, 151
Autoimmune, lesions in liver, 125
   lymphocyte circulation in autoimmune NZB mouse, 124, 125
Autoradiography, 21
Azide, effect of sodium azide on lymphocyte migration, 91

B lymphoblasts, fate in gut mucosa, 118
B lymphocytes, adhesion, 187
   distribution of labelled B lymphocytes:
      in the lymph node, 56, 57
      in the Peyer's patch, 56, 57
      in the spleen, 57
   ^{3}H-uridine labelling characteristics:
      in the mouse, 56
      in the rat, 56, 57

migration of leukemic B lymphocytes in man, 155
paucity of, in peripheral lymph, 102
tempo of circulation from blood to lymph, 44
BALT, 112, 113, 115, 121
development of, in absence of antigen, 113
Blood flow, changes during the immune response, 10–12, 107
shunt flow, 12
velocity v. sectional area, 2
Bone marrow, fate of cells labelled *in vitro*, 47
fate of cells labelled *in vivo*, 49
fate of fractionated bone marrow cell populations, 47, 48
Bordetella pertussis, effect of treatment with supernatants on lymphocyte migration in the mouse, 95, 96
lymphocytosis infection, 95
Brain, metal implants and lymphocyte infiltration, 209
Bronchial mucosa, lymphocytes in, 111, 113
monocytes in, 111
Bronchus, associated lymphoid tissues, *see* BALT
Bursa of Fabricus, fate of cells labelled *in situ*, 53, 54
fate of cells labelled *in vitro*, 53, 54
germinal centre localization of bursa cells, 53
migration of young bursa cells, 77
migration of old bursa cells, 78

C3, effect of lowering levels on lymphocyte migration, 96
Chemotaxis, in patterning of pigmented cells, 184, 185
in recognition, 164, 178
of psoriasis scales, 143
CNS diseases, 149–152
aseptic meningitis, 151
multiple sclerosis, 149
Coeliac disease, foecal loss of labelled lymphocytes, 136
intraepithelial lymphocytes in, 120
Colchicine, effect of lymphocyte adherence to HEV, 199
effect on lymphocyte migration, 92
Colostrum, cytotoxic T lymphocytes in, 111

immunosuppressive effect of cell free, 206
lymphocytes in human, 111
Concanavilin A, effect on lymph node cell migration, 85, 86
Connective tissue diseases, progressive systemic sclerosis, 148
rheumatoid arthritis, 144
systemic lupus erythematosus, 146
Contact guidance, in regeneration of the optic nerve, 167
Contact inhibition, 173
Contact promotion, 173
Contact sensitivity, blood flow and lymphocyte migration in, 107
lymphocyte migration to sites of, 104–106
Crohn's disease, autotransfusion of labelled lymphocytes, 120
B and T cells in sections of resected tissues, 134
faecal loss of lymphocytes, 134
peripheral blood T lymphocytes before and after surgery, 134, 135
T cell lymphopenia in, 134
Croton oil, 106
CVF, effect of injection of, on lymphocyte migration in different species, 96–98
Cyclic AMP stimulators, effect on lymphocyte migration in the mouse, 92
Cytochalisin A, impaired lymph node entry of treated cells, 91
Cytochalisin B, effect of treatment of lymphocytes on lymph node entry, 91
effect on lymphocyte adherence to HEV, 199

DCR, histochemical features, 29
ultrastructural features, 30
Dextrans, effect of dextran sulphate on lymphocyte migration, 89
effect of neutral, 89
Diseases, chronic liver, 136
CNS, 149–152
connective tissue,
Crohn's, 134
Hodgkin's, 131
Kaschin–Beck's, 209–211
leprosy, 209
murine leprosy, 126–128
Newcastle virus (NDV), 126

pulmonary with pleurisy, 152
skin, 139–143
Dome areas, antigen and particle entry through, 113
of Peyer's patches, 112
ontogeny of T lymphocyte appearance in, 113
M cell in, 112
Duodenum, blood flow, 117, 203
IgA producing cells in, 117, 203
iron absorption, 203
mesenteric lymphoblast migration to, 117

E-rosette forming cells, in CSF in multiple sclerosis, 151
in liver biopsies, 137
in spleen in Hodgkin's disease, 132
infiltrating tumours, 154
Ecotaxis, 45–57
Ecotaxopathies, 129–161
Efferent lymph, cell output after antigen, 57
role of cells in, on propagation of immune response, 72
Embryogenesis, 168
Endothelium, ultrastructure of different types of, 2
Enzymes,
effect on lymphocyte migration: neuraminidase, 79–81
Phospholipases, 82
trypsin, 82
β-glucoronidase activity in high endothelium, 7
lactic dehydrogenase activity in high endothelium, 7

Ferritin, biochemistry, 213
synthesis by lymphocytes, 215
Foetus, lymphocyte migration to the liver in the foetal lamb, 204
lymphocyte recirculation in the foetal lamb, 40

GALT, 112, 113, 117
development in absence of antigen, 113
Gastro-intestinal (GI) tract diseases,
coeliac disease, 120
Crohn's disease, 120, 134
giardiasis, man, 120
mouse, 120

Glomerulonephritis, thoracic duct drainage in severe, 161
Granuloma, cell numbers in afferent lymph draining chronic granuloma in sheep, 103
Gut,
antigen free grafts, IgA producing cells in, 118
intraepithelial lymphocytes in, 118
Gut mucosa, B lymphoblasts, 118
B lymphocytes in, 110
failure of peripheral blast cells to enter, 116
IgA containing cells in, 109, 115, 117
IgD containing cells in, 109
IgE containing cells in, 109
IgG containing cells in, 109
IgM containing cells in, 109
intraepithelial lymphocytes, 109, 110
lymphocytes in biopsies of human colon, 110
ontogeny of lymphocyte appearance in, 113
T lymphoblasts in, 116
T lymphocytes in, 109, 115

Hepatitis, activated T cells in blood and liver in alcoholic and chronic active, 137
HEV, adhesion of lymphocytes to, 198–200
histochemistry, 7
in granuloma, 10
in Peyer's patches, 112
morphology in T cell depletion, 9
permeability, 8
^{35}S-sulphate uptake by, 7
ultrastructure, 6
Hodgkin's disease, lymphopenia, 131
maldistribution of T lymphocyte subsets, 132
peripheral blood and spleen cell responses to PHA stimulation, 131
peripheral blood response to PHA after splenectomy, 134

Ia, positive cells in T cell areas, 33
IDC, histochemistry, 29
in lymph nodes, 33
in skin in T cell lymphomas, 201
in spleen, 29, 30
ultrastructure, 30

IgA, containing cells in gut, 109, 117
  in biliary secretions, 122
  in milk, 121
  in saliva, 121
Ileum, lymphoblast migration to, 203
  lymphocyte infiltration in Crohn's disease, 134
Immune deviation, 66
Immune response, role of recirculation in initiation of, 69
  role of recirculation in propagation of, 71
Immunological memory, role of recirculatory lymphocytes in, long lived cells and, 72–75
Infection, IgA antibodies in milk in *S. typhimurium*, 121
  lymphoblast migration to gut in *T. spiralis*, 119, 121
  murine leprosy, 126–128
  Newcastle disease virus, 126
  Nippostrongylus brasiliensis, 203
  tuberculosis, 152
Interaction modulation factors, 186–189, 193
  H-2 restriction, 193
Iron, absorption, 203
  microbial cell growth, 216
  overload and lymphoid cell traffic in the mouse, 129
  synovium in rheumatoid arthritis, 208
  tumour cell growth, 216
Irradiation, effect of high doses on antibody responses after cell transfer, 92–94
  effect of *in vitro* irradiation on T and B cell migration, 93
  of spleen, 69
  thoracic duct cell output in irradiated rats, 93
Isoproterenol, effect of treatment on lymphocyte migration in the mouse, 92

Jejunum, blood flow, 117, 203
  mesenteric lymphoblast migration to, 117, 203
  IgA containing cells in, 203

Kaschin–Beck's disease, 209–211
Kidney allografts, cell output in, 102
  changes in cell composition of afferent lymph in, 103

Kidney transplants, thoracic duct drainage in man, 161

Lactation, IgA concentration during, 205
  lymphocyte migration to the mammary gland, iron in milk during, 205, 206
  milk lymphocytes, 205
  T lymphocyte numbers during, 205, 206
Lacteals, lymphatic drainage of, 113
Lactoferrin, biochemistry, 212
  receptors for, on macrophages, 214
  regulator of CFU–C differentiation, 213
Lamina propria, T cells in, 109
Leprosy,
  human, metals in skin, 209
  murine, impaired lymphocyte recirculation in, 126–128
Leukaemia, 155–161
  autotransfusion of labelled lymphocytes in, 155–157
  impaired lymphocyte recirculation in CLL, 157
  T and B lymphocytes in peripheral lymph of leukaemic patients, 159
Lichen planus, cutaneous infiltrate in, 143
Lifespan, B lymphocytes in thoracic duct lymph, 74
  distribution in lymph nodes of long-lived cells, 56
  distribution in lymph nodes of short-lived cells, 56
  distribution in spleen of long-lived cells, 55, 56
  distribution in spleen of short-lived cells, 55, 56
  T lymphocytes in thoracic duct lymph, 74
Lipopolysaccharide, effect on lymph node cell migration in the mouse, 88
Liver, auto-immune lesions caused by neurominidase treated lymphocytes, 125
  D-galactose recognizing lectin-like receptors in, 82
  lymphocytes in afferent lymph, 100, 101
  lymphocytes in biopsies, 137
  neuraminidase treated lymphocytes in, 79, 80, 125
Liver diseases, activated T cells in, 137
  alcohol related, 136
  chronic active hepatitis, 137
  primary biliary cirrhosis, 137

Locomotion, of peripheral and mesenteric blasts *in vitro*, 118
LPS, effect of *in vitro* treatment with, on lymphocyte migration in the mouse, 88
Lung, bone marrow cells in, 47
  Con A treated cells in, 86
  Dextran sulphate treated cells in, 89
  IgA producing cells in, 121
  lymphocytes in lavage fluid, 111
  slow circulation of B lymphocytes through, 45
  slow circulation of thymocytes through, 49
  tuberculosis, 152
Lupus erythematosis, lymphopenia in, 146
  thoracic duct cannulation in one case, 162
  see also SLE
Ly system of cell surface antigens, discovery of, 24
  distribution of Ly positive T cells in tissues, 25
Lymph, cell composition of afferent, 101
  cell composition of efferent, 101
  cells in peripheral lymph in man, 159
  renal in hydronephrosis, 103
Lymph node, arteriovenous shunts, 4
  B cell nodules, 32
  blood flow during the immune response, 10–12, 107
  cortex, 32
  efferent lymph, 57, 72
  high endothelium venules, see HEV
  IDC in, 33
  medulla, 32
  microvasculature, 4
  microvasculature changes during the immune response, 10
  morphology, 32
  paracortex, 32
  pig, 32
  postcapillary venules, 5, 32
  reticulum cells, 29
  T lymphocytes in, 33
  thymus-dependent area, 32
  ultrastructure in human lymphomas, 35
Lymph node cells, fate of cells labelled *in vitro*, 56
Lymphatics, initial and collecting, 13
  spleen, 3
  thoracic duct, 13
Lymphoblasts, migration of T, to sites of inflammation, 104
  migration to lamina propria, 116, 118
  migration to skin in cell-mediated immunity, 106
Lymphomas, germinal centre origin, 35
  Hodgkin's, 130
  lymphocytes in peripheral blood and spleen in, 131
  non-Hodgkin's, 35, 157
  T cell origin, 34

M cell, in Peyer's patch, 112
Mammary gland, lymphocyte migration to the, 121
Marginal zone, capillary network, 3
  dextran sulphate treated cells in, 89
  macrophages of, 31
Memory, see Immunological memory
Meningitis, viral aseptic, lymphocytes in cerebrospinal fluid, 151
Mesenteric node, in IgA production cycle, 115
  traffic of T blasts from, 116
Metals, effect of metal implants on lymphocyte infiltration of brain, 209
  lymphocyte migration in iron overload, in the mouse, 129
  migration of iron treated lymphocytes, 91
Milk, IgA antibodies, 121
  inhibition of the PHA response by, 206
  T lymphocytes, 111
Mitogens, Con A, effect of on lymphocyte migration in the mouse, 86
  LPS, 88
  PHA, effect of on lymphocyte migration in the mouse, 86
Mucosa, see Bronchial mucosa, Gut mucosa
Mucosal lymphocytes, as effector cells, 111
Multiple sclerosis, 149–151
  B cells in blood, 150, 151
  B cells in CSF, 150, 151
  Immunoglobulins in CSF, 149
  T cells in blood, 150, 151
  T cells in CSF, 150, 151
Mycosis Fungoides, 139–143
  helper T cells, 142
  IDC in skin, 140
  IgA levels in, 143
  IgE levels in, 143
  null cells in blood, 139
  reduced T cells in blood, 139

Neuraminidase, effect of neuraminidase treatment on lymph node recovery, 80, 81
  neuraminidase treated lymphocytes in liver, 80
NZB, 77, 124

Oxazolone, lymphocyte migration to skin in response to, 104
Oxidation, of sodium periodate on lymphocyte migration in the mouse, 88

^{32}P, use as lymphocyte label, 19
Patterning systems, 166–170
Periodate, effect of sodium periodate oxidation in lymphocyte migration, 87
Peyer's patches, B cell area, 34
  IgA precursor cells in, 113, 114
  morphology, 34
  thymus derived lymphocytes in, 35, 112, 114
Phenotype, influence of on lymphocyte distribution, 75
Phospholipases, 82, 85
  PLA$_2$, 84
  PLA–C, 85
Picryl chloride, 106
PL–A2, effect on lymphocyte migration, 84
PL–C, effect of on lymphocyte migration, 84
Pleurisy, T and B cells in pleural fluid, 152
Pokeweed mitogen (PWM), effect on cell input and output from draining node, 61–63
Polysaccharides, effect of sulfated polysaccharides on lymphocyte migration, 88
Positioning, control mechanisms of, 166–170
  during embryogenesis, 168–169
Post capillary venules, in lymph nodes, *see* HEV
Preemption, 66
Psoriasis, chemotaxis of scale extracts, 143
PSS, action of extracts of skin *in vitro*, 149
  T lymphocytes in skin in, 146
Pulmonary diseases, 152, 153
  malignancy, lymphocytes in peripheral blood and pleural fluid, 152, 153
  tuberculosis, lymphocytes in pleural fluid and blood, 152, 153

Recirculation, discovery of lymphocyte in the rat, 16–21
  in the foetal lamb, 39, 40
  transit time from blood to lymph, 39
Recognition, cell–cell systems, 163–166
Rheumatoid arthritis, activated T cells in synovial fluid, 145, 146
  B cells in blood, 144, 145
  B cells in synovial fluid, 144, 145
  iron in lymph nodes, 207
  iron in synovium, 208
  macrophages in synovial fluid, 145
  T cells in blood, 144, 145
  T cells in synovial fluid, 144, 145
  thoracic duct drainage in, 162

^{35}S Sulphate, incorporation by high endothelial cells in lymph node, 199
S. typhimurium, IgA antibodies in milk of infected subjects, 121
Scleroderma, *see* PSS
Skin, activated T lymphoblasts in, 102
  changes in cell composition of afferent lymph, 103
  diseases, 139–143
  lymphocyte migration to in cell mediated immunity, 106
  specific migration of primed blast cells to peripheral sites of antigen deposition, 108
SLE, 146–148
  antilymphocyte antibodies and lymphopenia, 146, 147
  cold-reactive antibodies in, 146
  lymphocytes in peripheral blood, 146, 147
  T cell lymphopenia during active disease, 147
  T cell subpopulations in, 146
  thoracic duct drainage in, 162
Specific recruitment, of antigen-reactive cells, 66–69
Sphingomyelinase, 84
Spleen, antigen reactive cells in, 68
  arteries, 4
  B cell, lymphatics, chicken, marginal zone, 30
  chicken, 28
  macrophages, 31
  microvasculature, 3
  morphology, 26–32
  recovery of Con A-treated cells in, 86
  red pulp, 31

reticulum cells, 29, 30
T cell areas, 29
white pulp, 28
Spleen cells, fate of cells labelled *in vitro*, 54
    fate of cells labelled *in vivo*, 54
Splenectomy, migration of Con A-treated cells in splenectomized mice, 87
    migration of phospholipase treated cells in splenectomized mice, 84
    migration of trypsin treated cells in splenectomized mice, 82
    persistence of sodium azide treated cells in blood of splenectomized mice, 91
    persistence of trypsin treated cells in blood of splenectomized mice, 82
Superoxide dismutase, levels in selected lymphocyte populations, 202
Synovial fluid, T and B lymphocytes in, 145

T_6 chromosome marker, discovery and first application, 14–16
T lymphoblasts, migration to lamina propria, 119
    migration to sites of inflammation, 102
T lymphocytes, distribution in lymph nodes, 32
    distribution in spleen, 29
    high numbers of afferent lymph, 102
    tempo of circulation from blood to lymph, 44
T. spiralis, migration of lymphoblasts to gut during infection, 119, 121
Theory, discussion of common mucosal, 121, 122
    hypothetical models of cell adhesion, 105
    interaction modulation, 178, 179–181
Thoracic duct drainage, in glomerulonephritis, 161
    in kidney transplantation, 161
    in rheumatoid arthritis, 162
    in SLE, 162
Thoracic duct lymph, B lymphocytes, 42, 43
    enrichment of long lived memory cells in, 74
    IgA producing cells in, 115

    lymphocyte output in the foetal lamb, 39, 40
    lymphocyte output in the normal rat, 43
    lymphocyte output in thymectomized animals, 41–45
    output of labelled lymphocytes in human leukemia, 157
    recovery of B lymphocytes in, 45
    recovery of T lymphocytes in, 44
    reduced capacity to induce GVH of passaged parental lymphocytes through F_1 hybrids, 67
    T lymphocyte sets in mouse, 25
Tonsil, 112, 121
Tonsillectomy, reduced response to Salk vaccine after, 121
Transit times from blood to lymph, in different species, 39
Thymocytes, in liver, 52
    in lymph node, 53
    in Peyer's patches, 53
    in spleen, 52
    low density in spleen, 52
    high density in spleen, 52
Thymus, effect of antigen on thymus-derived labelled cells, 53
    labelling in situ with ^{3}H thymidine, 53
    lymphocyte migration in thymus aplasia, 123
Thymus cells, *see* Thymocytes
Transferrin, association with lymphocytes, 214
    receptors on activated lymphocytes and cell lines, 215
Trypsin, effect of treatment on lymph node entry, 82
    recovery of effect, 82
Tumours, lymphocyte migration in animals after MSV inoculation, 154, 155
    suppression of growth by T. TDL, 75
    T and B lymphocytes in peripheral blood, 154
    T and B lymphocytes infiltrating, 152, 154, 155

Vascular permeability, unrelated to lymphocyte extravasation into tissues, 104
Veiled cells, in afferent lymph, 33
Viral diseases, meningitis, 151, 152
    Newcastle disease virus (NDV) infection, 126